Lunatic Hospitals in Georgian England, 1750-1830

Routledge Studies in the Social History of Medicine

EDITED BY JOSEPH MELLING, *University of Exeter*
AND ANNE BORSAY, *University of Wales, Swansea, U.K.*

Lunatic Hospitals in Georgian England, 1750-1830

Leonard Smith

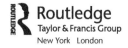

Routledge
Taylor & Francis Group
New York   London

Routledge
Taylor & Francis Group
711 Third Avenue
New York, NY 10017

Routledge
Taylor & Francis Group
2 Park Square
Milton Park, Abingdon
Oxfordshire OX14 4RN

First issued in paperback 2014

Routledge is an imprint of the Taylor and Francis Group, an informa company

© 2007 by Leonard Smith

ISBN 978-0-415-37516-0 (hbk)
ISBN 978-0-415-75918-2 (pbk)

Library of Congress Cataloging-in-Publication Data

Smith, Leonard D., 1947-
  Lunatic hospitals in Georgian England, 1750-1830 / Leonard Smith.
    p. ; cm. -- (Routledge studies in the social history of medicine ; 28)
  Includes bibliographical references and index.
  ISBN 978-0-415-37516-0 (hardback : alk. paper)
    1. Psychiatric hospitals--Great Britain--History--18th century. 2. Psychiatric hospitals--Great Britain--History--19th century. I. Title. II. Series.
    [DNLM: 1. Hospitals, Psychiatric--history--England. 2. History, 18th Century--England. 3. History, 19th Century--England. WM 27 FE5 S654L 2007]

  RC450.G7S633 2007
  362.2'10941--dc22   2006037464

Visit the Taylor & Francis Web site at
http://www.taylorandfrancis.com

and the Routledge Web site at
http://www.routledge.com

To those who have experienced the ravages of insanity and to those who have striven to bring relief.

Contents

Illustrations

Tables

Acknowledgments

Like so many aspiring historians, I owe a very considerable debt to the late Roy Porter. I never had the privilege of being a student of Roy's, although I did hear his erudite lectures and presentations on several occasions. I was one of a remarkably large number of people who received direct assistance from him in the form of references, advice, encouragement, and constructive criticism. That assistance was invaluable in the completion of my previous book, *'Cure, Comfort and Safe Custody'; Public Lunatic Asylums in Early Nineteenth-Century England*. It was largely the inspiration gained from Roy's work that stimulated me then to take my researches backwards into the eighteenth century.

There are many people whom I would also like to thank for encouragement and advice. Particular mention should go to one of Roy Porter's foremost disciples, Jonathan Andrews, whose own excellent work has shown how disparate eighteenth-century sources can be best utilised in reconstructing a realistic picture of people and events. Considerable gratitude is also due to Joseph Melling, who gave his editorial backing to the preparation of this book and then much helpful criticism and advice in the latter stages towards its completion.

The Centre for the History of Medicine at the University of Birmingham Medical School has provided an invaluable academic base, and my gratitude goes to its director, Bob Arnott, and also to Jonathan Reinarz for helpful discussions and comments on chapter drafts. Other people elsewhere who have assisted, advised or encouraged in different ways include Chris Philo, Pamela Michael, Anne Digby, Christine Stevenson, Hilary Marland, Jane Adams, David George, Michael Brown, Peter Bartlett, David Wright, Andrew Scull, Akihito Suzuki, Elaine Murphy, Matthew Hilton, Tom Harrison, Wendy Webster, Leonard Schwarz, and Daniel Smith.

The staffs of various archives offices deserve thanks for their assistance, including those of the London Metropolitan Archives, Tyne and Wear Archives, the University of York Borthwick Institute, and the record offices of Devon, Northumberland, Leicestershire, Herefordshire, Staffordshire, Nottinghamshire, Lincolnshire, and Liverpool. Thanks are also due to the staff of several libraries. In London, these include the British Library, its Newspaper Library at Colindale, the Wellcome Institute Library, the Guildhall Library, and the Goldsmiths Collection at the University of London. In the provinces, I must thank the staff of Birmingham University's excellent Barnes Medical Library, as well as the reference libraries of Manchester, York, Newcastle, Birmingham, Hereford and Gloucester, the West Country Studies Library in Exeter, and the special collections at the libraries of the Universities of Birmingham and Cambridge.

In some instances original documents have remained at the institutions that generated them, or their successors. Thanks are due to those who look after the archives of the Manchester Royal Infirmary, Cheadle Royal Hospital, and the Warneford Hospital in Oxford. My special gratitude is due to Sylvia Mannering at St Luke's Hospital, Woodside, in north London, for enabling me to have ready access to the St Luke's archives and to the splendid board room in which to study them, in addition to all her other practical help, support and cups of tea. Robert Leon, who acted as voluntary archivist at St Luke's for many years, also gave valuable assistance. Whilst this book has been in the final stages of preparation, the voluminous St Luke's archives have been transferred to the London Metropolitan Archives, which is only right and proper, though there must be some sadness at their final separation from the parent institution after 250 years.

I am grateful to the Wellcome Trust for providing assistance with a research expenses grant in the early stages of the preparation of this book.

Service users and my professional colleagues in the Metropolitan Borough of Sandwell's mental health services have provided a continual grounding, by constant reminders of the essential continuities over time in the presentation of mental disorder and how we attempt to treat and manage it.

My appreciation is due to my partner and to my family for their patience and forbearance whilst I have been unavailable for an inordinate amount of time.

Abbreviations

BPP   British Parliamentary Papers
DNB   Dictionary of National Biography
CRO   County Record Office
DCRO Devon County Record Office
LCRO Record Office for Leicestershire Leicester and Rutland
LRO   Liverpool Record Office
MRI   Manchester Royal Infirmary
MSS   Manuscripts
ODNB Oxford Dictionary of National Biography
RO   Record Office
SC   Select Committee
SCRO Staffordshire County Record Office
SLH   St Luke's Hospital

Introduction

In England, as in other countries, the late twentieth century has witnessed the rapid demolition and deconstruction of the mental hospital, or lunatic asylum, and its replacement by arrangements that are ostensibly more sophisticated. The speed of this phenomenon, and the evident unbounded enthusiasm for its achievement, has been quite remarkable. It will no doubt intrigue the social and medical historians of the future. They will seek to understand why an institution whose history stretched back to the seventeenth century and beyond, and which was for long the dominant element in the management of mental disorder, became so universally regarded as ineffective and obsolete. A serious multi-pronged attack on the lunatic asylum began in the early nineteen sixties. It is no coincidence that there has been an upsurge of historical interest in the asylum since that time. Historians have tended to concentrate much of their attention on the institutional developments of the nineteenth and early twentieth centuries. This was the period of the great expansion of asylumdom, when an ideal developed into a huge system, with all its attendant phenomena. The great 'museums of madness', as Andrew Scull so aptly characterized them, were to form much of the legacy that is being systematically discarded and consigned to the annals of history.[1]

In seeking to understand the emergence of the network of lunatic asylums that were characteristic of late-Victorian England, it is essential to place them in proper historical context. These asylums were mostly built under the provisions of the key mandatory legislation of 1845.[2] They were, though, part of a continuing evolutionary process. The model for the county pauper lunatic asylum had been previously established under the provisions of the County Asylums Act (Wynn's Act) of 1808, which enabled county authorities to provide an asylum.[3] This legislation had, in turn, been based on an intention to promote the dissemination of asylums on a system that had evidently been successfully developed in the later eighteenth century – the lunatic hospital founded and furthered by public charitable subscription.

Between 1750 and 1810 lunatic hospitals, or asylums as they gradually became known, were either built or projected in several major English cities. Historians of psychiatry, including even Roy Porter, have generally under-played their significance, allocating them a relatively minor role in the developing fabric of provision for the insane.[4] That significance, how-ever, has to be measured not only in regard to the number and size of the institutions and the numbers of patients who passed through them, but also in terms of what they symbolized. They represented a critical development not only in actual material provision, but also in philosophy, attitudes, and policy in relation to the treatment and management of mental disorder and its victims.

A number of varied influences coalesced to bring about the formation and subsequent development of these specialist hospitals. Not the least of these influences was the developing idealogical context, exemplified by changing ideas and conceptions about the nature of madness and how it ought to be managed, depicted by Scull as a shift in 'cultural perceptions'.[5] Rather than being an animal-like state that was beyond control, insanity was increas-ingly being accepted as a disease, with origins that might be often discerned in a physical disorder, and that could be amenable to treatment with a view to a cure. The excesses of madness could conceivably now be tamed and manageable. In Enlightenment discourse, unreason might be confronted and reason and rationality restored. The madman, hitherto characterized as a brute, could even be brought back toward proper participation in fam-ily and community.[6] The practical results apparently being achieved by Bethlem and St Luke's Hospitals and other institutions, demonstrated in their published cure rates, furthered this new optimism. So also did the writings of a new group of evident experts in the diagnosis and treatment of mental disorder, like William Battie, John Monro, Thomas Arnold, and William Pargeter.[7] The idea that madness could be both brought under control and treated, like other diseases, formed a central argument in the appeals for public support for new hospital projects.[8]

Coincidental to the emergence of a new optimism about the outcome of treatment, there was a perception that insanity was on the increase and that its ravages were spreading. Various epidemiological, social and economic reasons could be adduced to explain the advance of the 'English malady' and related complaints.[9] Calls to action referred to the possible risks to the local social order, as well as to the increasing threats of nuisance and even danger both to individuals and to communities. Underlying these anxieties were the fear and scarcely-veiled disgust associated with the disorderly poor, who would be even more alarming if unpredictability and chaotic behaviour were added to their defects. At the same time, it was apparent that mental disorder was far from being a preserve of the lowest classes. Its presence among the middling, and even the higher ranks was a growing cause of con-cern, which would assist in the mobilization of a charitable response.

There had been perceptible and significant developments in approaches to insanity and the insane in the late seventeenth century and the first part of the eighteenth. The most prominent manifestation was the commissioning, construction and opening of the great edifice of the new Bethlem Hospital in 1676. There could hardly have been more material acknowledgement that madness existed, that it had to be contained, and that there was a public responsibility to undertake the task.[10] However, Bethlem remained a unique institution, at least until the founding of the Bethel Hospital at Norwich, England's then second city, in 1713.[11] In parallel to the charitable response that these two hospitals represented, there was an emerging private sector offering various options of care and treatment. Most notably the 'madhouse', providing sequestration for lunatic relatives of the wealthy, was becoming a more apparent phenomenon both in London and the provinces.[12] It would be later in the eighteenth century before some madhouses catered also for parish paupers. In the mean time, those of the poorer classes whose behaviour necessitated removal from home and community, and who could not gain admittance to Bethlem, were likely to be incarcerated in poorhouses or penal institutions. The creation of a legislative framework, albeit a relatively crude one, by means of specific provisions relating to the care and control of lunatics in the Vagrancy Acts of 1714 and 1744, was further acknowledgement of the acceptance of public responsibility. Significantly, the latter Act contained a stated expectation that there would be some attempt at curative treatment.[13]

Notwithstanding these various developments, it was still the case that most people deemed 'lunatics' or 'idiots' remained within their families or communities.[14] By the second half of the eighteenth century, however, committal to some sort of institution was becoming the response of choice in dealing with the insane. Partly this was pragmatic, because of the perceived need to protect others from the excesses that mad people might display. There was also, though, a therapeutic rationale which was increasingly being advanced. The process of cure was seen to require removal of the sick individual from the 'morbid associations' that had contributed to his disorder. The patient had to be separated from family and friends and confined in a safe place where unwelcome influences could be kept away. As the century progressed this idea attained the status of a doctrine, accepted as an essential element in the successful management of insanity.[15]

The growing adherence to the institutional solution created raised expectations as to the amount of provision that was required. This put pressure on the specialist facilities that were available, in particular Bethlem Hospital, as it became unable to accommodate the increasing numbers of people being referred from all round the country. A portion of the demand, at least for the financially better-off sufferers, was being met by the private madhouses. These were among the numerous manifestations of the highly sophisticated consumer-orientated economy that characterized eighteenth-century English society.[16] However, the madhouse was already acquiring the taint of commercial exploitation allied to poor practice.[17] This was contrasted with what might be achieved by the philanthropy being brought to bear in other areas of social need. In a self-consciously enlightened and prosperous age, there was a perceived responsibility on leading members of the community to ensure disinterested provision for victims of disadvantage.[18] When charitable intent coincided with a desire to display conspicuous civic munificence, the motivation to provide a facility like a hospital for the insane became greatly strengthened.

The phenomenon of 'urban renaissance' in eighteenth-century England has been carefully delineated by Peter Borsay. A coalescence of commercial prosperity and a growing cultural sophistication among the middle and upper classes, rooted in Enlightenment attitudes, transformed the material fabric of towns and cities throughout the country.[19] A significant element of this urban renaissance was the creation of a range of new civic and philanthropic institutions. The financing and development of many of these institutions utilized the mechanism of public subscription. Prominent among them were the voluntary hospitals which, from the 1720s onwards, were established in growing numbers in London and the provinces.[20] The foundation and setting up of an hospital not only brought demonstrable practical benefits but also gave clear exemplification of the enlightened munificence of the leading figures of town and county. Once the effectiveness of the public subscription method had been demonstrated in the establishment of general hospitals, it could be seen as potentially applicable to other more specialist types of medical facility. A means for financing the replication of Bethlem had, therefore, become available.

For ideas and ideals to come to fruition, people were needed who were motivated to provide the leadership and expertise to develop care for the insane making use of the model offered by the voluntary hospital. Fundraising efforts tended to be led in London by members of the merchant and commercial classes, and in the provinces by the local aristocracy, gentry and clergy. In almost every instance, however, the intellectual leadership and the practical direction were provided by a physician. Lunatic hospitals were developed within a clearly medical context, consistent with the concept that madness was a disease whose relief or cure required medical intervention. In this construction, the claim of medical men to responsibility for the management of insanity was self-evident and not amenable to argument, at least until the challenge of the York Retreat at the end of the century.[21] However, their involvement was not solely a question of the promotion and maintenance of professional integrity. There was an evident liberal conception as to the physician's role. The medical men at the forefront of lunatic hospital development exhibited an acceptance of a duty to develop a broad and eclectic practice, in a way that encompassed ministration to a particularly unattractive and disadvantaged group of patients.

The dominating influence of the physicians became one of the characterizing features of the lunatic hospitals. Their central role both reflected and reinforced the conception that insanity had to be treated within a medically orientated environment. In several instances, as in Manchester, Liverpool and Leicester, this contributed to the development of a lunatic hospital as a direct appendage of an existing infirmary. Where the decision was taken to establish a lunatic hospital as a separate entity, it was still likely to be a physician attached to the general hospital who was the prime mover, retaining close links with both institutions. The medical model was, however, much more pervasive than the role of the physicians. The overall management arrangements, medical and administrative, of the lunatic hospitals conformed closely to those of the infirmaries, whether or not the one was the off-shoot of the other.

There were, though, significant ways in which the lunatic hospital diverged from the general hospital. One of these was the financial basis on which they operated. Where the general hospital normally provided in-patient care free to the recipient, provincial lunatic hospitals were never able to do so, despite the occasionally expressed aspirations of their governors.[22] They depended on regular payments from parishes, from relatives, or from the charitable funds to cover the maintenance and medical costs of patients who might require lengthy periods in the hospital. Partly for financial reasons, the governors of lunatic hospitals began to accept private patients, whose payments could help to subsidize the charges for those with limited means. These sorts of arrangements brought a distinctly commercial element into the running of institutions promoted as an alternative to the less desirable private madhouses. The presence of paying patients was likely to lead to some ethical and professional dilemmas for the physicians and other medical men, whose services were normally given free to the general hospitals but who found themselves part of a 'medical market-place' as regards their treatment of the insane.[23] The manner in which these dilemmas were addressed and resolved could significantly affect the nature of the lunatic hospital's operation.

There was an even more significant limitation to the similarities between the two types of institution. Because of the nature of insanity, and the attendant risks to the sufferer and to others, a lunatic hospital or asylum was seen to require a commensurate level of security. This took the predictable form of high walls, strong doors, and barred windows. These architectural features would be supplemented by the means used to restrain potentially threatening individuals, in the form of chains, locks, strait waistcoats, and so on. Taken together, these manifestations of control meant that a public facility for the insane had a good deal in common with a penal institution. This highlighted the great paradox in the care and management of mental disorder. In order to provide security for the public as well as treatment for the individual sufferer, the lunatic hospital had to provide features of both prison and hospital. The attempt to reconcile apparently conflicting requirements and objectives epitomized the 'custody versus cure' dilemma which has continued to influence the provision of mental health services down to the present day.[24]

One issue that has exercised historians of psychiatry and of the asylum, whether they are perceived to adhere to a 'whiggish', a radical, or a revisionist perspective, is that of 'reform'. Although scholars may have differed as to the meaning and significance of events, there is a general consensus that profound changes took place in the management of insanity and the insane in the first half of the nineteenth century.[25] The main public manifestations were the official investigations of 1807, 1815, 1827, and 1844, and the key legislation passed in 1808, 1828, and 1845. The lunatic hospitals formed a central element in the early stages of the lunacy reform process. Aspects of the management of the York Lunatic Asylum and practices at St Luke's Hospital proved extremely influential in the deliberations and conclusions of the 1807 parliamentary select committee, which led on to the legislation that followed in 1808.[26] St Luke's was again investigated extensively, and more critically, in 1815–16.[27] It was, however, the crisis of the York Asylum (along-side that of Bethlem Hospital) that was made to exemplify the failures and flagrant abuses of an *ancien regime* that had to be swept away and replaced by something more rational, orderly and humane. The voluntary lunatic hospitals had to respond to a profound threat to their integrity and their rationale. At the same time they also had to meet the challenges posed by a new generation of asylums financed through the county rates.

There has long been an acceptance that the voluntary general hospitals that emerged in the eighteenth century constituted a 'system' that formed the basis of the present-day national network of hospitals.[28] My main objective in this book will be to ensure that the voluntary lunatic hospitals are accorded their own rightful place in the historical development of provision for mentally disordered people. In the chapters that follow I will examine their origins and rise, and will consider what sort of institutions they were, how they operated and were managed, who were some of the leading figures, who were their patients, and what methods and means were employed to treat and 'cure' those patients. Along the way, a number of other significant questions have to be addressed. What was the nature and extent of the relationship between lunatic hospitals and the previously established voluntary hospitals? How influential were medical men, and in particular physicians, in the direction of the lunatic hospitals and in the determination of policy and practices? Was the purpose of these institutions to provide primarily for the insane poor of the locality, or did they acquire a wider remit? How did the lunatic hospitals and their physicians respond to the challenges and opportunities presented by an active private sector in the wider medical market-place? How did they reconcile conflicting expectations, and in particular the dilemmas associated with trying to accommodate the means for both custody and cure? Were there significant developments in treatment practices, and how influential were the emerging ideas and techniques of 'moral management'? Responses to these important questions will help to demonstrate the significant place of the voluntary lunatic hospital in the evolution of the institutional management and treatment of people deemed to be insane.

1   St Luke's Hospital for lunaticks

The opening of Robert Hooke's 'New Bethlem' at Moorfields in 1676 presented a powerful visual message. The City elite had not just financed and constructed a magnificent building, destined to become one of the sights of London. They had created a material acknowledgement of the place of the insane within society, and of its duty to manage and care for them appropriately. The sheer scale and grandeur of the edifice, likened by contemporaries to a palace, illustrated conclusively that the victims of insanity were now to be openly included within the charitable arena. Its external beauty indicated that they were to be treated with respect and sympathy, whilst its imposing physical presence conveyed the impression that madness and its excesses could be contained and controlled. Whether by design or by accident, the governors of Bethlem had laid down a clear standard for future institutional provision for the insane.[1]

Attitudes toward insanity and those who suffer from it have always tended to be complex and ambivalent. The dual perception was succinctly expressed in a fund-raising appeal for the York Lunatic Asylum, which described mad people as 'objects of terror and compassion'.[2] Through the course of the eighteenth century there was a slow shift in the emphasis. The 'terror' element persisted, exemplified in the perpetuation of custodial methods of treatment and patient management. However, the 'compassion' came increasingly to the fore, illustrated in the rise of some of the better-managed private madhouses, as well as public lunatic hospitals with an avowed curative intent. Whether the prime object was custody or cure, however, removal to a specialist institution had become accepted as the most appropriate means of providing it.

England's commercial prosperity in the eighteenth century was bringing new wealth to an ever-widening middle class, whilst also enhancing that of the gentry and upper classes. Prosperity brought opportunities for indulgence in many forms of luxurious consumption, some newly available in an increasingly sophisticated market for goods and services. It also brought new possibilities to offer aid and comfort to those less fortunate, which could include people who also had the potential to become disruptive to the social order. The century witnessed a singularly remarkable upsurge of charitable endeavour. A confluence of aristocratic duty and conspicuous philanthropy expressed itself in a consciously developing enlightened approach to the relief of social ills.[3] A growing acceptance that disadvantaged or deviant groups of people were best managed or looked after in institutions accorded well with the desire of philanthropists to create visible manifestations of their charitable works.

As historians like Paul Langford and Kathleen Wilson have shown, among the most significant of these philanthropic endeavours were the new hospitals or infirmaries that were projected, commissioned, and built by public subscription.[4] The success of the first ventures, by the 1740s, led the elites of many cities and counties around the country to follow suit. The next stage, after a general hospital had been established and operational for some time in a town or city, was for them to consider the addition of more specialist types of hospital. One significant category among these might be a hospital for the insane, who had hitherto been largely excluded from admission to the general institutions on account both of the stigma attached to them and the particular management problems they could pose.[5] In London and in several provincial centres these were precisely the deliberations that took place and which eventually produced material outcomes. The processes and developments that occurred in the provinces will be outlined in chapter two. The present chapter will concentrate on the emergence and early history of St Luke's, the first and arguably the most important of the voluntary lunatic hospitals.

THE INSTITUTIONAL CONTEXT

In 1750, Bethlem Hospital constituted almost the sole, and certainly the most substantial, public institutional provision for mentally disordered people in England. It could claim a history of some 500 years, dating from the foundation of the original priory of St Mary of Bethlehem in 1247.[6] Its emergence as a specialist hospital for the insane was gradual and largely took place during the course of the fifteenth century.[7] In 1547 management was taken over by the City of London, and Bethlem's administration was combined with that of the Bridewell house of correction. It remained, however, a relatively small institution; there were only twenty inmates in 1598 and thirty-one in 1624.[8] Despite this, Bethlem had attained a degree of prominence and notoriety by the mid-seventeenth century, with its developing alter ego image of 'Bedlam' reinforced through literature and drama.[9] Even by 1650, though, the hospital was still providing for less than fifty patients.[10] With the sustained growth of London, and its material prosperity, this was no longer adequate. The projection of the new hospital, and its opening in 1676, represented a fundamental transition in several ways. Quite apart from the symbolism of the spectacular building, the actual provision was now on a significantly larger scale. Bethlem was to be more than a hospital for some of the lunatic poor of London. It was a major City institution, and its catchment was becoming nationwide.[11]

Bethlem's position was consolidated during the first half of the eighteenth century. Administrative arrangements became more sophisticated, with sub-committees of the governors taking responsibility for particular aspects of the hospital's operation. Clear medical management, under the leadership of members of the Monro dynasty, was maintained. Bethlem's role was widening; although its primary rationale continued to be as a curative hospital, wards were developed to provide for more than one hundred 'incurable' patients. Its role as a public institution had several aspects. Whilst it continued to be a focus for voluntary and philanthropic endeavour, it also became a notorious place of public resort. As Jonathan Andrews has shown, however, visitation was more than an excuse for voyeurism and entertainment. It fostered charitable giving, as well as providing some check on the sort of abuses that could occur in a closed institution. Behind the imagery of 'Bedlam' and its less savoury features, the hospital's governors were attempting to provide genuine care and treatment for its inmates.[12]

Although Bethlem remained the only really significant public lunatic hospital, two other institutions were opened in the early eighteenth century.[13] The first of these was at Norwich, England's then second city. The Bethel Hospital was established in 1713, founded and funded by Mrs Mary Chapman, the widow of a clergyman, primarily to cater for the insane poor of Norwich and the county of Norfolk.[14] After her death in 1724 it became a public charity administered by trustees. The original building was fairly small, consisting of two stories with two wings. Despite various enlargements and alterations, the number of patients remained between twenty and thirty up to 1750. The admission policy does not appear to have been as strict as Bethlem's, but the intent was primarily to achieve cures.[15] It was the lack of provision in London for various types of 'incurable' patients that led to the setting up of a female ward adjoining Guy's Hospital in 1725, which accepted people discharged from Bethlem for whom there were 'small Hopes of their Cure'. This was a relatively small-scale facility, still only providing for twenty women in 1815.[16]

Whilst charitable lunatic hospitals formed an important element of the developing fabric of institutional provision for mentally disordered people, a notable development from the latter part of the seventeenth century onwards was the rise and multiplication of private madhouses. They were, in part, a market response to the shortage of public provision, though more a means of meeting the growing demand for confinement of the insane relatives of members of the middle and upper classes. Evidence as to the number and dispersal of these houses, and how many people they contained, is sketchy for the early eighteenth century. However, the increasing significance of madhouses in the emerging pattern of care is clear, particularly in London but also in the provinces, even before the upsurge of large licensed houses later in the century.[17] Their very presence, as well as the not entirely favourable reputation they were gaining, raised challenges to those who looked askance at the intrusion of the profit motive into the care of the damaged and vulnerable.

THE VOLUNTARY HOSPITALS — A MODEL FOR EMULATION

The public subscription funded voluntary hospitals of the first half of the eighteenth century marked a significant advance, both as examples of the management of charitable endeavour and as means of care for the sick. The earliest of the hospitals were established in London, with the Westminster in 1720, Guy's in 1724, St George's in 1733, and the London Hospital in 1740. The example had eventually been taken up in the provinces, with the opening of the Winchester County Hospital in 1736, to be followed by the Bristol Royal Infirmary in 1737, the York County Hospital in 1740, and the Royal Devon and Exeter in 1741. The evident effectiveness of this model led to widespread imitation. Between 1735 and 1775, twenty-one hospitals were opened, and by the end of the century a pattern of provision had been clearly established, with hospitals or infirmaries in most major cities or county towns.[18] The Manchester physician, John Aikin, could justifiably proclaim in 1771 that in less than half a century 'numerous edifices' had been built throughout the country, 'dedicated to the support of the poor under the severe afflictions of disease and want'.[19]

The voluntary hospitals represented a new form of charity. Their predecessor chartered institutions had depended on the gifts of wealthy benefactors and the income derived from the original endowments. The new hospitals were financed largely by voluntary contribution or regular subscription, which might involve a large number of individuals giving or subscribing widely varying sums of money. They were the product of communal effort in the city or county, which brought together people from different social classes. The county aristocracy and gentry normally took a leading role in the ventures, frequently with the active support of clergymen. In some cities, the impetus came more from the merchant and industrialist classes.[20] Several writers have argued that the subscription hospital constituted an updated expression of *noblesse oblige*, reinforcing authoritarian paternalist structures whereby the privileged fulfilled their duty to provide for casualties of the poorer classes.[21]

The motivations for establishing a hospital combined altruism with practical self-interest and class interest. A typical fund-raising advertisement, for the General Infirmary at Bath in 1737, spoke of a 'glorious opportunity' for 'assisting and relieving their distressed fellow-creatures'.[22] Projectors and subscribers sought to provide a practical means of poor relief for those unable through sickness to maintain themselves. At the same time, propaganda proclaimed intentions to promote economic utility, by offering the opportunity for cure of people who could then return to productive work. The Bath Infirmary's plans spoke of the lofty aim to deliver the poor 'from beggary and want, to a capacity of getting an honest livelihood, and comfortable subsistence'.[23] In the wider context of the period, advocates of charitable benevolence were increasingly arguing the importance of mercantilist principles, drawing the clear link between relief of the disadvantaged, employment, and the wealth of the nation.[24]

The subscribers and donors were not only creating an institution that was of clear benefit to the sick and the poor. It also provided the opportunity for conspicuous philanthropy. With the regular publication of subscription lists in annual reports and in the county press, they enhanced their own prestige and standing. Members of the nobility and gentry felt obliged to make significant donations and be prominent on committees, in order to demonstrate that they were fully playing their part in the community and carrying out their social duty. For the middle classes, presence on the lists and in the committee room was an important means of staking a claim to presence among the local social elite. The hospital provided a genuine opportunity for the various classes, and for people of differing religious denominations and political persuasions, to work and mix together and, incidentally, to pursue business contacts.[25]

A significant additional advantage for subscribers was the right to nominate patients for admission to the hospital, according to the level of their donation or subscription. It became the norm that prospective patients required the recommendation of a subscriber (or group of subscribers, if a society or a parish) in order to gain admittance. The patient required certification that he was a 'proper object of charity'. This mechanism constituted a form of direct patronage.[26] For most hospitals the catchment area was based on their hinterland, primarily the town and county, though some accepted people from a wider area. Generally, although they sought to provide for poor patients, parish paupers were not accepted. The emphasis was primarily upon the rural and urban working poor. Admission policies tended to be similar between hospitals, with particular categories of people excluded, such as children and those suffering from fever, venereal diseases, or, significantly, those 'disordered in their senses'.[27]

The management arrangements of the voluntary hospitals resembled, in some ways, those of a joint-stock company. The institution was controlled by the votes of subscribers, who elected a management committee from among themselves. Substantial donors, normally those paying an annual amount in excess of £25, would become subscribers for life, and might earn an automatic right to a seat on the board of governors.[28] The committee or board of governors would determine overall policy. They would also provide for the more routine aspects of administration and patient management, in a set of rules. These would prescribe strict guide-lines for conduct, with prohibitions against behaviours like cursing, gambling, smoking, drinking, and so on. Patients would be required, according to capability, to assist with domestic work in the hospital.[29] The emphasis was on the maintenance of proper moral and religious standards.

Medical attendance on the hospitals formed a key aspect of the charitable endeavour. Unlike in the earlier endowed hospitals, physicians and surgeons would be appointed to honorary posts and were expected to provide their services without payment. This was viewed as their appropriate contribution to the relief of the sick poor. Although potentially an onerous commitment, the burden of unremunerated work would be offset by the prestige gained and by the potentially lucrative patronage and private consultation work to be attracted from among the hospital's subscribers.[30] The physician occupied the key supervisory role in directing treatment and in prescribing medicines, through his regular ward rounds. Much of the day-to-day responsibility, however, tended to rest with the house apothecary. Working under the direction of the physician, he would prepare medicines, carry out bleedings, blisterings and other physical treatments, and supervise the use of equipment. Normally a salaried officer, the apothecary's role became pivotal to the effective operation of the hospital.[31]

By the middle of the eighteenth century the voluntary public subscription hospital model had already proved itself. It offered a mechanism for provision of service that could be adopted in any substantial town or populous district. More than that, the fine building that was normally erected served as an ornament to the town and county, as well as a symbol of the munificence, sophistication, and progressive spirit of their leading citizens. The model could now conceivably be adapted to provide for sufferers from other specific complaints, not least victims of those conditions which led to exclusion from the existing hospitals. Indeed, the establishment of a charitable institution for the restoration of the stigmatized insane could conceivably offer practical demonstration of the particularly high degree of enlightenment of those who sought to pursue so laudable a goal.

FOUNDATIONS

The profound influence of the voluntary hospital movement on the projectors of St Luke's was evident from the outset. Although, unlike some of its successors, St Luke's did not originate directly from an existing hospital, the example was explicitly stated. The group of City merchants who assembled at the Kings Arms Tavern in Exchange Alley in June 1750 noted that London already abounded with hospitals and infirmaries 'calculated for the Relief of almost every Distemper attending the poor'. To provide 'an Hospital for the immediate Reception and Cure of Poor Lunaticks' would be to extend 'this sort of Charity...one step farther'.[32] An address issued shortly afterwards contended that the 'Usefulness and necessity of Hospitals in general' was so well understood that it was needless to explain. What was being proposed was 'a new Design of this sort' specifically for the relief of 'Poor Lunaticks'.[33] In other words, this was not to be a completely new departure, but rather a logical extension of existing provision, and a response toward addressing one of the range of requirements of a great city like London.

While the London subscription hospitals provided the inspiration and the practical points of reference, it was the increasingly apparent limitations of Bethlem that gave the impetus toward decisive action. It was plain to critics that, although a 'noble and extensive Charity', it was 'incapable of receiving and maintaining the great Number of melancholy Objects' who applied for relief. This meant some people spending long periods on the waiting list, and others not receiving 'the proper and necessary Means of Cure' unless paid for at great expense elsewhere.[34] There were also, in certain quarters, major idealogical concerns and moral qualms about Bethlem. A writer in the *Gentleman's Magazine* in 1748 had highlighted the most serious of these, deploring the activities of those people who were so low that they would:

> resort to an hospital, intended for the reception and cure of unhappy lunatics purely to mock at the extravagancies that deface the image of the creator, and exhibit their fellow creatures in circumstances of the most pitiable infirmity, debility, and unhappiness.

He called for action from people with the power to prevent the 'enormity' of Bethlem serving as a spectacle, 'by which our country is disgraced' and the intent of the charity defeated.[35] The hope was that any new hospital would be established on a rather different footing.

In appealing to the public for funds for a hospital for poor lunatics, the committee who met at the Kings Arms carefully stressed both the unique tragedy of insanity and its associated hazards:

> there is no Disease to which human nature is subject, so terrible in its Appearances, or so fatal in its Consequences; those who are Melancholy often do violence to themselves, and those who are raving, to Others, and too often to their nearest Relations and Friends...

Particular provision was required for these 'ungovernable and mischievous Persons', comprising 'seperate (sic) apartments'. In this hospital they were to have 'the proper means of Cure early administered to them', which were most effectively provided when the patients were 'under the Management of strangers'.[36] Several key elements had therefore been emphasized. The insane were entitled to sympathy and pity. Their condition rendered them hard to manage, due to the risks they posed to those around them and to the wider public. They required specialist treatment and management by people with whom they were not familiar. Finally, it was considered to be of considerable therapeutic importance to remove the person from home to a properly equipped place, with facilities for isolation. These themes constantly recurred in the literature emanating from all the subsequent lunatic hospitals.

The plan was brought to fruition relatively speedily. Subscriptions were opened and arrangements agreed for the hospital's government. A committee was chosen to carry the project into effect. By November 1750 a lease had been agreed with the City authorities for a 'spot of ground' on the edge of Moorfields, near Windmill Hill, adjoining an old building known as 'The Foundery', in use as a Wesleyan meeting house.[37] George Dance, the City Surveyor, gave his services gratis and drew up plans for the building. A sub-committee was delegated to frame the hospital's bye–laws, and arrangements were made to publish 3,000 copies of the 'Address to the Public', along with a further statement of the governors' intentions.[38]

This new statement explained and amplified the rationale for providing a second major lunatic hospital, and put forward some significant new arguments. It pointed out that lunatics were 'incapable of providing for themselves and families', and were excluded from admission to other hospitals. Private charity could not meet the expense, as they required 'Servants peculiarly qualified', and for each patient a 'seperate Room, and Diet, most of them, equal to persons in Health'. The expenses of confinement and 'other means of Cure', which generally required several months to complete, were too much to bear even for people in 'middling circumstances'. The plan was to provide for 'proper Objects' and, 'for the sake of the Publick as well as themselves', to admit them without delay and 'without Expense also'. They anticipated, however, additional significant benefits, indeed 'some Advantages of a very interesting Nature to the good of all Mankind', with the prospect of increased medical and scientific knowledge:

> for more Gentlemen of the Faculty, making this Branch of Physick, their particular Care & Study, it may from thence reasonably expected that the Cure of this dreadful Disease will hereafter be rendered more certain and expeditious, as well as less Expensive.[39]

This phrase laid out a key element of St Luke's claims to be adopting a progressive approach to the treatment of insanity. It was also, incidentally, another way in which the promoters of St Luke's carefully distanced themselves from practices at Bethlem.[40]

Another paper, published shortly afterwards, dwelt on the inadequacies of present provision, and particularly of Bethlem. The 'Expence and Difficulty' of gaining admission to Bethlem had discouraged many applications, particularly from 'the more necessitous objects' and from those living in the 'remote parts of the Kingdom'. The delays and exclusions had the result that 'many useful Members have been lost to Society', with some patients falling into the hands of the unskilled or those who sought their own advantage by neglecting the means of cure. Delays in placing people in specialist care had led to the 'most fatal Acts of Violence' on themselves, their relatives, or their attendants. The most telling censure of Bethlem, however, was in the manner of the reinforcement of St Luke's intention to encourage more 'Gentlemen of the Faculty' to study and practice the treatment of 'one of the most important Branches of Physick'. This had been, it declared, 'already too long confined (almost) to a Single Person.' That person, who allegedly was seeking to retain a monopoly of perceived knowledge, could be none other than Dr James Monro, the long-serving physician to Bethlem.[41]

The appointment in October 1750 of Monro's professional rival, Dr William Battie, as St Luke's first physician was, therefore, of considerable significance.[42] He immediately became involved in the practical steps necessary to prepare for its eventual opening, preparing a dietary table and a list of the drugs and medicines that would be required.[43] He was probably involved in the appointment of a keeper, nurse, and 'Under Maid Servant' in March 1751, and in the drawing up of the Rules and Orders ordered to be published in June.[44] He certainly was to take on a key role in the admission and discharge of patients, as well as in directing treatment. The first admissions to what was to be called 'St Luke's Hospital for Lunaticks' took place on July 29th 1751, only just over a year since the meeting at the Kings Arms.[45]

George Dance's hospital building was a plain, functional structure, rather austere in appearance.[46] According to a contemporary description, it was 'a neat but very plain edifice: nothing is here expended on ornament'. It was 'of considerable length', with the brickwork covered in plaster and painted white. It exhibited a series of small square windows 'on which no decorations have been bestowed'.[47] Situated as it was on Moorfields, only a short distance from Bethlem, the deliberate plainness of St. Luke's (see Figure 1.1) was, as Andrews and Scull have argued, in clear and unambiguous contrast with the ostentatious grandeur of its illustrious neighbour.[48]

There were, therefore, some significant features about St Luke's Hospital. Much of the early publicity surrounding it was concerned with Bethlem. That hospital offered a model for comparison and partial imitation. Its perceived shortcomings provided examples of pit-falls to avoid, and inspiration for trying new approaches. One particularly important aspect of St Luke's was that it was designed expressly to provide for the poor. Although Bethlem was also intended primarily for poor people, including paupers, it did cater for some who were better off.[49] At St Luke's, admission was to be free of charge, other than for parish paupers for whom there was a nominal charge of £1.12s for bedding. There were no ongoing charges for the patient's keep or medical treatment.[50] The costs were to be met by the earnings from interest payments on its growing investments. This adherence to the ideal of an hospital providing free care was only possible

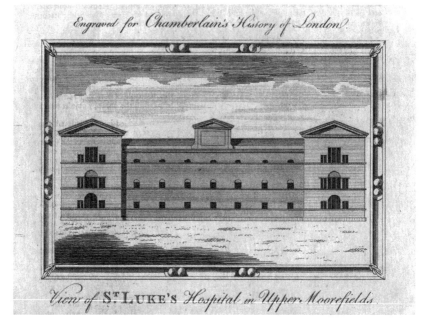

Figure 1.1 The first St Luke's Hospital, Windmill Hill.
Source: Copy of engraving in author's possession.

because of the charity's steadily increasing wealth, and it was a luxury that none of its successor lunatic hospitals was able to enjoy.[51]

FROM MOORFIELDS TO OLD STREET

St Luke's initial accommodation was for twenty-five patients. This soon proved insufficient to meet the demand, particularly as in February 1752 the governors agreed in principle to immediately re-admit any patient who relapsed within two months of having been discharged 'cured'. They also agreed to fit up more of the building, increasing the capacity to fifty, and by August 1752 there were forty-seven in the house.[52] Expansion highlighted the building's deficiencies. One common room adjoining the kitchen was serving for all of the patients, and in early 1754 another had to be provided to facilitate separation of the sexes.[53] At the same time a significant alteration to policy was made, which recognized that the optimistic hopes that St Luke's could achieve a break-through in treatment might not be fully realized. Provision was to be made initially for up to ten patients who either had been previously discharged as incurable or who were approaching the end of their year's treatment but were not showing sufficient signs of recovery. Unlike the curable patients, their 'friends' were to pay a weekly charge of five shillings for their 'Lodging Physick Diet and all other Necessaries'.[54]

By the end of 1755, twenty cells were being provided for incurables, and they were being recorded separately in the hospital's statistical returns.[55]

The pressure to expand the hospital, to accommodate ever more patients, was almost inexorable. In early 1763 it was decided to erect an additional building to provide for a further thirty, including ten incurables. Within two years St Luke's had capacity for one hundred patients.[56] By 1770 the governors were seeking ways to accept still more people, 'so as to render this Charity more extensive'. They considered various options, including additional buildings adjoining the hospital, the provision of temporary out-relief to some 'proper Objects', and even a drastic plan to make an agreement 'with some proper Person who is accustomed to the Care of Lunaticks'— in other words to contract with a private madhouse proprietor.[57] Following advice from the hospital's physician Dr Thomas Brooke (who had succeeded Battie in 1764) that the site was already too confined to be healthy for the patients, the governors rejected the idea of further buildings, though they did agree to rent two nearby houses 'for the Reception of Sick Patients'. They also rejected the other options, because the patients would be outside the governors' sphere of control and might also be liable to 'the greatest Impositions'.[58]

Piecemeal solutions, however, could no longer meet the necessity created by a continuing demand for the accommodation of the unmanageable insane poor of the metropolis and its surrounding counties. The main beneficiaries were the proprietors of the large private madhouses of London's East End, at Hoxton and Bethnal Green.[59] The original building was becoming increasingly inadequate, as well as dilapidated. One topographical writer described it as being 'so much decayed' that replacement was going to be required, and according to the prison reformer John Howard it had become 'old and inconvenient'.[60] By 1775 it had been concluded that the only realistic response was to move to a much larger new building and, with the funds in a very healthy state, explorations and negotiations to locate a site began in earnest.[61] In August 1776 agreement was reached with St Bartholomew's Hospital to lease from them a three-acre parcel of land on Old Street, known as the 'Bowling Green', together with some other buildings and tenements including the 'Fox and Goose'.[62] George Dance junior, son of the architect of the first St Luke's Hospital, was commissioned to design and build the new hospital at a projected cost of just over £17,000.[63] Unlike the 1751 building, however, the completion of the second St Luke's was plagued by delay and it did not finally open to receive its transferred patients until January 1787.[64] The final cost worked out as being in excess of £35,000.[65]

George Dance's design for the new St Luke's was heavily influenced by Robert Hooke's New Bethlem.[66] Dance had also designed Newgate Prison, which was reflected in the combination of 'harmony of proportion with unity and appropriateness of style' of St Luke's.[67] Its façade comprised features that were simultaneously imposing and austere, dispensing with any undue ornamentation rather like its predecessor building. Various elements combined to give it a forbidding aspect — its considerable length and height; its closeness to Old Street, over which the building loomed; and, particularly, the high arched windows, largely bricked up, with small apertures at the top for lighting and ventilation.[68] The new St Luke's building (see Figure 1.2), like Hooke's Bethlem before it, became a place for visitors from around the country and from overseas to come and admire. As the journal *The World* noted in 1787, shortly after it opened: 'the foreigners who have seen the new St Luke's Hospital are loud and lavish in their good report of the architect'.[69] Not all commentators were so favourable, however. Prior to the hospital's opening, a newspaper correspondent referred to the 'heavy mass of melancholy architecture' which rendered the building a 'gloom-inspiring edifice'.[70] He went on to criticize George Dance, suggesting that the genius evident in the design of Newgate had 'failed him' in St Luke's. In a building designed to provide for 'the most affecting infirmity of human nature', there was no reason for 'marking to the eye, and fixing on the mind of those who pass it, the cell of an irrecoverable maniac.'[71]

The new building's internal arrangements were carefully described by John Howard, two years after the hospital opened. There were three floors, each with 'three long galleries and wings, with opposite cells for the patients'. Accommodation for officers and staff was in the centre. Male patients were housed on one side and women on the other. Every gallery contained thirty-two arched cells, thirteen feet in height, each with a high external window and a large aperture above the door. These were pro-

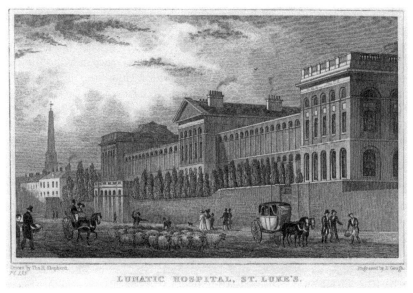

LUNATIC HOSPITAL, ST. LUKE'S.

Figure 1.2 The second St Luke's Hospital, Old Street.
Source: Copy of engraving in author's possession.

tected with iron bars, latticed 'to prevent accidents'. The galleries, into which the cells opened, were fifteen feet wide.[72] They were, in fact, slightly narrower than those at Bethlem, but were well provided with windows, offering views out of the building, in marked contrast to the sleeping cells.[73] The inter-relation of single cells and large galleries brought together the features of prison and hospital which were to become so characteristic of asylum architecture.[74]

One problem which the St Luke's governors did not have to face was a lack of resources. The hospital continued to receive substantial donations, including a bequest of £10,000 from a Mrs Betenson in late 1788. With the funds standing at over £100,000, St Luke's was declared to be one of the wealthiest hospitals in London.[75] Patient numbers climbed steadily in the new hospital. In February 1787 there were 106 in the house, increasing to 120 a year later.[76] The west wing was opened to receive patients in February 1788, and by the following February numbers had risen to 170.[77] By June 1794 the numbers stood at 250, and in January 1800 St Luke's was virtually full with 305 patients.[78] The old division into curable and incurable patients had been perpetuated. Significantly, however, it was the provision for incurables which expanded at the greater rate. The new hospital initially provided for thirty incurables.[79] By 1791, there were seventy-two, increasing to 120 in 1800.[80] There had been a marked shift from the policies and plans of the original projectors of 1750. The provision for incurables in St Luke's was clearly meeting a demand. In August 1800 the hospital was declared 'full of both Curable & Incurable Patients', with a 'considerable number of both description of Objects' on the waiting list. Initial discussions even began about further expansion.[81]

From modest beginnings, within half a century St Luke's had become one of the foremost hospitals in London, and had attained and consolidated a position of prominence in the institutional management of the insane. It still retained its roots in the voluntary hospital sector as regards its financing, its organization, and its management structures. Essentially, the projectors and governors had utilized the mechanisms of the public subscription hospital and its techniques of attracting funds and support in order to launch and establish their specialist lunatic hospital. Once that was achieved, St Luke's had been able to move on and forge an independent identity. Its other key point of reference had been Bethlem Hospital, although the intention of the St Luke's governors and of William Battie had always been to operate quite differently to Bethlem. Rivalries between the two hospitals did persist, with the St Luke's governors continuing for several decades to reproduce, rather defensively, the contentions of 1750 about the inadequacies and shortcomings of Bethlem and why an alternative institution was required.[82] As Andrews and Porter have suggested, however, actual practices may not have been so different. Indeed, as time went on the relationship between St Luke's and Bethlem, and between their respective medical officers, became reasonably cordial and co-operative.[83]

The completion and opening of the huge new St Luke's on Old Street gave it a location and a presence in the City that was comparable to Bethlem's, and within a few years it would contain more patients than its erstwhile rival. There was no longer any real need for self-justification.

The significance of St Luke's was considerably greater than its own achievements. It had further raised the profile of insanity and of the effectiveness of both a public charitable and a medical response. Crucially, it provided the example and the model for the successful establishment of several voluntary lunatic hospitals in the provinces.[84] Despite its evident shortcomings and the criticism it received, the younger George Dance's building was perceived as the epitome of institutional provision for lunatics at the time, and it remained highly influential on subsequent public lunatic asylum construction. The influence of St Luke's, however, was considerably wider than its important architectural contribution, for its pretensions to be at the forefront of progressive practice were exceeded only by the York Retreat.[85] When parliament was considering reforms to lunacy provision in 1807 and again in 1815, it was almost taken for granted that comprehensive evidence would be taken from St Luke's, and from its long serving 'Master', Thomas Dunston, in particular. The patient management systems adopted there were promoted as worthy of emulation and as being greatly superior to those of increasingly discredited Bethlem.[86] By this time the first of the new generation of county lunatic asylums had been opened, at Bedford, Nottingham, and Thorpe St Andrew, near Norwich. In each case, the stamp of St Luke's on both building design and operational policy, had been clearly evident.[87]

2   The provincial lunatic hospitals

The successful development of St Luke's, based on the mechanism of funding by public subscription, gradually attracted attention in the provinces, where concerns had evidently been growing about the problems associated with the insane poor. In the same way that the voluntary hospital model, once properly established, had become steadily disseminated around the country, the lunatic hospital idea was taken up in several towns and cities. There was an element of imitation, and even competition, as county and urban elites reacted to developments in other centres as well as responding to their own local pressures to provide for the lunatic poor. However, some notable differences were evident in the manner of foundation of their lunatic hospitals, as was to be expected in cities and regions with distinctive traditions and circumstances. There were, though, some important commonalities, particularly because all the lunatic hospitals in some way emerged out of an existing voluntary hospital.[1]

Reflecting these common origins, there were similarities in the early planning of the lunatic hospitals and the manner in which their projectors sought to attract support and funds. Crucially, the hospitals shared a similar philosophical base, one key aspect of which was an acceptance that they were fundamentally medical institutions, to be administered and operated accordingly. Almost as significant, the lunatic hospitals were constituted to combine both curative and custodial ideals. Patients were to be actively treated with a view to their recovery and eventual discharge, but in conditions that ensured the safety and security of officers and staff as well as the wider public. There was one additional element, though, common to all the provincial lunatic hospitals but which clearly set them apart from St Luke's. All their patients, whether 'curable' or 'incurable', had to pay (or have paid on their behalf) a weekly rate for maintenance. This was essentially a consequence of the charities' relatively meagre subscription bases, in comparison to their wealthy London predecessor.

It was significant that steps to establish a lunatic hospital were more likely to be taken in towns and cities whose distance from London meant that placements at Bethlem and St Luke's were inconvenient and problematic, quite apart from all the difficulties associated with actually obtaining a vacancy. It was certainly not accidental, therefore, that the first four provincial lunatic hospitals to open were all in the north of England, at Newcastle-upon-Tyne (1764), Manchester (1766), York (1777), and Liverpool (1792). Over the next three decades or so the axis shifted towards the midland counties and the west. Lunatic asylums, as they had now become known, opened at Leicester (1794), Hereford (1799), and Exeter (1801), later followed by Lincoln (1819) and Oxford (1826).[2] This geographical pattern was even further reinforced if we include also those early county asylums that began originally as voluntary projects but subsequently became joint ventures under the provisions of the legislation of 1808.[3]

Two distinct types of lunatic hospital provision emerged in the eighteenth century. St Luke's had been founded as an independent institution, having no formal relationship with any of the voluntary hospitals that had been established in London, albeit that it was organized and managed in similar manner to them. In the provincial centres, although the lunatic hospitals invariably had their origins in a local voluntary hospital, the subsequent relationship between the two differed markedly. In Manchester, a completely new model of provision was adopted. Its lunatic hospital was, from the outset, set up in close conjunction with the town's infirmary and remained largely integrated with it. The Manchester example proved highly influential and Liverpool, Leicester and Hereford all subsequently followed suit. Elsewhere, the governors implemented a model more like that of St Luke's, opting for an independent facility completely separate from the general hospital. This was the approach to be followed in Newcastle, York, Exeter and later Lincoln. Each type of institution retained some distinct advantages and each would have its articulate advocate, in the persons of James Currie and Alexander Hunter.

RATIONALES

The promoters of St Luke's had explained very clearly to the public, and to potential subscribers, what were the reasons for seeking to set up a specialist lunatic hospital. Their provincial counter-parts, with the later exception of Exeter,[4] chose not to copy the St Luke's arguments, although there were some inevitable similarities. One of the most telling reasons that could be adduced for establishing a hospital specifically for lunatics was that they had been directly excluded from admission to the voluntary general hospitals. Those hospitals tended to adopt sets of rules similar, often identical, to one another.[5] One of those rules stated clearly, as in Rule 45 of the Manchester Infirmary founded in 1752, that 'No Persons disordered in their senses' were to be admitted.[6] The constitutions of the York County Hospital and the Liverpool Infirmary operated a similar bar on their admission.[7] The exclusion of mentally disordered people from general hospitals was due to a number of linked factors. Because of their unpredictable and possibly noisy behaviour, they were seen to have considerable potential for disruption of the smooth running of the hospital, therefore posing difficult management problems. Not least, they were seen to require a specialist approach, in respect of the nature of their accommodation, medical oversight, and staffing.

Appeals for donations and subscriptions toward the establishment of lunatic hospitals argued for the special circumstances attached to madness, which made it very distinct from other types of illness, and entitled its victims to particular consideration. The initial appeal in Newcastle, for example, argued that they were 'for the most Part, poor and helpless to an extreme Degree.'[8] According to the trustees of the Manchester Infirmary in 1763, 'no cases can be more truly deplorable than those of poor Lunaticks', referring to them variously as 'unhappy Wretches', 'miserable Objects', and 'distress'd Creatures'.[9] Perhaps worse, without proper care and attendance, lunatics were likely to continue as 'publick Spectacles of the deepest Misery'.[10] Similar sentiments were expressed at York in 1772; the 'unhappy sufferers' were justly entitled to the compassion of the benevolent.[11] The Leicester appeal in 1794 called on public sympathy for 'that most helpless and pitiable class of mortals, poor lunatics'. It contended that 'Every Species of it produces a State of Distress and Degradation, peculiarly humiliating to Human Nature.'[12] All of these appeals emphasized the uniquely pathetic tragedy of insanity, inferring that, more than any other condition, it warranted a charitable response.

It was almost as if the advocates for lunatic hospitals in the different cities tried to outdo one another with the affecting persuasiveness of their appeals to public compassion. In Liverpool, the project had the especially influential and eloquent support of the physician James Currie, who had become active in local literary and radical political circles.[13] Currie argued that that there was no evil to which men were subjected 'so dreadful as insanity', for madness 'destroys all that makes life valuable'. He emphasized its all-pervasive consequences:

> It is not a single enjoyment of which it bereaves us, nor a single blessing that it carries away. It preys not on the gifts of fortune, but on the attributes of reason, and strikes at once at all the powers and privileges of man!'

The 'hapless victims' were entitled to 'our pity and our succour'. An asylum would protect them 'from the dangers of life, and from the selfish contempt of an unfeeling world'.[14] Currie had carefully articulated the essentially humanitarian element of the discourse of lunatic hospital foundation.

There was, however, another significant element to the discourse. Even more than the calls for public sympathy, the promoters of lunatic hospital projects dwelt increasingly on the risks associated with madness, both to the sufferer and to other people. The initial appeal in Newcastle in 1763 concentrated particularly on the danger to the sufferer. As a disease, insanity merited 'equal attention' to others, but 'when upon a closer Examination we find that Self-murder but too often arises from it', unlike in any other condition, it had to be accorded 'the Preference'.[15] Elsewhere, the emphasis was at least as much on the nuisance and danger posed to other people. At Manchester, the 'great Concern and Terror' caused to neighbours was invoked.[16] The dangerous aspect was emphasized at York a few years later. The public was warned that shortcomings in provision and the neglect of proper treatment had led to 'the most fatal acts of violence' toward relations and attendants, as well as to sufferers.[17] The appeal made at Leicester in 1794 similarly dwelt on the fear of harm to close relatives as well as to the lunatic himself:

> Surrounding Friends deeply partake of the Calamity, and in Addition to the Feelings which the present State of the Lunatic must excite, are subject to the alarming Apprehension of those common Effects of mental Derangement, Outrage to themselves or others, or the Suicide of the unhappy Sufferer.[18]

Such assertions were bound to strike a chord with public perceptions and prejudices, and were calculated to convince their audience that appropriate solutions were required.

In order to provide for the particular needs of the insane, and to confront the evident risks, it was contended that there had to be specialist facilities. The argument of 'mad-doctors' like William Battie that successful treatment depended on the removal of the patient from his home environment, and separation from family and friends, had gained wide currency.[19] Segregation from society and family was allied to 'confinement' as the means to provide a therapeutic environment for the patient, as well as security for others. Battie went as far as to suggest that 'confinement alone is often-times sufficient' in the successful treatment of the insane.[20] This was something on which he and his great rival John Monro could agree, the latter talking about the 'necessity of *confining* such as are deprived of their senses', and that in many cases it had restored people to reason without further medical intervention.[21]

Separation and confinement, however, did not in themselves require a public lunatic hospital. The specific argument advanced by proponents was the desirability of specialized care and management, based on knowledge of the particular needs of the insane. Thomas Arnold, the Leicester physician who played a key role in the establishment of the Leicester Asylum, argued that a 'particular management' was required, in a 'house adapted to the purpose'. Those in charge of the patients had to be 'furnished with the requisite conveniences for their government and safety'.[22] The point had been made fairly crudely some years earlier by the advocates for a Newcastle Lunatic Hospital, in advising the public that 'Mad People in general, require a very close Attendance'.[23] The trustees of the Manchester Infirmary were a little more sophisticated, arguing that the insane required a 'proper Place for their reception', which meant ensuring a 'suitable Guard and Attendance upon their Persons'.[24] This entailed not only a suitable building with the necessary facilities, but also its staffing by 'Servants, whose whole Care would entirely be taken up in guarding and securing these unhappy Persons from those Violences which they frequently commit upon themselves and others.'[25] The emphasis was decidedly custodial, albeit within a context of lunatic hospitals being designated as medical institutions.[26]

There were, of course, other types of specialist institutions for the insane becoming available, notably within the expanding private madhouse sector. Concerns had been growing about the exploitative nature of some of these houses, and the promoters of public lunatic hospitals actively sought to position their proposed institutions as a more moral and humane alternative, particularly for the vulnerable middle classes. This motive was spelt out quite explicitly by the Manchester Infirmary trustees, both in their initial appeal for funds and support and in subsequent publicity:

> The last, but not least, Consideration is, the Assistance which they reasonably hope to give to many Persons of middling Fortunes, who may unhappily have Relations thus terribly afflicted — by preserving them from the Impositions of those who keep private Mad-Houses, and thus supplying what is so much Wanted in this part of the Kingdom, an Hospital for Lunaticks, upon the most benevolent and modest Terms.[27]

One of the early annual reports of the York Lunatic Asylum went so far as to claim that it had been 'erected with a view to lessen the number of private Madhouses'.[28] Both at Manchester and York the decision had been taken to extend access to the lunatic hospital beyond the poorest classes. To this end, the public was assured that the institution was to be managed by 'men of principles and honour', who would provide for 'the most humane and disinterested treatment', in direct contrast to what was offered by the 'mercenary keepers' of private madhouses.[29]

In Liverpool, the radical Dr James Currie went even further in advocating the extension of the facility to those outside the ranks of the poor. He insisted that 'the interests of rich and poor are equally and immediately united', for with other diseases the rich could be treated in their own homes, but with insanity they would have to seek relief in a specialized establishment. Consequently, an asylum would have two objects – 'to provide accommodation for the poor suitable to their circumstances, and to make provision for those of superior stations who are able to remunerate the expense.'[30] By 1789, when Currie was writing, eligibility for admission to a lunatic hospital in relation to class, poverty, and wealth had become a live issue, particularly in York.[31] In fact, it proved problematic in most of the cities where lunatic hospitals were established. In Newcastle, the initial plan had been to include provision for some private patients, but the great demand for places for the poor made that policy highly controversial in the city and it had to be changed after a short time.[32] Only in Leicester was the question not raised as an idealogical matter, no doubt because the city already contained a substantial private madhouse, under the proprietorship of Dr Thomas Arnold, the infirmary physician who was to oversee the development and management of the public asylum. The Leicester Lunatic Asylum would provide primarily for paupers, while the wealthier patients were accommodated in Arnold's Bond Street madhouse.[33]

An important motivating factor for the proponents of lunatic hospitals was civic and county pride. This had been a significant element in the garnering of support for general hospitals and infirmaries, and led to the design and construction of prestigious buildings in prominent positions.[34] The same reserve of pride was mined for the foundation of a lunatic hospital, which could be represented as a distinguishing symbol of achievement by a particularly enlightened and altruistic local elite. In Newcastle, for example, the contention was that a subscription for the purpose would 'do Honour to this Part of the Kingdom'.[35] James Currie argued that a public asylum would 'reflect credit on the munificence of Liverpool'. The city's 'honours will be increased' as its system of charities was completed.[36] In other words, the establishment of a lunatic hospital could be construed as confirmation of the liberal, progressive and benevolent credentials of a city and its surrounding region.

Finally, there was the question of geography. Distance from London, and from Bethlem and St Luke's, would be cited as a primary reason for initiating projects in provincial centres. The issue was taken up from the outset in Manchester, with the infirmary governors declaring it to be too far from London to benefit from the 'two noble Hospitals established there'.[37] It was not only a question of distance and the associated travel costs and inconvenience, but also the practical difficulties surrounding the need to find a London resident prepared to nominate to the waiting list and act as surety for a person from some far-flung place. Even if this hurdle could be overcome, the likelihood was that Bethlem and St Luke's would be full with a waiting list.[38] At York it was emphasized that the consequence of the lack of access of Yorkshire patients to the London hospitals, as well as to those in Newcastle and Manchester, was that 'many useful members have been lost to society'. This held the fearful consequence that the illness might progress to a stage where it was 'beyond the reach of medicine', or that the sufferer could fall into the hands of 'those utterly unskilled in the treatment of the disease'.[39] In the north of England, the evident limited access to Bethlem and St Luke's was almost certainly the decisive factor in precipitating practical action toward establishment of the lunatic hospitals.

THE NORTHERN CITIES

The first successful foundation of a lunatic hospital by public subscription was in Newcastle-upon-Tyne, the city furthest distant from the capital.[40] The Newcastle Royal Infirmary had been opened in 1751.[41] Moves to develop a separate 'well regulated Hospital for the Relief of Lunatics' began in May 1763, with the initiation of a subscription, to be collected in the city's coffee houses.[42] Subscriptions were initially quite limited. The largest contributor was the Newcastle Common Council, which committed itself to £50 per annum. Despite the sluggish arrival of funds the governors decided to make a start, albeit on a modest scale. The 'Hospital for Lunatics for the Counties of Durham, Newcastle, and Northumberland' opened in July 1764, in a large adapted house, with capacity for nineteen patients.[43] In a significant break from the practices at Bethlem and St Luke's, presumably because of funding problems, a charge of three shillings per week for paupers was initiated, with private patients to pay according to the discretion of the governors. The hospital was to provide for both incurables and 'those whose Complaints may admit of Relief'. Poor patients were to be attended by a physician and a surgeon, appointed by the governors, who would make use of all means 'for the Recovery of their Reason'.[44] Dr John Hall, also physician to the Newcastle Infirmary, was from its inception a central figure in the lunatic hospital's development.[45]

The Newcastle Lunatic Hospital quickly exceeded its governors' expectations. The nineteen places proved insufficient, for within six months it was full with a waiting list and recognized as being 'too small and very insufficient for the purpose'. In August 1765, they resolved to develop a new and larger building, and in October the common council agreed the lease of a parcel of land in an undeveloped area outside the city walls near the Westgate, at a nominal yearly rent of 2s.6d.[46] There was, however, clear dissension among the governors as to what should be the proper nature of the hospital. Dr Hall sought to ensure provision for private patients, whose payments could subsidize the cost of admitting more poor patients. His proposal for the addition of a storey to the new building to accommodate the extra patients was rejected by the governors, who insisted on the hospital's integrity as an institution solely for the poor. They advised Hall to open a private madhouse for his paying patients, which he subsequently did. Nevertheless, even after he opened 'St Luke's House', and despite his public quarrel with the governors and the city's other medical men, he continued in the role of physician to the lunatic hospital.[47]

The second Newcastle Lunatic Hospital opened in 1767, with capacity for more than thirty patients.[48] A new and detailed set of rules was produced for its management and operation. The charges for pauper patients were revised upwards to four shillings per week.[49] The building itself was later described by an observer as 'elegant...with a neat pediment in the centre and spacious gardens'.[50] The architect William Newton's design shows a fairly modest structure, eighty feet in width at the front. The exterior resembled that of a large house. Inside, on the ground floor, there was a kitchen and pantry, accommodation for the keepers, and cells for twelve patients, six of which adjoined an enclosed court.[51] With some modifications and additions, this building remained in operation for upwards of sixty years. The difficulties which would eventually befall the Newcastle Lunatic Hospital will be considered in chapter seven.

Although Newcastle was the first of the provincial lunatic hospitals to actually open, moves had been simultaneously taking place in Manchester. Here, however, matters proceeded somewhat differently. Where the projectors in Newcastle had followed the model of St Luke's and opted to establish a hospital that was independent of the main infirmary, in Manchester the lunatic hospital was set up wholly under the auspices of the Manchester Infirmary, and was effectively an appendage to it. A new model of provision was thereby established that would prove very influential in Liverpool, Leicester, and elsewhere.

The Manchester Infirmary had opened in 1752 in a converted house, moving in 1755 to more imposing premises on Piccadilly.[52] The infirmary trustees had found it 'extremely inconvenient' to admit poor lunatics, and its rules consequently excluded them.[53] They evidently grew increasingly uneasy about the exclusion, which did not sit comfortably with the progressive image they sought to convey for the hospital and for the town itself. Discussions began in earnest in 1763 on the idea of making distinct provision for lunatics. After strong representations from 'a Number of pious and charitable Persons', the trustees decided to abolish Rule 45 and began a subscription to provide additional wards specifically for the insane.[54] The appeals for funds adopted the format that became standard, seeking public sympathy for the insane poor, whilst also promising protection of the public by building dedicated wards that would offer specialist care and treatment.[55] Donations and subscriptions were supplemented by funds raised by other means, such as charity sermons.[56] The necessary minimum sums accrued mainly through a large number of relatively small contributors, though there were some larger subscribers of £100 each. The cost of the building was £1500 by the time that it opened in May 1766.[57]

From the beginning Manchester's lunatic hospital (see Figure 2.1) venture was fully inter-linked with the infirmary. Infirmary trustees automatically became governors, their numbers augmented by the few who subscribed over £50. Rather than erect a completely separate building, the trustees chose to provide a 'large Wing for the Reception of Lunatics' immediately adjoining the infirmary proper. Food and 'Physick' were to be supplied from the infirmary. The only differences were to be in the type of accommodation and in the separate staffing, in the form of 'an experienced Governor and Governess' and 'proper Servants' to attend on the patients.[58] Until 1771 the finances and accounts were managed jointly, to

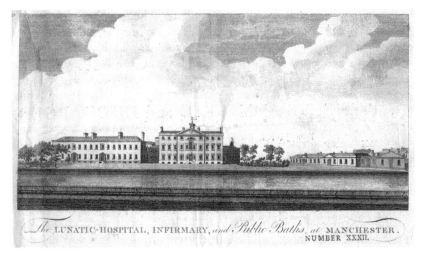

Figure 2.1 Manchester Infirmary and Lunatic Hospital, late 18th century.
Source: Copy of engraving courtesy of Chetham's Library, Manchester.

the extent that the lunatic hospital was treated as 'a separate ward of the Infirmary'.[59]

Although the Manchester Lunatic Hospital's status as an adjunct of the infirmary distinguished it from its predecessors, some ideas were nevertheless taken up from them. The initial intention had actually been to adopt the rules of the Newcastle Lunatic Hospital.[60] However, the governors subsequently decided to develop their own rules, based on those of Bethlem and St Luke's.[61] Unlike at Newcastle, custom built up very slowly at first. Places for twenty-two people had been provided, but only four were admitted during the hospital's first month of operation.[62] By late June 1767, one year on, thirty-two had been admitted and thirteen remained.[63] A year later, it still only contained sixteen people, but the infirmary trustees were able to express guarded satisfaction with the outcomes:

> The Lunatic Hospital....has been accompanied with the signal Blessing of the Almighty: For though yet in its Infancy, little known to the World, of Consequence but slenderly provided for; we have been happy enough to find seventeen poor Creatures in most lamentable Situation, discharged absolutely cured, and eight more greatly relieved, within the last Year.

They were, however, clearly still concerned about a lack of funds, and appealed to the public for more money in order to keep down the weekly charges.[64]

The financing of the Manchester Lunatic Hospital had been problematic from the outset. The amount of money subscribed, in comparison to St Luke's, was small and offered no scope to form a fund sufficient to defray the costs of treatment, care, and residence. The infirmary trustees were not prepared to contemplate diversion of any money raised, hitherto or in the future, from the main hospital.[65] They reluctantly recognized from the outset that there would have to be charges, as at Newcastle, with the minimum initially set at seven shillings per week. They could do little more than express an intention to provide free care for the poor at some future time, or at least gradually to lower the charges for paupers, either by accumulation of a fund or by subsidy from the income received from private patients. The significant question was posed to the public, however, whether an institution that had to levy charges really merited the name of 'hospital'.[66]

By the time that steps were initiated in York, in 1772, to develop provision for 'poor lunaticks' for the city and county, the 'excellent Establishments' at Newcastle and Manchester were there to provide 'noble Examples' for imitation.[67] A public meeting was held at York Castle in late August, a committee established, and a subscription launched. It was determined that the project could not proceed until a sum of £5000 had been pledged.[68] In September an address published in support of the appeal, with words borrowed from Manchester, detailed the reasons why a public lunatic hospital was needed and what it was hoped to achieve.[69] In order to ascertain the likely level of demand, and the scale on which the hospital should be built, requests were issued to all the corporate and parochial authorities in the county to submit numbers of those 'furiously mad' and likely to need admission.[70] Unresolved ambiguities about the determination of who appropriately fell into the category of 'poor lunaticks', however, were to create the basis of later disputes in York.[71]

Although the arguments put forward bore a close resemblance to those previously advanced in Manchester, the York committee eventually opted to provide their lunatic hospital on a different footing. The York County Hospital had been established more than thirty years before.[72] One of its physicians, Dr Alexander Hunter, was the prime mover in the lunatic hospital project.[73] He and his colleagues on the committee had initially wanted it built next to the main hospital, as in Manchester, but problems of land acquisition prevented this. The locating of a separate site near Bootham Bar proved a significant factor in ensuring that the lunatic hospital became a distinct and independent entity, like St Luke's and the Newcastle Lunatic Hospital.[74] Hunter himself would go on to become an enthusiastic advocate of autonomy.

Early fund-raising was relatively successful, though the committee was far from satisfied with progress. The target of £5000 had been achieved by July 1773, less than a year after the initial appeal. Members of the county aristocracy and gentry and leading people from the city of York were prominent on the subscription list, but their support was augmented by that of less exalted individuals, local firms, and societies such as 'The Social Club at the Black Dog'.[75] In August 1773 the governors took the significant decision to re-name the proposed hospital the York Lunatic Asylum.[76] It was the first to be given this title, clearly distinguishing an institution for treating insanity, intended to offer refuge and seclusion, from a hospital for people with specifically physical ailments. The site was acquired in 1774, at a cost of £1000.[77] The county's leading architect, John Carr, designed an imposing building, similar in design to his Leeds Infirmary.[78] It took three years to complete. The whole project was to prove rather more expensive than anticipated. A good deal of controversy ensued, with accusations of extravagance and misconduct. It was alleged that cheaper land would have been available nearer to the county hospital, and that the governors deliberately sought for the erection of a 'Sumptuous Edifice' for purposes of conspicuous ostentation.[79] These differences of opinion over the levels of initial expenditure on the land and the building proved to be only the start of what would become bitter and recurring disputes about all aspects of the financing of the asylum.

Carr had designed his building for fifty-four patients.[80] However, a combination of the unplanned level of costs, and lack of adequate subscriptions to meet the excess, meant a scaling down of the initial provision. The York Lunatic Asylum (see Figure 2.2) opened on 20 September 1777, with accommodation ready initially for only ten patients, though with the intention of providing for a further twenty shortly afterwards.[81] As had been the case with its predecessors, its beginnings were fairly modest. In 1779 there were twenty-three patients in the house, rising to twenty-eight in 1780 and reaching forty-three by 1785.[82] From the outset it had been determined that the asylum would be primarily 'an Establishment for the County of York', with limitations imposed on the acceptance of patients from elsewhere.[83]

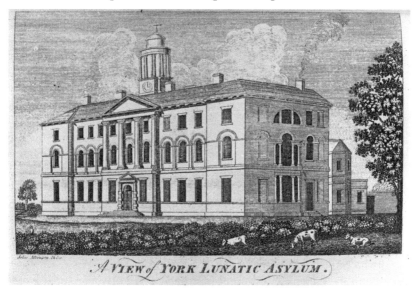

Figure 2.2 York Lunatic Asylum.
Source: Sotheran's York Guide, 1799, copy courtesy of York Reference Library.

Charges for patients' board were accepted as inevitable. The costings at Newcastle and Manchester had been studied in some detail, and produced a calculation in 1774 that six shillings a week would provide for a break-even situation.[84] However, this had to be revised upwards to eight shillings by the time the asylum opened in 1777, though, like at Manchester, there were expressions of regret and of intention to reduce the charges when this became possible.[85] This issue would also become the focus of later controversy.

Fifteen years were to elapse after the opening of the York Asylum before the next lunatic hospital project came to fruition in Liverpool. The Liverpool Infirmary had been opened as long ago as 1749,[86] but it took more than forty years for the town's leading citizens to begin practical steps toward augmenting it with a lunatic hospital. This is perhaps even more surprising when contrasted with the example set by their neighbours and rivals in Manchester as early as 1766.[87] The presence of the Manchester Lunatic Hospital may actually have delayed activity in Liverpool, for it was accepting patients from throughout Lancashire and the north-west, and had received a number of admissions from Liverpool.[88] It was inevitable, though, that a thriving and expanding city like Liverpool would come to require its own facility.

With two proven types of provision to consider, an independent institution or one connected to the infirmary, Liverpool opted to follow the Manchester example. As had been the case there, the initial impetus came from the infirmary governors. The plan to erect a 'Building...for the reception of Lunatics' was set in motion at a meeting of 'Gentlemen, Clergy & Merchants' held at the infirmary on 7 August 1789. The proposed institution was to be 'under the direction of the Officers & Faculty' of the infirmary. They formed the nucleus of the committee set up to carry the plan into effect, which met ten days later and agreed a proposal for a building large enough to accommodate sixty patients. It was to be financed by voluntary subscription, in a fund kept distinct from that of the infirmary proper.[89] A decision was quickly taken to build on the garden belonging to the infirmary and on some adjoining land currently leased out as a ropery.[90]

As elsewhere, the driving force behind the asylum's projection and establishment was one of the infirmary's senior physicians, Dr James Currie.[91] A man of not inconsiderable political and literary skills, Currie proved an excellent publicist, eloquently laying out the case in two extended letters to the Liverpool newspapers.[92] The first, written shortly after the initial public meeting, was intended to raise awareness of the philosophical and humanitarian grounds for establishing a lunatic asylum. Currie restated some of the familiar arguments, though without entering into much actual detail about the project, other than suggesting that the ability to provide for the poor could be increased by accepting some paying private patients.

Currie's second letter, published in October, dealt much more with practicalities. It came in the wake of some evident criticism of the scheme.

Opponents had condemned the proposed expense, and had questioned whether an asylum was actually needed and even whether insane paupers were entitled to specialist care outside the poor house or the city's new gaol. Others had argued that, though they favoured an asylum, it ought to be separated from the infirmary and preferably sited outside the city, with space for recreation and occupation as well as the benefits of purer air. Significantly, Currie had been in correspondence with Dr Alexander Hunter of York, who had strongly argued the case for separation. Currie conceded the validity of this, but pointed out the prohibitive expense. He countered that union with the infirmary would carry a number of advantages. There would 'not only be an immense saving of expense in the building itself, but in the annual disbursements', due to the prospect of sharing the apothecary and other officers as well as the administration. The arguments were not solely economic, however. Currie was a strong adherent to the conception of close linkages between mental and physical disorders, both as regards their origins and the means required to manage and treat them:

> The discipline of an Infirmary and of a Lunatic Asylum have similar objects, and require the same habits, and nearly the same degree of watchfulness and attention. The institutions themselves are closely allied in their nature; the first affords relief for diseases of the body, the second to diseases of the mind.

He acknowledged concerns that noise emanating from the lunatic wards might disturb other infirmary patients, but contended that information from Manchester, and also from Dumfries where a lunatic ward adjoined the hospital, showed such anxieties to be unfounded. A separation of fifty yards would deal with any possible problems, he suggested.[93] Ultimately, though, it was primarily the financial constraints that steered Currie and his colleagues toward the Manchester rather than the York model.[94]

Currie's letters were acknowledged as highly influential in gathering practical support for the project. Subscriptions were collected at various coffee houses and at the offices of Gore's, the publisher of one of the main Liverpool newspapers. In early December, the infirmary's General Quarterly Board formally adopted the scheme.[95] The local press assisted as best it could, publicizing the gruesome suicide of a carpenter's apprentice, who had 'frequently before shewn signs of insanity', and suggesting that he might have been prevented from committing this 'horrid deed' had there been a lunatic asylum where the 'unhappy wretch' might have been cured. For good measure, the paper added that there were currently twenty-nine insane people in the workhouse, some being 'public spectacles of the deepest misery'.[96]

As had been the case elsewhere, the preparedness of the Liverpool middle classes to stump up the necessary funds did not apparently match the projectors' enthusiasm. Currie had received advice from Hunter at York that the cost of an asylum for thirty to forty patients should be between £4,000 and £5,000.[97] The infirmary governors apparently took this to mean £4,500. By March 1790 only £2,000 had been raised, but the committee were nevertheless directed to carry out the plans 'with all prudent dispatch'.[98] A year later, the amount subscribed had only increased to £2,800. Things were clearly not going as smoothly as Currie and his supporters had hoped. The governors were trying to persuade a reluctant public that the 'plan and situation' had been highly approved by 'gentlemen of first character for abilities and experience' in the care and management of the insane. They referred to 'a collision of opposite judgments' that had occurred and trusted that any 'partial objections' would be overcome by the 'authority' of these 'competent judges', enabling support for the scheme to resume.[99] However, their hopes were disappointed and no more money was forthcoming. Being committed to proceed, and without adequate pledged subscriptions, finance had to be found from elsewhere. Some money was transferred direct from the infirmary funds, and the difference was made up by a substantial loan of £3,000 from Liverpool Corporation.[100]

The infusion of funds rescued the project. The asylum opened to accept patients in September 1792, but on a much smaller scale than envisaged, and it struggled for a few years. Despite capacity for sixty patients, there were only five in the house in March 1794, by which time thirty-two had been admitted and nineteen 'cured'.[101] A year later there were still only five patients remaining in the house, with twenty having been admitted in the course of the year. The Governors announced that they had brought in 'an experienced and approved' keeper and matron from St Luke's Hospital in London, and were now confident that the asylum 'promises speedily to realize the hopes of its friends'.[102] Their optimism was finally borne out, for sixty-three people were admitted during 1795 and thirty-six remained in March 1796.[103] By the end of the decade, the number of patients in the Liverpool Lunatic Asylum had risen to a respectable fifty.[104]

THE MIDLANDS AND THE WEST

With the opening of the Liverpool Lunatic Asylum in 1792, the network of voluntary lunatic hospitals in the north of England was effectively completed. Meanwhile, however, the model had been attracting attention further south, particularly in some of the midland counties. The governors of the infirmaries in several towns had initiated tentative steps toward the provision of a lunatic hospital, though in most cases there was a very long gestation period before anything materialized. The first project to actually reach fruition was in Leicester. The origins of the Leicester Lunatic Asylum were somewhat inauspicious.[105] Its checkered early history reflected several of the elements that proved problematic in the general development of lunatic hospitals. There were difficulties in raising the necessary funds, which was partly the consequence of the stigma associated with mental disorder. Professional rivalries and jealousies were endemic in the city's medical circles, and these were part cause and part effect of the uneasy relationship between private practice and public charity that characterized the nature of provision for the insane in Leicester. These factors came together to lead firstly to protracted delays, and later to the problems of maladministration and dubious practice that were to surface in several lunatic hospitals.

The pattern of development in Leicester followed Manchester rather than York. The Leicester Infirmary had opened in 1771.[106] Its admission rules had comprised the usual exclusions, amongst which were the insane. Agreement to remedy the situation was reached at the annual general meeting of the infirmary governors in June 1781.[107] They advised the public that they were 'anxious to render that Receptacle for the indigent Sick, more extensively useful than its present Establishment will admit of', and to erect 'an additional Building for the admission of LUNATICS'. The plan was for a building large enough to accommodate twenty patients.[108] The governors quickly put their proposals into effect, advertising for architects to prepare plans. A Mr Harrison was appointed in October, and contracts were made with builders to complete the construction.[109] As elsewhere, the driving force behind the project was one of the senior physicians to the Leicester Infirmary, Dr James Vaughan.[110] He had advocated strongly for adding a separate building to the infirmary itself, and was instrumental in attracting a specific bequest of £1000 for the purpose.[111] Vaughan provided ongoing advice to the governors, traveling north in early 1782 to visit and report on the operation of the lunatic hospitals at Manchester and York.[112]

The construction work proceeded comparatively quickly, and in late October 1782 the governors announced that 'the building of the HOSPITAL intended for the reception of LUNATICKS' was nearly completed.[113] Plans were being made for a full opening at the end of the Leicester races in June 1784.[114] The optimism, however, proved misplaced for something was going badly wrong. An eventful meeting of the general board of the infirmary on 17 June 1784 decided to postpone the opening of the lunatic hospital 'untill further orders shall be given concerning the same'. Thereupon Dr Vaughan resigned as physician to the infirmary, and three other physicians were elected, including Dr Thomas Arnold.[115] One problem had been the singular lack of success in raising the requisite funds.[116] However, of at least equal significance was Arnold's role and the bitter rivalry and hostility that had evidently developed between him and James Vaughan.[117]

Arnold was to become the pivotal figure in the later development of the Leicester Lunatic Asylum. The son of William Arnold, proprietor of a substantial private madhouse, he was sent by his father to Edinburgh University to study medicine, with the intention that he would take over the running of the madhouse. After gaining his M.D. in 1766, young Arnold duly returned to Leicester to join his father.[118] He was an early subscriber to the proposed Leicester Infirmary and became joint physician along with

Vaughan when it opened in 1771.[119] Relations between them were already strained when Arnold resigned his infirmary post in 1776, leaving Vaughan as sole physician.[120] The prospect a few years later of a charitable public facility in Leicester posed a distinct threat to Arnold's business, at a time when he was clearly seeking to establish himself as a respectable maddoctor. In early 1782, whilst the lunatic hospital was under construction, Arnold published the first volume of his book *Observations on the Nature, Kinds, Causes, and Prevention of Insanity, Lunacy, or Madness*[121], which he hoped would establish his reputation as an authority on insanity and its treatment. It is very conceivable that Vaughan's enthusiasm for setting up a lunatic hospital had been partly motivated by a wish to pose a serious challenge to Arnold and his madhouse. Arnold responded by becoming re-involved in infirmary affairs, and he was closely associated with the decision in June 1784 to indefinitely postpone the opening of the lunatic hospital, which directly precipitated Vaughan's resignation.[122]

The practical consequence of these unedifying events was that the lunatic hospital building was left standing empty for several years as a 'useless and disgraceful pile'.[123] John Throsby, the local historian, posed the contrast between the infirmary as 'a noble monument of the liberality of the present age' and its unoccupied section that may have been 'built to gratify the desires of one gentleman, or shut up to serve the purposes of another'.[124] There was no doubt locally that Throsby was referring to Vaughan and Arnold respectively, leading people to conclude that the pursuit of individual over public interests was largely responsible for the scandal.

The shelving of the plan to open the lunatic hospital worked very much to Thomas Arnold's advantage. The private asylum on Bond Street attracted growing custom, placing Arnold in a position where he could make a magnanimous gesture which he hoped would show that a lunatic hospital was both unnecessary and a waste of money. In May 1785 he announced a plan to admit ten poor patients at 8s per week, comparable to the rates charged at the lunatic hospitals of Manchester and York, and a further two patients at no charge whatsoever. He pointedly claimed that this initiative constituted a 'HOSPITAL for LUNATICS'. Any patient admitted under the scheme had to be 'a proper object of the charity', with preference given to those nominated by infirmary governors.[125] The infirmary board was sufficiently impressed to issue a public thanks to Arnold for his 'generous and patriotic Institution', which was 'similar to the plan of the ASYLUM' which they had intended to open.[126] Arnold's apparent benevolence did not rest there, however, for in June 1790, 'having had frequent reason to lament the difficulty with which the insane poor obtain the necessary relief from their respective parishes', he expanded the remit of his 'charitable Asylum' to accept parish paupers on the same terms as other poor people deemed 'proper objects'. Furthermore, he increased the number of patients admitted at 8s from ten to fourteen, and doubled the numbers of those admitted free of charge from two to four.[127]

It was Arnold's hope, no doubt, that his apparently public-spirited gestures had obviated the need for the infirmary governors to persevere with their asylum project. The empty building, however, remained a source of continuing embarrassment. It was periodically used for other medical purposes, such as to house women with venereal disease.[128] After years of apparent inertia the infirmary governors finally agreed in 1792 to take some action. At their annual meeting in September they decided to ascertain the likely expense involved in opening and operating 'the building intended for the reception of Lunatics'.[129] They naturally called upon the expertise close at hand, and commissioned Thomas Arnold to prepare a plan of what was needed to render the asylum 'in a proper state' to open and receive twenty patients. Within a few days, Arnold had presented a comprehensive report on the necessary building alterations, detailing the furniture, equipment and staffing required. He projected the likely cost of the essential work as being a minimum of £300. He also produced estimated running costs, and sought to demonstrate that these would be at a level the charity would be unable to sustain until some future time when its funds were in a healthier state. Nevertheless, and doubtless with a view to dispelling any suspicion that he may be counseling abandonment for reasons of self-interest, Arnold concluded his report with an offer, when the time came, to 'most willingly and cordially undertake the management' of the asylum, promising that 'no attention or exertion shall be wanting on my part' to ensure its 'efficacy'.[130]

The governors were undeterred by Arnold's caution and equivocation. They prepared detailed estimates, based on his proposals and on information obtained from the lunatic hospitals at Manchester and York as to their scales of charges. New appeals for funds were launched, though still with only moderate success.[131] By September 1793 it was determined to undertake the building alterations, and contracts were advertised.[132] As work went on through the spring of 1794, efforts to extract money from reluctant subscribers continued.[133] Despite ongoing financial problems the governors were anxious to proceed, and a special meeting on 15 August agreed to a partial opening.[134] The Leicester Lunatic Asylum finally opened to receive ten patients in late September 1794, a decade after the building's initial completion, with an expressed intention to increase numbers at some future point when finances permitted.[135]

Dr Thomas Arnold's role remained, at best, ambiguous. His offer to superintend the operation of the asylum had been gratefully accepted by the governors. He was involved in all aspects of the preparations — furnishing and equipping the building, drafting of the rules, and the appointment of staff.[136] Yet, starting in March 1794 and through the spring, when the asylum was being prepared for opening under his oversight, Arnold continued to advertise simultaneously the charitable facilities on offer at his own 'hospital for lunatics' in Bond Street, emphasizing its extensive provision for the poor.[137] The new asylum's remit to provide 'expressly for the reception of pauper lunatics & others of the insane poor' meant there was virtually no competitive threat to Arnold's lucrative private business.[138] Indeed, the public asylum catered for a much smaller number of patients than the madhouse, and it continued to operate on a relatively modest scale. Every year, in the annual reports, the infirmary governors were lamenting 'the want of an adequate Fund from Donations and Annual Subscriptions' and urging greater 'benevolence' from the Leicester public.[139] The intention to utilize all of the twenty places did not materialize; in 1795 the numbers 'admissable' were increased to twelve, and by 1799 the capacity had only been raised to fourteen.[140] The long saga could hardly be said to have culminated in a successful outcome.

Hitherto, all the successfully established lunatic hospitals had been sited in large and populous towns or cities. Hereford, however, was little more than a substantial market town, at the hub of a large rural county. The origins of the Hereford Lunatic Asylum were not dissimilar to those of its provincial predecessors. Its subsequent history, though, was rather singular. As in Leicester, there was an apparent collision between aspirations of public charity and private medical interest. In Hereford, this did not significantly delay the plans to open an asylum. What resulted, though, within a comparatively short period of time, were profound changes in its constitution and methods of operation.

The Hereford Infirmary had been established in 1776.[141] Proposals to develop a lunatic hospital in the city appear to have been considered by the infirmary governors shortly afterwards.[142] A supportive correspondent to the *Gloucester Journal* in March 1777 suggested that, other than the normal reasons for establishing an hospital for the insane, there was an important factor peculiar to the locality, associated with its excessive consumption of alcohol. The 'cyder-counties', he contended, 'unfortunately abound with the greatest numbers of these objects of compassion'.[143] A public subscription was initiated under the auspices of the infirmary, but the money proved slow to come in. It was not until October 1792, following 'several large Benefactions' which brought the fund to over £1,300, that the governors agreed to proceed. They adopted the Manchester model of close linkage to the infirmary, and a committee was formed to execute the plan to build a lunatic asylum on adjoining ground.[144] The architect John Nash, still at an early stage of his illustrious career, was commissioned to design and prepare estimates for the erection of 'Lunatick Apartments' for twenty patients. Plans and information were sought from elsewhere, notably the new Liverpool Asylum.[145]

Delays occurred, connected with fund-raising difficulties. From the beginning the infirmary governors were clearly equivocal about managing a specialist facility for the insane, and the physicians and surgeons sought to protect their own financial interests. In April 1798, with the asylum being prepared for opening, consideration was given to leasing it at a nominal rent to three of the medical men, the physicians Dr Blount and Dr Campbell and surgeon Mr Cotes, to operate as a private establishment, advertising for and receiving patients 'upon the Usual & Customary Terms'.[146] This curious idea was soon shelved, being found after 'mature consideration' to be 'difficult in its execution'. However, the physicians retained effective control with the appointment of a committee of the 'Gentlemen of the Faculty belonging to the Infirmary' to oversee the asylum's opening. Dr Campbell was given particular responsibility for the practical aspects and for the recruitment of a 'proper keeper' from Bethlem Hospital to take charge of the patients.[147]

The Hereford Lunatic Asylum finally opened, as a public charitable institution, in 1799. Following accepted practice, a set of rules for management of the asylum and its patients was published, including arrangements for referrals and admissions.[148] Within two years, though, the arrangements had broken down. Much of the blame was attributed to the shortcomings of David Davies, the keeper brought from Bethlem. A combination of Davies' alleged mismanagement and 'defects of the original building' had led to it rapidly becoming 'delapidated'. The medically dominated management committee concluded that the asylum 'could not be conducted according to the existing system'. The earlier ideas of privatization were revived, and the governors agreed in July 1801 to lease it at a nominal rent of one guinea per year to Dr William Blount and the surgeon Thomas Cotes, 'two of the Medical Superintendents of the Infirmary', who were to advance sufficient money to pay for necessary repairs and renovations. They in turn, with the governors' consent, assigned part of the lease to another surgeon, John Pateshall.[149]

The Hereford Asylum, in its short life as a public institution, was actually the last lunatic hospital directly attached to a general hospital. Its situation was now extremely anomalous, for it went on to operate in effect as a private madhouse and was eventually licensed as such by the magistrates. However, the infirmary governors did retain some residual powers of inspection and oversight, which they would occasionally exercise. Their continued reluctance to incur any financial burdens led to subsequent renewals of the lease.[150] The charitable funds accumulated for the asylum were invested at interest, and eventually made available for the future county asylum to accept poor non-paupers.[151] The unusual arrangement of a private asylum, situated within the infirmary grounds and operated for profit by some of its medical officers, persisted for several decades. The ills arising from a defective building were compounded by poor management, and the asylum was to become one of the less satisfactory examples of private provision. Serious concerns about aspects of its operation led eventually to a special parliamentary select committee investigation in 1839.[152]

The focus of activity had, by 1800, shifted further to the south-west. The Royal Devon and Exeter Hospital, opened in 1741, was one of the earliest provincial hospitals built by public subscription.[153] However, more than fifty years were to elapse before constructive steps were taken to provide a lunatic hospital for the region. The lead was taken by a group of clergymen, led by Reverend James Manning, in conjunction with one of the infirmary physicians, Dr George Daniell. The outline plan, prepared by Manning, was presented by the Bishop of Exeter to a meeting of the Grand Jury at the Assizes, held at Exeter Castle in March 1795.[154] The proposals were approved, and then published shortly afterwards. It was evident, though, that the process had actually begun some time before, for several hundred pounds had already been raised, and a provisional site near the county hospital identified and costed. Manning and his colleagues were concerned to demonstrate that the status and finances of the Royal Devon and Exeter would not be adversely affected, for 'each should be a distinct and independent Institution, standing on its own Foundation, and supported by separate and distinct Means'. They had been much influenced by the arrangements at the York Asylum. However, they went further than Hunter, arguing ambitiously that patients' weekly payments 'suited to their Circumstances' would 'render *Annual Subscriptions* unnecessary'.[155] The aim was, therefore, to provide a self-financing institution that would not drain charitable funds.

A subscription was opened after the March meeting. Rev. Manning and Dr Daniell personally approached 'some Gentlemen' for contributions.[156] Over £2,000 had been raised before the first subscribers' meeting at Exeter Castle in July 1795, which included several large contributions of £100 or more.[157] They resolved to establish a 'General Hospital, for the Reception of Insane Persons', in or near the city of Exeter. A committee was formed, with directions to obtain rules and regulations from similar institutions elsewhere, and to arrange for a building plan and estimates for fitting it out.[158] Local circumstances, however, were none too propitious for further fund-raising. In early 1796 the Devon and Exeter Hospital's finances were in a parlous state, with its governors having to sell off stocks to cover running costs and calling on the public for assistance.[159] Donations and subscriptions for the proposed Exeter Lunatic Asylum were clearly affected. After considering various unsatisfactory offers of building land, the committee concluded that they could obtain better value by renting and adapting a suitable existing building.[160] In November 1799, following some deft haggling, they bought Bowhill House, a long-fronted 'Gentleman's House' on the outskirts of the city, with over two acres of land attached, at a cost of just under £700. After the necessary adaptations, the total cost amounted to nearly £3,000.[161]

A detailed set of rules was published in 1801, later followed by a revised version in 1804.[162] Initial capacity was for fifteen people, the first patients being admitted in July 1801.[163] The expressed intention was to cater for those 'judged to be in Circumstances of restorable Insanity'. The asylum was to offer 'a most comfortable residence' for the pauper lunatic, which 'at the same Time that it guards him from a hopeless and miserable Treatment, holds out the consolatory Prospect of his Recovery'. However, it was not to be solely for paupers, but rather would provide for three classes of patients — 'Indigent Persons, dependent on the Charities of others'; 'Persons in moderate, but not independent Circumstances'; and, 'persons in affluent Circumstances'. As in predecessor lunatic hospitals, charges were determined according to ability to pay, with the payments of the more affluent subsidizing the costs of the poorer patients. Initial charges for the third or 'indigent' class were set at the relatively high level of 10s.6d per week, with an anticipation of reduction as the state of the funds improved.[164]

The first patients were admitted in July 1801. The fifteen places in the asylum rapidly proved insufficient, and by August 1802 the house had been full for some time.[165] In 1803, with more funds having been accumulated, an additional building was commissioned at a cost of a further £4,000. After its completion in the spring of 1804, forty-eight patients could now be accommodated. Following the original design to provide for people of varying levels of income, the rooms were 'neatly fitted up in a manner suited to their Ranks in Life'. There were four day rooms, and five 'extensive airing Grounds' separated by high brick walls and delineated according to gender and degrees of insanity. Hot and cold baths and showers were provided.[166] The enlarged asylum quite quickly gained a good reputation further afield.[167] In 1807 its governors were proclaiming that the proportion of people 'restored to the enjoyment of reason' at Exeter 'much surpassed' that at any other asylum. Patients were being attracted there from beyond Devon and the other western counties.[168] By 1812, further expansion plans were being set in motion.[169]

The idea of establishing a lunatic hospital by public subscription may well have received consideration in most major towns with a voluntary hospital. In several, particularly across the midlands, a subscription was launched. In Nottingham, Gloucester, and Stafford, efforts that began in the eighteenth century did not bring quick results, but they eventually came to fruition after the legislation of 1808. In Nottingham, where the county hospital had been established in 1782,[170] moves to add 'an Asylum, for Lunatics' were initiated around 1789.[171] Funds accumulated steadily and some land was leased from Nottingham Corporation, but it was not until October 1803, with a sum of £5,500 available, that practical steps were initiated. A new committee was formed, under the auspices of the Nottingham General Hospital and including three of its physicians. They communicated with Dr Alexander Hunter at York Asylum, and with Atkinson, one of its architects, who prepared some plans.[172] It was probably Hunter's influence that diverted them from a location adjoining the county hospital. Acquisition of a suitable alternative site proved problematic, however, and it took until July 1808 to conclude the purchase of land at Sneinton, on the edge of the city.[173] The whole project was given a huge boost by the passage of Wynn's Act in 1808, with its clauses encouraging county justices to unite with voluntary subscribers to construct and operate a joint asylum.[174] Agreement was reached in October 1810, and the Nottinghamshire General Lunatic Asylum finally opened in early 1812.[175]

The Act of 1808 had followed from the Select Committee on the State of Criminal and Pauper Lunatics, which had met and reported in 1807.[176] The chief contributor to the committee's deliberations was the Gloucestershire magistrate and prison reformer Sir George Onisephorus Paul.[177] There is little doubt that Paul's intention in promoting the legislation had been to facilitate the development of asylums funded largely by subscription. He had formed a strong commitment to the model, based partly on correspondence with Drs Hunter in York and Currie in Liverpool. He was particularly interested in the establishment of financial arrangements whereby the payments of wealthy private patients could produce surplus funds to be utilized for the admission of poor patients. For many years Paul was the prime mover behind the scheme to develop a subscription asylum in Gloucester, which would provide for all the western counties.[178]

The process in Gloucester had followed the established pattern. The city's infirmary had been established as far back as 1755.[179] Its governors resolved in September 1793 to establish a 'GENERAL HOSPITAL, for the reception of INSANE PERSONS', adopting the York model of financing the scheme.[180] Subscriptions were initiated, and over £4,000 had been accumulated within a few months. Sir George Paul, who had taken charge of the project, prepared detailed plans covering finances, management systems, building lay-out, staffing, and the orientation of the treatment regime.[181] He had fully accepted Hunter's argument that the asylum should be entirely distinct from the general hospital, going so far as to quote a Hunter *dictum* on the first page of his pamphlet — 'An Asylum for Lunatics should always be a separate and independent charity; an union with an Infirmary is unnatural.'[182] Paul, however, was highly cautious in his approach, insisting that building work should not start until the funds were sufficient for its completion. The subscribers concluded by 1802 that they had enough money to proceed, but argument continued as to whether or not the asylum should be linked with the Gloucester Infirmary.[183] Although the 1808 Act, promoted by Paul himself, provided subscribers with the option to combine with the county, a succession of delays ensued. Paul continued a rearguard resistance to the establishment of a joint asylum, still nursing the hope that the subscribers could remain independent and set up a purely voluntary asylum.[184] It was not until 1823 that the Gloucestershire County Lunatic Asylum finally opened, based on partnership between subscribers and county justices.[185]

Wynn's Act had made available new options for the funding of a public lunatic asylum. However, the voluntary approach was not completely eclipsed for, almost twenty years after the Exeter Asylum, a new public subscription asylum opened in Lincoln in 1820. The Lincoln County Hospital had opened as far back as 1769,[186] but several decades passed before serious efforts were made to provide a separate institution for the insane. The scheme's actual start date is unclear, but there was a committee established and a subscription under way by June 1807, when the funds stood at nearly £2,400.[187] By late September they had risen to £3,800. Interestingly, the example cited for emulation was not the usual one of nearby York but Exeter, with its recent published claims of singular success in achieving cures.[188] Aristocratic support had been enlisted, with the Earl of Yarborough as president, and Lord Brownlow and the Bishop of Lincoln as vice-presidents.[189] By early 1809 the funds had grown to £6,500 and land was purchased in Eastgate. However, a succession of delays ensued. The architect Richard Ingleman's plans were approved in September 1809, but a year later the project was deferred when it was realized that costs were likely to exceed available finances.[190] In 1813 the county magistrates proposed a union with the subscribers to build a joint asylum under the 1808 Act, as had been accomplished in neighbouring Nottinghamshire.[191] Though attracted to the idea, the subscribers were unwilling to sacrifice their independence.[192] Finally, in March 1817, they concluded that their resources were sufficient to make it 'safe and expedient' to proceed independently to build an asylum for fifty patients.[193]

The imposing edifice of Lincoln Lunatic Asylum, fronted with Ionic pillars, was completed during 1819.[194] The building's grandeur matched its location, sited on top of the hill adjoining Lincoln Castle and commanding views over a wide area. There were, nevertheless, more delays, occasioned partly by a failure to recruit a medically qualified director at the low salary offered. The first patients were finally admitted in April 1820.[195] The asylum accepted pauper, charity, and private patients in similar fashion to others funded wholly or partly by subscription. As with its predecessors, patient numbers grew gradually, so that thirty were in the house by March 1825.[196] From the outset Lincoln Asylum operated as an independent institution, though its physicians were shared with the Lincoln County Hospital and some committee meetings were held there. That independence would later manifest itself in the innovative policies of patient management implemented from the late 1820s onwards, which culminated in Lincoln being the pioneer in the abolition of mechanical restraint. The celebrity which Lincoln Asylum and some of its medical officers attained might conceivably not have been possible if it had been anything other than a voluntary institution, unhindered by the constraints of magistrate superintendence.[197]

The voluntary model clearly still had something to offer for, by the time Lincoln Asylum opened, it had been taken up at two more county towns, Oxford and Northampton. In both places local factors influenced the decision to establish an institution by subscription rather than through the county rates. In Oxford as elsewhere the impetus came from an established general hospital, the Radcliffe Infirmary founded in 1770.[198] A governors' meeting in November 1812 noted the 'great public utility' of the 'lunatick asylums' established in various parts of the country and launched a subscription.[199] Specific proposals were adopted in April 1813. Considerable support came from several colleges as well as from clergymen and aristocrats in the locality.[200] Advice was taken from sources that included St Luke's, the Manchester Lunatic Hospital, and the Exeter and Lincoln Asylums, as well as from individuals like Sir George Paul, Reverend Thomas Becher[201], and Thomas Warburton, proprietor of the Bethnal Green madhouses.[202] Negotiations were opened with the county justices to combine under the Act of 1808, but these foundered due largely to the magistrates' reluctance to commit the county to a financial burden.[203] The subscribers decided to continue independently, and Richard Ingleman, the architect of the Nottingham and Lincoln Asylums, was commissioned to design the building.[204]

The Radcliffe governors initially sought a site within the vicinity of the infirmary, but this proved not to be affordable.[205] It was, therefore, primarily a financial rather than a therapeutic motive that led them to follow the Exeter precedent and locate at Headington, two miles outside the city. Even more noteworthy was the governors' proposed admission policy. Piqued perhaps by the county justices' rejection of the proposals to act in concert, they decided to exclude parish paupers and accept only private and charitable patients, members of the 'middling and inferior classes of society'.[206] The intention, as at Manchester, York, and Exeter, was to use the profits from the wealthier private patients to subsidize the costs of poor patients. To that end, they provided relatively high standards of accommodation. The Oxford Lunatic Asylum, as it was initially known, opened in July 1826.[207] As elsewhere, initial progress was slow, with only eleven patients having been admitted by the end of the year. The governors resorted to fairly extensive advertising to attract patents, in order to avert a financial crisis, and it was not until after 1828 that the asylum began to meet expectations.[208]

The Northampton Asylum, which opened in 1838 after an unusually long gestation period, technically falls outside the time frame of this book. However, its roots were clearly in the late eighteenth century. The town's first general hospital had been established as early as 1743.[209] In 1789, when planning a new building, its governors actively considered the inclusion of a lunatic hospital but rejected the idea on the grounds of potential noise disturbance to patients in the main hospital.[210] Active fund-raising began after a specific bequest in 1804 and a large donation in 1806, but progress was painfully slow. Despite this, the governors decided against making use of the 1808 Act to develop a joint asylum with the county magistrates, and opted to continue independently.[211] It was not until 1833, with the funds having reached the relatively large sum of £12,000, that they finally decided to proceed. The long saga finally ended in August 1838 with the opening of the Northampton General Lunatic Asylum.[212] It effectively constituted the last of the independently established voluntary lunatic hospitals.[213]

CONCLUSIONS

By the end of the Georgian era, the plan adopted by the subscribers of St Luke's in 1750 had proved extremely influential, having been followed in upwards of ten centres in the provinces. Although there were considerable variations in how these provincial lunatic hospitals were developed, due to local or regional circumstances, the essential elements remained consistent. At the heart were the funding arrangements, based on donation and subscription. Here the contrast between the situation in London and elsewhere was greatest. The governors of St Luke's apparently had little difficulty in raising very substantial funds. Its assets had reached £100,000 by 1787, and in 1794 one single individual donated £5,000, an amount sufficient to build and open a provincial lunatic hospital.[214] In some regional centres there were serious difficulties in raising sums that were even a fraction of what St Luke's had accumulated. Evidently, conspicuous charitable giving was more likely to focus on a high profile metropolitan institution. Provincial philanthropists and donors, it would seem, were far more constrained by concerns around the stigma of insanity than their more openly progressive London counter-parts.

The chief consequence of these disparities in funding base was that, where St Luke's could provide its services free of charge to 'fit objects of charity', the provincial lunatic hospitals were never able to do so. From the outset they were reliant on weekly payments by, or on behalf of, their patients. Although there were some expressed intentions to remedy the situation in the future as funds permitted, in reality these were little more than hopeful aspirations. What emerged were increasingly sophisticated charging systems, tailored according to financial means and social class. The ostensible rationale to gain currency was that the costs of treating the poor should be subsidized by payments received from the better off. Developed under Dr Alexander Hunter's guidance at York, and given the seal of approval by Sir George Onisephorus Paul, these arrangements were brought toward perfection at Exeter, where there were eventually seven divisions of classes.[215]

The issue of the lunatic hospital's degree of independence became particularly significant. In every case there had been at least some initial link to an existing voluntary hospital, and this had offered the intellectual and practical impetus required to support their early development. Beginning at Manchester, several of the provincial institutions emerged directly out of parent hospitals and remained inextricably linked with them. The close connection with an infirmary provided clear financial and managerial benefits, as well as a degree of respectability from being attached to an established charity in the town or city. For some reason, however, this model of provision was not adopted again after the failure of the Hereford experiment.[216] Ideals of self-sufficiency and autonomous control had evidently gained greater favour among those interested in financing and governing an institution for the insane. Independence offered some clear advantages, not least the opportunities to innovate in administrative and financial arrangements, as at York, and in treatment and patient management practices, as would be illustrated at Lincoln from the 1820s onwards.

The associations with general hospitals highlighted the extent to which the lunatic hospitals were perceived and developed as institutions driven by medical principles and medical expertise. This was underlined by the involvement of physicians at all stages of their development. Men like William Battie, John Hall, Alexander Hunter, Thomas Arnold, James Currie, and George Daniell played a pivotal role in first initiating, and then directing the affairs of their lunatic institutions. The growing emphasis on achieving high rates of cures, illustrated in annual reports and appeals for financial support, was a clear reflection of the medical influence. The curative orientation of lunatic hospitals, however, continued in parallel to overtly custodial features. The stark and solid building of the second St Luke's, and the walled enclave of the Leicester Lunatic Asylum within the grounds of the Leicester Infirmary, articulated the continuing expectation of secure confinement and control of the insane.

There was a striking geographical dimension to the development of the provincial lunatic hospitals. As has been highlighted, the first few to be opened were all in the north of England, in response to perceptions that the access of lunatics from Newcastle, Manchester and York to the hospitals of Bethlem and St Luke's was severely restricted. Once the northern network was established, the focus moved southwards. Projects were initiated in most of the major midland county towns, though with varying outcomes.[217] There was also a notable western element around the turn of the century, first with Hereford and then Exeter shortly afterwards. One significant region, however, remained virtually untouched by the movement to establish a lunatic hospital — the south east of the country. The main explanation was relatively simple for, as the admission registers of St Luke's clearly demonstrate, it was functioning from the outset as a facility primarily for the London area and the surrounding counties.[218] An additional factor was doubtless the extensive private madhouse sector that had developed in London, which also catered for a wide geographical catchment area.[219]

The relative success of the voluntary lunatic hospital movement, acknowledged in the report of the 1807 select committee, was reflected in the continually rising demand for places for admission of new patients. The combination of this demand with the steady accumulation of chronic or 'incurable' patients resulted in several of the hospitals becoming filled to capacity within a few years of opening, as numbers continued to grow apace.[220] Consequently there emerged a recurring pattern of insufficient capacity leading to over-crowding, which would be followed by extensions, adaptations, and additional buildings, which was to become so characteristic of later generations of public lunatic asylums in the nineteenth and twentieth centuries.

To a large degree, the rationale for the purely voluntary model of provision was superseded by the County Asylums Act of 1808.[221] By empowering county justices to build an asylum, funded through the county rates, a much more reliable means of finance had been made available. However, the 1807 select committee had clearly been impressed with Sir George Paul's arguments in support of subscription asylums. The succeeding legislation actively sought to stimulate voluntary provision in its clauses enabling combination between county justices and subscribers. Existing subscribers in Staffordshire and Cornwall, as well as those in Nottinghamshire and Gloucestershire, who had been experiencing serious difficulties in raising enough money to start building, now found themselves able to proceed, with the prospect of an infusion of county funds.[222] Far from being rendered obsolete, the voluntary subscription model had been given an important boost. Its continuing resilience was exemplified not only by the completion of the joint projects, but also by the new lunatic asylums financed solely by public subscription that later opened at Lincoln, Oxford and Northampton.

3   Management and staffing

The efficient operation of a charitable organization like a hospital necessitated a suitable framework for its direction. The governors of lunatic hospitals, however, normally lacked knowledge and experience in the field. In developing their systems of management they therefore took account of the precedents that had been set elsewhere, at Bethlem, at the voluntary hospitals, and at predecessor lunatic hospitals. In several instances financial structures, constitution, rules and regulations were largely copied from other institutions and adapted to meet any local or other special circumstances. The consequence was that there was some degree of similarity in the ways in which the lunatic hospitals were constituted. However, as was emphasized in the previous chapter, two distinct types of lunatic hospital developed — the independent charity, and one that was integrated with a general hospital. There were increasingly clear distinctions in *modus operandi* between these two models, and management arrangements needed to respond accordingly.

The key dynamics influencing and determining the nature of operation of the lunatic hospital were located in the interactions between the main power and interest groups, particularly the lay and the medical. The official authority over the management of the institution, its staff, and its patients, would reside with the lay governors. Their composition was similar to that of the governors of the voluntary general hospitals, comprising a mixture of aristocracy, gentry, clergy, and people from the disparate ranks of the middle classes. Individual reasons for becoming a subscriber and a governor might range from the philanthropic, through the desire for social esteem, to the wish to establish or consolidate business connections.[1] With their differing motivations to take on the role, governors would vary markedly in the level of commitment they were prepared to offer to their duties, even if they possessed the necessary knowledge and skills. There was an inherent risk that a board of governors might gradually lapse into becoming a complacent and ineffective oligarchy.

Where there was a management deficiency because of the lack of involvement by the governors, it was likely to be filled by medical men, and in particular the physician. Indeed, the most conscientious governors would recognize their own limitations and look to rely upon the knowledge and professional expertise that was seen to reside with the medical officers. Some physicians, in particular, considered themselves entitled, by virtue of their qualifications and experience, to determine not only the treatment of the patients but also the main operational policies of the hospital. In several of the lunatic hospitals a physician came to exercise a dominant influence over most aspects of the management of the institution. This was certainly recognized to be the case with Dr Alexander Hunter at York, in particular, but a similar phenomenon became evident elsewhere.

There was also a third group, nominally dependent upon and subservient to the other two, who could wield considerable influence. These were the salaried managers of the lunatic hospitals, designated variously as 'governor', 'keeper', 'master', or 'matron'.[2] The level of responsibility accorded to them varied between institutions. Their power lay partly in the day-to-day management of the other staff, as well as the authority they could wield over the patients. In certain cases, like that of Thomas Dunston at St Luke's, the role became absolutely pivotal, with much of the power to manage the hospital and its patients falling into his hands. Elsewhere the position was much more subservient, either to the governors or the physician, or both. In some of the independent provincial lunatic hospitals it was largely superseded by the appointment of a house apothecary, in imitation of the voluntary general hospitals.

The last part of the chapter will consider the situation of the more junior staff, usually denominated the 'servants'.[3] They too were not without power, for they were the people in most constant contact with the 'objects' to whom the lunatic hospital was intended to minister — its patients. Their role was crucial in ensuring the proper running of the institution. They carried out the orders of the physician and the governor or keeper, and provided the direct care and control of the patients. Few in numbers and poorly remunerated, their role was invariably an onerous one. Yet their calibre and their qualities, or the lack of them, were key in determining the true nature of the lunatic hospital's regime.

CONSTITUTION AND CONTROL

Formal governance arrangements were largely adapted from what had come into being in the voluntary hospitals. In these emblematic manifestations of 'urban renaissance', to be a governor was considered both a privilege and a duty, as well as a practical expression of the achievement of a place within the local social hierarchy, particularly for members of the middling classes.[4] Governors, or trustees as they were designated in some places, would acquire their status either by commitment to an annual subscription to the charity or by a substantial donation to its funds. These contributions would entitle the donor to participation in the active management of the hospital, through meetings of its board of governors and sub-committees. Hospital governors would also be entitled to nomination rights of patients, the numbers of these determined by the level of subscription or donation.[5]

The example of the voluntary hospitals' system of governance was applied both to the independent lunatic hospitals and to those constituted as part of an established voluntary hospital. In the latter, the constitutional arrangements would be, in effect, an extension of what had been developed for the parent hospital. This was the principle adopted at Manchester, the first of the voluntary hospitals to set up a division for lunatics. It was laid down from the outset in 1766 that trustees of the infirmary were automatically governors of the lunatic hospital.[6] This arrangement was subsequently confirmed in 1771, and again when the rules were revised in 1791.[7] The infirmary governors were clearly intent on consolidating their authority over their offspring, and made it even more explicit in 1773 by resolving that 'the Rules for the Government of the Public Infirmary shall be established in the Lunatic House where they can be Subservient to it.'[8]

Similar arrangements were adopted at the other attached lunatic hospitals. When the Leicester Lunatic Asylum finally opened in 1794, the expectations could not have been made more clear in the first sentence of its Rules — 'The Governors of the Leicester Infirmary, in consequence of subscription or benefaction to the same, shall, of course, be governors of the Leicester Lunatic Asylum'.[9] When the asylum was subjected to a programme of reform in 1815, this inter-connection was reinforced.[10] At Liverpool also the infirmary trustees were, by definition, trustees of the lunatic asylum.[11] Comparable arrangements were instituted at Hereford in 1799, for the short period that the lunatic asylum operated as a public facility, with infirmary governors made governors of 'this Institution'.[12]

There were normally, though, additional means by which one could become specifically a governor of the lunatic hospital, without having to be involved with the main hospital. At Manchester, a contribution of £50 or more would acquire the privilege.[13] In 1791, the requirements were amended, so that a benefactor of only twenty guineas would be a trustee of the lunatic hospital, and additionally of the infirmary itself, an arrangement subsequently adopted in Liverpool.[14] At Hereford also, benefactors to the asylum of twenty guineas or upwards were entitled to be governors.[15] The situation at Leicester was slightly more complex. A benefaction of £50 or upwards earned a governorship for life, whilst a subscriber of two guineas per annum was entitled to be a governor during the period of their subscription.[16]

At St Luke's, the voluntary hospital model was not the only point of reference. As in other aspects of its establishment, the example of Bethlem was considered and then discarded in favour of something different. It was noted that 'no Benefaction to Bethlem how great soever necessarily constitutes the donor a Governor of that Hospital'.[17] The St Luke's founders group consequently decided that 'Subscribers only should become

Governors of this Charity'. They resolved that a single payment of twenty guineas or more, or an annual subscription of five guineas, would entitle the subscriber to be a governor. A version of the hospital's constitution published in 1790 shows that these qualifications remained unchanged.[18] The considerable wealth that St Luke's had by then accumulated potentially meant a very large number of governors.[19]

At the independent provincial lunatic hospitals, the financial requirements for governorship were invariably more modest than at St Luke's, though there were marked variations between them. At Newcastle, the expectation was a payment of £20 or an annual subscription of £1.[20] At the York Lunatic Asylum, the sole qualification was a donation or benefaction of £20 or upwards, an annual subscription not being a requirement.[21] This was also the case at the Exeter Asylum, where the criterion to be a governor was a donation of ten guineas or upwards.[22] With the benefit of examples from several predecessors, the founders of the Lincoln Lunatic Asylum in 1819 agreed that benefactors of twenty guineas or subscribers of three guineas annually would be governors, arrangements that were confirmed when the rules were revised in 1832.[23]

In the voluntary general hospitals, one of the main advantages of being a subscriber and governor was the acquisition of rights to nominate patients for admission.[24] In most of the lunatic hospitals, the right was not written into their constitutions, though this does not necessarily mean that it did not exist. Governors of those lunatic hospitals that were part of a general hospital may well have acquired the privilege from their governorship of the parent institution. Only at Leicester were nomination rights made explicit, and they were quite complex. A benefactor of £300 or more was entitled to be a governor for life, and to have 'at all times' one patient in the asylum, if there were a vacancy. Other benefactors could 'recommend' patients, according to the level of their contribution; £50 paid for two annually, £100 paid for five, and anything more brought unlimited recommendations. There was a similar scale for annual subscriptions; two guineas paid for two recommendations, three guineas for three, and five guineas for recommendations without limitation.[25] Among the independent institutions it was only at York that there was, from the outset, a prescribed right of nomination of patients. A governor, having paid his £20, became entitled to recommend 'as many patients as he may think proper'.[26] The right to recommend, however, may not have been a great advantage in itself, for it did not supersede the normal certification requirements for admission of a patient.

Governors varied widely in the extent of their preparedness to provide direct input into the running of the institution. In those hospitals with large numbers of governors it would not have been practical for them all to participate actively. Administrative arrangements had to be put in place to facilitate the routine management of the hospital. The chief decision making occasion would always be the annual general meeting of the board of governors, which for many would be the only time they put in an appearance. In the general hospitals quarterly boards and weekly boards, often with small attendances of particularly committed governors, would usually be responsible for the ongoing decision-making. The more detailed administration might be delegated to a sub-committee, known as the house committee.[27] At the lunatic asylums in Liverpool, Leicester, and Hereford, the management of affairs was overseen by the infirmary's board and committee meetings.[28] It would appear that, for a long time, it was only at Manchester that a sub-group was set up specifically to manage the lunatic hospital. Its 'immediate care and management' was devolved to twenty-one people chosen from the infirmary trustees, with five being sufficient to constitute a 'Board' empowered to transact business.[29] A similar arrangement was eventually established at Liverpool in 1820.[30] However, it was clear in both cases that the ultimate power over major decision-making remained with the infirmary board of governors.[31]

The independent lunatic hospitals adopted various management structures. At St Luke's these were quite elaborate. The chief management body was the general court, which met twice yearly, in February and August, and comprised at least nine governors. It was responsible for the election of the key office-holders of president, vice-presidents, and treasurer, and, perhaps more crucially, of the medical officers. The general court's powers, however, appear to have been largely symbolic. The main responsibilities were delegated to the general committee, which consisted of the main office-holders, the five original founding governors, and a further twenty-four governors elected by the general court. The general committee met on a monthly basis, or more frequently if needed, with a minimum of five governors required to transact business. The committee held key powers, such as to 'hire, govern, and discharge the domestick Servants of this Hospital', and to ensure the maintenance of the building and oversight of the purchase of provisions, furniture, and equipment. It was in charge of administrative and financial affairs, including the receipt of subscriptions and other revenues, and the careful investment of surplus income. It was responsible for the admission and discharge of patients. Not least, the general committee were empowered to 'make such Rules for the Management and Oeconomy of the Hospital as they shall find necessary'.[32] Most of these powers were, in practice, delegated to a powerful house committee.[33]

The administrative provisions at the small Newcastle Lunatic Hospital were naturally somewhat different. Its management was vested in the hands of a president, three vice-presidents, a treasurer, and the governors. The court of governors met quarterly, and dealt directly with the senior appointments — physician, surgeon, secretary, keeper, and matron. The ongoing practical business was delegated to a committee of five governors, meeting on a weekly basis. They were accorded authority to 'direct all Matters whatsoever, which may relate to the receiving, rejecting, or discharging of Patients or which concern the Expenses, Government, or Conduct of the

Hospital, and of all the officers belonging to the same'. These potentially wide-ranging powers were strengthened by the committee being given responsibility for appointing the 'Nurses and common Servants', and the power to dismiss them in the event of misconduct. However, they could only suspend the keeper and matron, whose misdemeanours would then have to be dealt with by the court of governors.[34]

At the York Asylum the management responsibilities appear to have been retained, at least nominally, by the governors. It was laid down before the asylum opened that the court of governors would meet quarterly, on the Wednesday of each assize week, with a general meeting on the Wednesday of York Races week.[35] In actual practice the governors became increasingly factionalised. The assumption by Dr Alexander Hunter of much of the actual power of managing the asylum was partly cause and partly consequence of the splits that emerged. Although the governors did periodically attempt to assert their authority by making orders and passing new regulations, these actions generally took place within the context of the institution's political in-fighting.[36] The situation steadily deteriorated, the extent of the problem being highlighted by the indignant Yorkshire magistrate Godfrey Higgins before the 1815 parliamentary select committee:

> There was no visitation of the Asylum at all by any of the governors, or the magistrates in the neighbourhood? — I never heard that there was any visitation by governors, except at the quarter days, and the annual day; and the magistrates had no authority whatever.
>
> At these quarterly and annual meetings, did the governors who visited examine into the conduct and management of the house? — I never heard that they went over it to examine it at those periods.[37]

Dr Charles Best, some of whose other evidence was disparaged by the committee, confirmed the governors' lack of direct involvement in overseeing practices in the asylum.[38] The circumstances that transpired at York may well have represented the extreme of governors abdicating their responsibilities in deference to an all-powerful physician. It is doubtful, though, that this was a completely unique phenomenon, especially as something similar evidently happened at the Leicester Asylum.[39]

At the Exeter Lunatic Asylum the overall system was established similar to that at York, based on a general court of governors that met four times per year. The ongoing work of the institution, however, was delegated to a management committee, which met each Tuesday.[40] When Lincoln Asylum opened in 1820, its subscribers had the benefit of the experience of predecessors as well as that of the county hospital. They developed a quite sophisticated system of management, detailed in comprehensive published rules. The president (Lord Yarborough) was assisted by up to twelve vice-presidents, chosen from the subscribers and benefactors. The general board of governors met quarterly and took responsibility for inspecting the accounts, amending the rules, and for key appointments. Much of the ongoing business was transacted by weekly boards, with a quorum of three governors, to whom wide powers were delegated. They oversaw the work of the director, having the power to suspend him or any other officer for misconduct or incompetence, and to dismiss any 'Nurse' or 'Servant'. They regulated admissions and discharges, and determined the level of patients' weekly payments. They also examined the expenditure and monitored the condition of the 'House and Furniture'. Issues for major decisions, though, had to be laid before the general board.[41] In the Lincoln Asylum's later history, the system of general and weekly boards became problematic, as the two bodies became arenas for dramatic confrontation, allowing powerful individuals and factions to fight out bitter battles over the proper means to treat the insane and manage the institution.[42]

The situation that later transpired at Lincoln demonstrated the extent to which governors could become actively involved and influential in key decisions if they chose. In reality, however, whether the lunatic hospital was an independent entity or was attached to an infirmary, most governors did not participate actively. Crises in the institution's affairs, or an actual or potential scandal, would bring about an upsurge of interest and attract large attendances to board meetings. Such manifestations did occur from time to time, for example at York in the late 1780s and in the years from 1813 to 1815, at Leicester in 1815, and Liverpool in 1826.[43] Otherwise it was the small group of men that constituted the house committee, or turned up at weekly boards, who would involve themselves in the ongoing management. However, even if they had the time and the interest, they were likely to be constrained by an absence of specialist knowledge of the treatment of insanity. Much of the direct management of the lunatic hospitals therefore passed to, and remained in the hands of, those who claimed the expertise — the medical officers and, in particular, the physicians.

MEDICAL MANAGEMENT

> Was there any committee or visitors who looked after the affairs of the Asylum? — No; the physician had for many years been the sole physician, sole visitor, and sole committee, and had the whole management of the Institution. — Godfrey Higgins, to the *Select Committee on the State of Madhouses*, 1815[44]

In virtually all of the lunatic hospitals the physician emerged as a key figure in the direction of the institution's operation. In most instances he had taken a lead in its projection and establishment, before going on to dominate its management over an extended period. Oversight of the treatment and care was clearly a major element of his responsibilities.[45] The physician's role, however, became a good deal wider, encompassing both policy formation and practical administration. The extent to which he concerned himself directly in the hospital's affairs did vary, especially as the position was honorary and usually unpaid. Several of them were powerful personalities, whose drive and single-mindedness proved highly influential in determining the manner in which their institutions developed.

The physicians' prominence in the workings of the lunatic hospitals had been established from the outset. The status and position that the Monro's had acquired at Bethlem Hospital formed the basis for the role accorded to William Battie at St Luke's.[46] The recruitment by the St Luke's governors of a prominent physician like Battie lent a certain prestige to the new hospital, and he was to exercise a strong influence both in the processes of setting it up and in the formulation and application of policies and procedures.[47] Others followed suit elsewhere, a combination of their apparent expertise with individual energy and sheer force of personality bringing them to the forefront. Drs John Hall, Alexander Hunter, James Currie, and Thomas Arnold were all intimately involved with the establishment of the lunatic hospitals in their respective cities, and without their active participation it is likely that those at Newcastle, York, Liverpool, and Leicester respectively may never have successfully materialized.[48]

The lunatic hospitals were acknowledged without question as medical institutions. It followed, therefore, that the physician took overall responsibility for the direction of the methods of treatment and their implementation. This meant oversight of the hospital's therapeutic regime, as well as individual prescription and case supervision. In practice, however, these responsibilities were translated into a management role that was likely to be much wider. Sir George Onisephorus Paul confirmed the reality of this when, before the 1807 select committee, he praised the example of the York Lunatic Asylum which had been 'under the excellent management of Dr Hunter'.[49] Paul had, in fact, previously indicated his approval of the physician's leadership of the lunatic hospital in his plans for an asylum at Gloucester. The draft rules laid down that the 'care and treatment of the patients and the controul of the officers and servants' would be vested in an attendant physician.[50]

Paul's influence was evident in the formulation of the constitution and rules of the Exeter Asylum. Nowhere was the extent of the physician's management powers and responsibilities laid down more explicitly. It was stated firmly that the 'Physician alone' was to direct the 'Treatment and Management' of the patients. He would 'possess a controul over the Officers and Servants of the House'.[51] In regard to the patients, he was in complete charge of their dietary intake, for none was allowed 'Tea, Sugar, Wine, Spirituous Liquors, or Strong Beer', unless by the 'particular Direction' of the physician. Patients were only allowed to exercise in the airing grounds as often as weather permitted and 'it shall be judged proper by the Physician'. He had to be informed about patients who were particularly refractory, and only he could give the necessary directions 'concerning the Method to be pursued with such Patient'.[52] The physician's authority was largely enforced, however, through his direct management of the house apothecary. The apothecary was required to make up and deliver medicines according to the physician's direction, and to report regularly on their effect on the patients. He had to provide the physician with information in writing regarding new admissions, as well as various other tasks that confirmed the differentiations of professional rank.[53]

Dr Thomas Arnold had offered to the Leicester Infirmary governors in 1792 that he would 'most willingly and cordially undertake the management' of the lunatic asylum that would soon open.[54] The governors accepted his tempting offer, and Arnold subsequently wrote the rules for the asylum.[55] The powers these gave to the physician were not as comprehensive as those subsequently implemented at Exeter. However, Arnold was careful to insert clauses that provided considerable authority over everyone else, including even the infirmary governors. Its surgeons were only to assist in the asylum when called upon by the physician. Nobody other than the physician, the apothecary, or staff of the asylum was permitted to 'see, or converse with the patients', except by permission of the physician. Governors could only enter 'on special occasions', by express order of a board meeting, but their opportunities to visit were severely constrained and granted only with the 'advice and approbation of the Physician'. His claim to a monopoly of expertise was underlined, for he was 'the only proper judge when, and in what manner, they may safely be visited; so that they may not be disturbed, nor their cure impeded, by improper, and unseasonable visitations.'[56] This virtual prevention of inspection by the governors would later prove to be a source of abuses. Arnold also ensured that the physician controlled other aspects of the asylum's operation. For example, no discharge of a patient could take place without his direction, albeit supported by an order of the house committee if it met.[57] He also was the final authority for decisions about patients' exercise in the courts, and whether and for how long they were allowed visitors. The physician's power over the 'servants of the house' was absolute, for they were liable to 'immediate dismissal' for disobedience or neglect of his 'orders and directions'.[58]

The physician's leadership role was not necessarily enshrined in the institution's rules. Those at St Luke's, for example, were not explicit about the various responsibilities accorded to him.[59] In practice, though, Battie's dominance of most aspects of the hospital's affairs was clear. Having been appointed before it opened, he took the lead in determining important practical arrangements, such as preparation of the patients' dietary table and the list of drugs and medicines required.[60] He exercised much of his power and influence through assiduous attendance at the house committee, where he was the main arbiter for both admissions and discharges. He determined who was a 'proper object', particularly in regard to the curability criteria, and would recommend refusal of admission if a person appeared to have been 'Lunatick more than Twelve Calendar Months'.[61] For those whose condition had improved in the hospital, it would be for Battie to decide they were 'recovered & fit to be discharged'.[62] However, in many cases he ordered discharge for other reasons, such as when he judged a patient to be 'an Ideot and uncapable of receiving any Benefit from this Charity', if there were complicating physical symptoms, or if he 'hath not discovered any symptoms of Lunacy'.[63] Battie's influence, however, was far greater than deciding on individual cases. He was behind key policy decisions, such as the celebrated proclamation that medical students were welcome at St Luke's in order to learn about the treatment of insanity.[64] Certainly, part of Battie's authority derived from his personal prestige. His successors, Thomas Brooke and Samuel Foart Simmons, were never able to attain the same degree of leadership of St Luke's.

At Manchester the medical involvement in management was not as clear cut, by virtue of there being no single designated physician for the lunatic hospital. Rather, the three physicians of the infirmary acted in rotation, restricting the scope for any individual to dominate, even though Manchester Infirmary's physicians at different times included prestigious figures like John Ferriar and Thomas Percival.[65] Nevertheless, the physicians were still accorded a considerable amount of authority, to judge from rules issued in 1791 and 1816. They retained control of patient discharges and of visiting, as well as oversight of exercise arrangements and the direction of methods to control refractory patients.[66] Important decisions would be passed to the physicians, such as the recruitment and selection of a new governor/keeper in 1807.[67] They showed a willingness to act collectively in urging important policy changes, such as proposals in 1801 to separate the lunatic hospital from the main infirmary and move away from the city centre.[68] Similar rotation arrangements among the infirmary physicians operated at Liverpool, and their powers over the lunatic asylum were comparable to their colleagues in Manchester.[69] However, the resulting diffusion of responsibility could prove a recipe for indecision rather than for a clear management lead. This, indeed, was a significant element behind a scandal that erupted in 1826 over the neglect and ill-treatment of patients by staff in the Liverpool Asylum, where the physicians' distinct lack of active involvement in the asylum's direction was apparent.[70]

Certain physicians became especially dominant in the direction of their lunatic hospital. William Battie's prominent role in the early years of St Luke's has already been alluded to, and Thomas Arnold held almost complete sway at Leicester for over thirty years.[71] At York Lunatic Asylum, which became the largest of the voluntary institutions outside London, Dr Alexander Hunter contrived to dominate most aspects of its affairs, from its conception in the early 1770s until his death in 1809.[72] A good deal has been written about the scandals surrounding the York Asylum in the years from 1813–15.[73] Contemporaries tended to highlight earlier circumstances, which appeared to have contributed materially to the institution's apparent long slow decline. They focused particularly on bitter controversies around the nature and purpose of the asylum, which came to a head in the late 1780s. Hunter was at the heart of those disputes, and his role and attitudes have not generally had a favourable appraisal.[74] Whatever the rights and wrongs, there is no doubting the singular position that he attained in directing the affairs of the York Asylum and in influencing its policies, procedures, and practices.

In a sermon in support of the York Lunatic Asylum in 1782, anticipating the opinion of Sir George Paul twenty-five years later, the Reverend R.B. Dealtry assured the York public that 'this Charity is under the management of an able Physician'.[75] It was only five years since the asylum had opened and Hunter's leadership position was already quite clear. He had evidently decided early on to concentrate his professional attention on the development of the asylum and, unlike the city's other leading physicians, opted out of any role with the York County Hospital. He was one of the original subscribers to the proposed lunatic hospital, and was directly concerned with negotiations for a suitable site and the decision to settle for a piece of land away from the county hospital. He was involved in the early planning meetings and in the formulation of rules and operational arrangements. Hunter's reward was his appointment in September 1777 as sole physician to the asylum.[76]

Hunter initially acted in a fully voluntary capacity, like his fellow lunatic hospital physicians elsewhere.[77] From the outset, as he later wrote, he 'paid a particular attention to the Government of the York Lunatic Asylum'.[78] He had some very clear ideas on its management and was able to prevail on the governors to carry these into effect. There were two key inter-connected elements to Hunter's vision for the asylum. Firstly, its charitable emphasis should be on providing for those in 'low and distressed circumstances', or members of the poorer classes who were not paupers. The former were, he considered, the 'real poor' who deserved to be aided, in contrast to paupers who ought to be relieved financially by their parishes.[79] The second element was that the money to pay for the charitably supported patients should come from the profits generated by the acceptance of paying private patients.[80] These formed the fundamental governing principles on which the asylum developed. Various other policies, usually initiated by Hunter, developed out of them. One of the more controversial, which followed the admission of private patients into the asylum from 1785 onwards, was the agreement to allow direct remuneration to the physician in the form of fees for his work with them. In 1787 this even led to the unprecedented step of Hunter being granted an actual salary of £200 per annum, though this experiment was discontinued a year later.[81]

Hunter conducted himself like a campaigning politician, writing provocative, polemical letters to the county press, and confronting his critics in forthright pamphlets.[82] According to his more outspoken opponents, his chief goal was personal advantage and he perverted the constitution of the asylum to that end.[83] His supporters, on the other hand, considered Hunter to be acting in a 'disinterested' manner, and they backed him in routing his adversaries in 1788.[84] The victory constituted, for Hunter, the vindication of his policies. With his power now greater than ever, he could declare confidently in 1792 that he continued to give 'unremitting attention to what appeared to me most conducive to the public good'.[85] Another unsuccessful attempt was made to challenge Hunter and his allies among the governors in 1794. Its failure seems to have finally quelled the anti-Hunter faction, and from that time his control of the asylum went virtually unchallenged. The visitation arrangements, whereby governors could enter the building and inspect it, had fallen into disuse.[86] Hunter gained agreement in 1799 to be allowed to accept pupils to study with him.[87] By this means he was effectively empowered to determine his own succession. Dr Charles Best commenced as his pupil in December 1804 and, following Hunter's death in July 1809, he was appointed sole physician to the York Asylum.[88] It was to be on his unfortunate head that fell much of the execration for the scandals that stemmed from many years of questionable management practices.[89]

Although the position attained at York by Alexander Hunter was exceptional, it exemplified the status of the physicians within the hierarchy of the lunatic hospitals. The other medical professions also played their part, but their role was generally more a supporting one, under the direction of the physician. In those lunatic hospitals attached to general infirmaries, the surgeons would have the same requirements of weekly attendance as in the main unit, with the additional expectation that they would attend on particular cases where surgical intervention was needed.[90] The independent lunatic hospitals would also normally have an appointed surgeon, with stipulations to attend a specified number of times weekly and additionally for emergencies.[91] The surgeons' role was clearly confined to medical matters. Their involvement in lunatic hospitals was in a purely professional capacity, without any direct managerial participation.[92]

Apothecaries, however, were likely to have a far more active role in the direct running of the institution. In the voluntary general hospitals the role of house apothecary was becoming established. As the only salaried full-time and resident member of staff, the duties could be quite arduous. His primary responsibility was the preparation and dispensing of medicines as directed by the physician. He would also be responsible for administering those medicines and for implementing some surgical techniques. Increasingly, however, the apothecary's duties widened to include general supervisory and administrative roles within the hospital. In addition, he was likely to have to undertake secretarial duties and also provide regular reports to the physician. As hospitals grew in size, so the apothecary's responsibilities increased accordingly.[93] Where a lunatic hospital was developed in conjunction with an existing hospital, as at Manchester and Liverpool, the apothecary's role would be extended to comprise it.

Several of the independent lunatic hospitals also appointed a house apothecary. St Luke's began in 1751 with six apothecaries acting in rotation. However, this cumbersome arrangement was replaced in 1754 by the appointment of a house apothecary at a salary of £30 per annum.[94] At the York Asylum, an apothecary post was established quite early. Matthew Wilcoxon, who had worked at Bethlem under Monro, occupied the post from 1777 until 1784, at a salary of £40.[95] The apothecary's duties at York were evidently quite extensive, and included significant management responsibilities. There were similar requirements as in the general hospitals in regard to the ordering of drugs, as directed by the physician, and supervision of the patients in taking their medicines. He was expected to take a written case history of new patients for the physician's attention. What stood out, though, were the supervisory aspects in relation to staff. For example, the apothecary had to see that the 'Servants' of the house 'do their duty' in cleaning patients' rooms and galleries, and in performing their 'other offices'. His relative subservience within the hierarchy was emphasized, however, for he was to 'strictly attend to the directions' given by the physician. He was also not permitted to absent himself from the asylum, except on 'proper occasions'.[96] After the investigations at York that culminated in the 1815 select committee, the role of house apothecary was re-evaluated. Rules published in 1820 made it clear that he was now to be the asylum's resident superintendent.[97]

Elsewhere, the house apothecary was increasingly being accorded the lead role in day-to-day management. Sir George Paul made this explicit in his detailed proposals for an asylum at Gloucester, in 1796, advocating the amalgamation of the role of apothecary and director, the duties to include 'attending the patients, the general economy of the house, and the keeping of the accounts.' He was to be 'engaged in no other occupation or business' and to be 'constantly resident in the house'.[98] Paul's ideas directly influenced the projectors of the Exeter Lunatic Asylum. Its plans stated the intention to choose 'a Person uniting in himself the Office of Apothecary and Director'. His primary duty would be to 'regulate the internal Oeconomy of the House', in addition to executing the directions of the physician in relation to medicines and the patients' diet.[99] The responsibilities were defined more fully in 1804. He oversaw individual diets, according to the 'regimen' directed by the physician. He had to 'go round the House every Morning at Eleven' to ascertain each patient's health, to check whether the prescribed medicine had been properly administered and its effects, and to report accordingly to the physician. His supervisory obligations included observation of 'the Behaviour of the Servants, towards the Patients', examination of cleanliness and ventilation, and monitoring the 'Comfort and Accommodation' of the patients. He was expected to ensure that patients were treated with 'Tenderness and Indulgence', not to use 'unnecessary Severity' and also not to 'suffer others' to do so.[100] In carrying out these responsibilities, the apothecary was answerable directly to the physician as well as to the governors.

At St Luke's, the role of director remained separate from that of apothecary.[101] Elsewhere, the creation of a salaried post that comprised both medical and managerial responsibilities became common practice in most public asylums developed after 1800. The medical qualification for the role was gradually raised from apothecary to surgeon. The first director of the Nottingham Asylum, a joint subscription and county asylum opened in 1811, was required to be an apothecary.[102] Within a few years the requirements were changing and at the Lancashire County Asylum (1816) a surgeon, Paul Slade Knight, was appointed as superintendent.[103] The precedent was followed two years later at Stafford, another joint subscription and county asylum, with the appointment of John Garrett as house surgeon, apothecary and superintendent.[104] However, at the next purely voluntary subscription asylum at Lincoln, the initial qualification required for the post of director was still that of apothecary. It was only after Thomas Fisher resigned in 1830, after bitter disputes with the physician Dr Edward Charlesworth, that the post was replaced with that of house surgeon.[105] At Exeter Asylum, the change had been made earlier, it being laid down in 1824 that the resident apothecary 'shall also be a Surgeon'.[106]

The incorporation of medical expertise into the role of director, or superintendent, was a recognition of the reality of medical leadership of the lunatic hospital or asylum. It meant, of course, a higher salary than had originally been the case. It also meant increased status and a greater level of authority for the post-holder. The inevitable consequence was a gradual shift in the balance of power away from the physician and toward the house apothecary, house surgeon, or director. The physician's role would revert more to the prescription and oversight of treatment for individuals, whilst the salaried man could attain the major influence over the regime that operated in the institution. There were, though, some individual physicians like Charlesworth at Lincoln who were not prepared to accept this new dispensation of power and fought hard to retain their dominant role in the management of the asylum.[107]

NON-MEDICAL MANAGEMENT

At several lunatic hospitals, the responsibility for day-to-day management of the institution and its patients remained in the hands of men (and women) who were not medically qualified. Certainly the physicians were likely to be influential in major aspects of policy and its implementation. They could not, though, be directly involved in the more practical and mundane elements of the hospital's operation. These would fall within the remit of someone whose title might be 'keeper', 'master', or 'governor', assisted by a 'housekeeper' or 'matron'. The archetypal lay manager was certainly Thomas Dunston, who occupied a dominant place at St Luke's Hospital for almost half a century until his death in 1830.[108]

The role originally delineated for the 'Man & Woman Keepers' at St Luke's was fairly modest, with a limited number of specified duties. The

'Mankeeper' was to weigh in the provisions and account for them, and jointly with his female counterpart, to oversee their distribution to the patients. He was to ensure the locking and unlocking of the house at the stipulated times, and was responsible for the care of furniture and equipment. In relation to the subordinate staff, he had to see that 'his Man Servants perform their Duty'. Regarding the patients, he was not to permit 'any strong Beer, Spirituous Liquors, Tea, or Provisions of any Kind' to be brought into them by their 'Friends' or other outsiders. The 'Woman Keeper' had the responsibility for care of the household linen, as well as having to oversee the washing. More importantly, and parallel to the male keeper, she was to see that the 'Maid Servants' performed their duties.[109]

The terminology could be somewhat confusing, for the term 'keeper' has also at times been used to refer to the more junior members of staff who cared directly for the patients.[110] At St Luke's the latter were described as 'servants', and the keeper was, in effect, the head keeper. The first post-holders were Joseph and Mary Mansfield, at an initial joint salary of only £30 per annum plus regular gratuities of about half that amount. Both had previously worked at Bethlem,[111] experience that was regarded as almost a pre-requisite for a senior post in a lunatic hospital. The Mansfields remained in post for thirty years until Joseph Mansfield was forced to resign through ill health in 1781.[112] They were succeeded by Mr and Mrs Pearson, whose tenure of office lasted only six months. Written complaints of abuses were investigated by the house committee, who found them guilty of a catalogue of misdemeanours, which included accepting bribes, replacing tradesmen with their own acquaintances, and allowing patients out to visit relatives without permission of the physician or the committee. There was a further and more graphic offence:

> instead of using the Chimney in the Yard for the purpose of burning the Waste Straw they have left the Straw a Dunghill in the Yard to the great Detriment & Health of the Patients in a Place where the Air and Room are already too much confined & have converted the Chimney from the Purpose for which it was intended into an Hogstye.

The Pearsons were dismissed immediately, and Mrs Mansfield was brought back to take temporary charge pending a new appointment.[113] What the episode demonstrated was the considerable range and extent of the keeper's authority, if it could provide such wide scope for potential corruption.

After the Pearsons' dismissal, in April 1782 Thomas and Sarah Dunston were appointed as male and female keeper, at salaries of £20 each. They too came from Bethlem Hospital, where they had worked for eight years.[114] With the growth of St Luke's, and the accompanying changes in responsibilities, the post's status was on the ascendant. This received acknowledgement in late 1786, with a significant change in nomenclature, from head keeper to 'Master' and from head woman keeper to 'Matron'.[115] This alteration was apparently in preparation for the hospital's move to Old Street. The Dunstons were to receive much credit for their 'great Care Attention and Assiduity' in organizing the smooth transfer to the new building, and were awarded the substantial gratuity of £50.[116] As the new hospital's patient numbers expanded, their position became yet more prominent. In October 1789, their salaries were doubled, to £60 and £40 respectively, although the customary annual gratuities were stopped.[117]

Undoubtedly, much of the authority attained by Thomas and Sarah Dunston within St Luke's was to do with their personal capabilities and capacities, combined with their longevity in post. In September 1805, tribute was paid to 'the very humane tender and proper behaviour' which they had shown 'at all times' to the patients.[118] Their salaries were periodically raised; in December 1811, in recognition of 'long and faithful service', Thomas Dunston received an increase from £100 to £150, and Sarah Dunston from £50 to £100 per annum.[119] By this time, Thomas Dunston had become the public face of St Luke's. If authoritative information was required on policies and practices within the hospital, it was Dunston who was called upon to give the necessary evidence, and he attained the status of expert witness to parliamentary select committees, with his opinions on the proper methods of treating and managing the insane accorded considerable weight, notwithstanding his lack of a medical qualification.[120]

Thomas Dunston took second place only to Sir George Onisephorus Paul in the prominence his evidence was accorded by the 1807 select committee. He outlined all aspects of the running of the hospital, as well as describing the different types of patients and their needs, and the facilities contained within the building. The intent of the questioning was clearly to ascertain how the experience gained at St Luke's could be replicated in future public lunatic asylums.[121] Dunston gave extensive evidence to the select committees of 1815–16. He was subjected to penetrating questioning as they sought to evaluate St Luke's reputation as a model institution and to ascertain whether it might be the site of similar abuses to those shown to be prevalent at Bethlem and the York Asylum. At his first interview in May 1815, the committee showed particular interest in the measures used to manage the most difficult patients. Dunston elaborated on the means and extent of restraint employed, along with his views on the subject. He made it apparent, with some evident satisfaction, that he had never referred to the physician when directing or authorizing that a patient be restrained.[122] Evidence given by the hospital's physician, Dr Alexander Sutherland, served to confirm that Dunston was indeed the main arbiter of patient management methods within the hospital.[123]

Dunston was recalled to the select committee in February 1816 and received a more incisive and hostile examination. He was questioned about the management of incontinent patients, about suicides and attempted suicides, about practices like gagging and force-feeding, and again about the use of mechanical restraint.[124] There were uncomfortable questions about a female patient who had become pregnant by one of the male 'servants'.[125] Dunston was particularly pressed about his dealings with the private sector. There was a suspicion that he was the proprietor of a private madhouse, which he denied though admitted that he was the landlord. He was also grilled about the arrangements whereby considerable numbers of incurable patients were moved to Warburton's madhouses in Bethnal Green after discharge from St Luke's.[126] From the tenor of the questions, some members of the committee appeared to have come to the view that aspects of Dunston's management of the hospital were corrupt. Some of his equivocal responses did little to dispel an impression that his power had become too great and was in danger of being abused.

Implicit criticism by the select committee notwithstanding, Dunston's position at St Luke's remained virtually unassailable. The extent of the master's responsibilities, and the difficulty of their being fulfilled properly by one man, had been acknowledged in 1814 with the appointment of James Tow as his assistant.[127] A visitor in 1818 to the 'noble hospital' detailed various aspects of its operation and spoke of how they did 'infinite honour' to the master. There was no mention of the role of governors or physician.[128] By this time, in fact, Dunston's position had been further elevated. In 1816 Mrs Dunston had died, and he tendered his resignation. The governors, 'desirous of availing themselves of his experience and abilities', responded by appointing him to the newly created role of resident 'Superintendent'.[129] James Tow was promoted to master, with Mrs Tow as matron. Tow was, however, receiving £100 to Dunston's £150, and over the following months it was clearly Dunston who continued to be the one making the decisions and carrying the responsibilities.[130] Dunston was still at the helm by the time of the 1827 select committee, though it was evident that, at the age of 76, his capabilities were declining.[131] He died in the hospital in 1830, having served St Luke's for just short of fifty years.[132]

The position that Thomas Dunston attained at St Luke's was unique. Although a similar post was established at several provincial lunatic hospitals, it was of a rather different nature and clearly subordinate to the physicians. In the planning stages of the Manchester Lunatic Hospital, the stated intention was to appoint an 'experienced Governor and Governess',[133] an aspiration rarely achieved. A report of 1770 indicated that the role of the 'Warder' was primarily to manage the patients. The infirmary trustees, in advancing his wages, noted the 'Importance of his Service' and the 'irksome Circumstances' under which he sometimes had to work.[134] Subsequent governors or keepers had a mixed record. In October 1773 Richard Wilding was dismissed and prosecuted for 'sundry Misdemeanours'.[135] A brief set of additional rules specifically for the lunatic hospital was then prepared by one of the infirmary physicians, Dr Peter Mainwaring. The 'Keeper of the Lunatic House' was required to attend each weekly board to give an account of the patients. He had to record the medicines given to them and describe their effects to the prescribing physician. Limits were placed on the extent to which the keeper could inflict physical punishment or restraint without the physician's direction, though he clearly could still exercise a degree of initiative according to circumstances.[136]

The early 1770s was evidently a particularly troubled period in the Manchester Lunatic Hospital's development, for within a few weeks of the new rules being confirmed serious violence had erupted in which a keeper lost his life.[137] Although the difficulties subsided, the role remained highly problematic. By 1781, William Day was the keeper and Mrs Betty Craddock the matron.[138] In the late 1780s problems with both keeper and matron led to a complaint and an investigation, resulting in their departure in early 1790.[139] The infirmary trustees, concerned not to repeat earlier mistakes, contacted Dr John Monro at Bethlem and Dr Samuel Foart Simmons at St Luke's for advice and help in recruiting a suitable keeper. This resulted in the appointment 'upon trial' in May 1790 of John Edwards from St Luke's, on Simmons' recommendation. Edwards, however, had several significant shortcomings for the responsibilities of the post, notably that 'he cannot write nor understands Accompts'. His initial salary of £35 per year was to rise to £40 if his 'Conduct' proved 'agreeable'.[140] Presumably he had to learn fast, for the revised rules of 1791 required the keeper to make a written request, accompanied with the necessary information, for the responsible physician to attend for each new patient admitted.[141]

Edwards did not last very long, for by 1794 Andrew Carter was keeper and Mrs Mary Bagshaw was matron.[142] Mrs Bagshaw remained in post until 1800, when she resigned due to ill health.[143] Carter left at the beginning of 1802 and the infirmary governors saw this as an opportunity to raise the qualifications and standards required for the post, now designated 'Keeper or Superintendent'. They optimistically promised preference to 'Any Person who has had a Medical Education & been in the habit of attending upon a similar institution.' He was also to be a single man of at least twenty years of age.[144] It is not clear to what extent the man appointed, David Haigh, met these criteria. However, by early 1807 he was in trouble for going absent without leave and other transgressions. The hospital's rules for the keeper and matron were tightened up and augmented. Not long after, in July 1807, Haigh resigned his post.[145] Still hopeful of enhancing the position's standing, the governors put out a similar advertisement to that of 1802. They delegated the actual selection process to the infirmary's 'Medical Gentlemen'.[146] The quality of applications, however, fell below expectations and the physicians adopted the old expedient of writing to Dr John Monro of Bethlem asking him to recommend someone 'whose acquirements correspond more nearly with the Conditions expressed in the advertisement'. Their request did not bear fruit, and the governors reluctantly appointed John Sanderson, the 'Still Man' from the infirmary, notwithstanding what the physicians called the 'obvious objection' of 'his deficiency in medical knowledge'.[147] Despite his shortcomings, Sanderson made a success of the post and remained in it for well over thirty years.[148]

Experiences at the Liverpool Lunatic Asylum were not dissimilar. When it opened in 1794, following established practice, an 'experienced and approved Keeper and Matron' were brought up from St Luke's.[149] John Squires and his wife remained in their posts until they resigned in 1812.[150] By this time, the title of the role had been amended to 'Governor' of the lunatic hospital and asylum. When the post became vacant in 1812 one of the infirmary physicians, Dr Renwick, contacted John Haslam, the Bethlem apothecary, for recommendation of 'a man and his wife proper to manage such a concern'. Haslam proposed Edward and Mary King, who were duly appointed.[151] King, however, was under something of a cloud as a consequence of allegations that, while acting as a keeper for the female patients at Bethlem, he had 'been too familiar with a female of great beauty'. These allegations, vehemently denied by King, were never proved or disproved and he was allowed the benefit of the doubt.[152] His tenure of office at Liverpool, though, was rather troubled. Within a few months of his appointment, he was being reprimanded by the 'Board of Oeconomy' for exceeding his authority, having arranged for the asylum's exterior to be painted and for employing tradesmen without permission.[153] King evidently did not learn much from this, for in early 1816 he was caught out for purchasing provisions and again employing tradesmen on his own initiative, as well as not keeping proper written records.[154] A year later he was in trouble for distributing wine to the patients without orders from the medical officers.[155] Nevertheless, it was to be another three years before the inevitable summary dismissal, in January 1820.[156]

To judge from the revised rules for the Liverpool Infirmary published in 1813, the governor, or keeper, of the asylum and the matron were acting in a clearly subordinate role to the physician and governors, whilst being responsible for oversight and direction of the 'Servants'. The responsibilities equated to those laid out at the Manchester Lunatic Hospital, and included giving written notice to the physician on the admission of each new patient, the bodily examination of newly admitted patients, and provision of information on patients to the infirmary's weekly board.[157] The existence of detailed rules, however, was of little apparent effect in restricting the activities of a keeper intent on abusing his position, as Edward King demonstrated.

Following the departure of the Kings, John and Eliza Davis were appointed as governor and matron in 1820.[158] They lasted for five years, until their resignation prior to the exposure in the local and national press of serious allegations of violent ill-treatment of patients in the asylum.[159] John Davis vehemently denied any part in what had occurred, and indeed claimed that the accusations were based on 'odious falsehoods' stemming from opposing factions among the infirmary governors.[160] There was strong evidence, though, that Mrs Davis and at least one male keeper had behaved violently toward patients on several occasions. John Davis was probably guilty of nothing more than poor management, apparently having little control over the keepers or his wife. Some of the physicians too were heavily criticized for negligence. The whole episode served to expose the general shortcomings of a management system that diffused power and responsibility between infirmary governors with little direct knowledge of the asylum or its patients, several physicians with only passing involvement in asylum affairs, and a salaried governor with limited authority to govern.

The unsatisfactory record of lay managers was replicated at most lunatic hospitals. At the Hereford Infirmary in 1799, the governors followed accepted practice by getting the physician Dr Campbell to apply to Bethlem Hospital for recommendation of a 'proper keeper' for their lunatic asylum.[161] Rules were produced which laid out the duties of keeper and matron, similar to those at Liverpool and Manchester, indicating the relationship between their roles and those of physician and house apothecary for the infirmary.[162] David Davies from Bethlem was appointed as keeper at a salary of £40 per annum. However, Hereford's experiment with a public lunatic hospital proved unsuccessful. Much of the blame for its failure was attributed to Davies's 'mismanagement', and this appears to have contributed materially to the decision to reconstitute it as a virtual private lunatic asylum in 1801.[163]

The role of keeper at the Exeter Lunatic Asylum was a somewhat lesser one, as the house's resident apothecary took on the more important managerial roles. The governors, as was the norm, opted for the Bethlem connection and contacted John Haslam for nomination of a suitable keeper and matron. The result was the appointment of William and Elizabeth Gillett, who were deemed 'fully qualified' from having lived and worked as keepers at one of Warburton's madhouses in Bethnal Green, as well as at Bethlem. They 'gave satisfaction' for a while, but Gillett gradually 'became irregular' and they were dismissed in 1804.[164] Gillett went on to open a private madhouse near Taunton. Edward Wakefield, visiting the house in 1814, was far from impressed with Gillett's treatment of his pauper patients and commented on his 'ignorant and brutal manners'.[165] He was replaced as 'head keeper' at Exeter by one of the original 'servants', described by Wakefield in 1814 as a 'humane and intelligent man'.[166] What singled out the management arrangements at Exeter was the precedence accorded to the matron, who received £30 per annum, in comparison to the head keeper's £25. She was expected to act as 'Housekeeper and Superintendent of the Female Wards'. In effect, she managed the female side and oversaw general domestic arrangements, complementing the house apothecary rather than the head keeper.[167] The aptly named Sarah Strong made the position her own, occupying it from 1806 until 1838.[168]

Part of the problem of the role of keeper, governor or matron was that there was rarely clarity as to what were the expectations placed on them and at what level they should be operating. Hospital or asylum governors and physicians wavered as to whether they wanted a proper house manager or merely a head keeper. With no requirement for particular qualifications, and the payment of relatively low salaries, the people appointed were generally of only moderate calibre. The key distinction was whether they were allowed to function as officers and accorded commensurate status, like Thomas Dunston at St Luke's, or whether they were deemed essentially as upper 'servants', with responsibility for the direction of those beneath them. In the provincial lunatic hospitals, it was the latter that appears to have become the accepted norm.

THE 'SERVANTS'

The trustees of Manchester Infirmary in 1766 assured the public that there were to be 'proper servants' to attend on the lunatic patients.[169] Implicit in the assurance was an acceptance that these servants had an important role to play in managing and caring for the inmates of the lunatic hospital. Similarly, in the proposals for the establishment of St Luke's, it was declared that lunatics needed to be placed 'under the Management of Strangers' for the curative process to succeed.[170] Those 'strangers' included the staff providing the direct care and control, in addition to the governor or master, the matron, and the medical officers.[171] However, although there was a degree of acknowledgement of the significance of the servants' role, there were no specified standards for recruitment, pay and conditions were usually unfavourable, and the quality of people employed was at best variable.

Andrews, in his study of eighteenth-century Bethlem, concluded that its 'basketmen' and maids were drawn from similar humble origins to those of most of the patients — small craftsmen, tradesmen, and domestic servants. They were often illiterate, and were selected partly on the basis of their physical attributes, their authoritarian demeanour, and their inclination to show obedience to their superiors. However, from the 1760s and 1770s onwards a better class was being attracted by higher wages, comparable to those paid at St Luke's.[172] The indications are that the staff recruited to St Luke's and the other lunatic hospitals were probably of a similar background to those at Bethlem.[173] Evidence for private madhouses and public asylums in the early nineteenth century tends in a similar direction, with domestic servants, agricultural labourers, and former soldiers, tradesmen and craftsmen providing the bulk of the 'keepers'. Internal promotion of washerwomen, house-maids and kitchen-maids, as well as the appointment of some recovered former patients, accounted for most of the rest. Where fortunate, new asylums recruited some keepers from other asylums.[174]

The servants' duties were extensive and onerous, comprising disparate elements. There were the menial tasks like the basic cleaning of the cells and galleries. The most significant part of the role was in the direct care and oversight of patients, which could vary from personally attending to someone in a weakened state to physically preventing people from harming themselves or others. There were the more general supervisory aspects, like ensuring that patients went to bed and rose at the specified times, and that they were relatively orderly at meal-times, in the day-rooms, and in the airing courts. There were also custodial responsibilities, such as locking and unlocking doors, administering the implements of mechanical restraint, and searching and examining patients on admission. The commitment was often for twenty-four hours a day and seven days a week, with servants expected to sleep in rooms adjoining the galleries.

The arduousness of the work was accentuated by generally low staffing levels. At the York Asylum, the initial provision in 1774 had been for three men and three women servants for fifty-four patients. By 1813, their numbers had only increased by one, but there were now almost 200 patients, and two of the keepers were almost exclusively looking after seventeen higher-class private patients.[175] In the early years of the Manchester Lunatic Hospital, there was apparently only one 'Man Servant' and one female 'Upper Servant' in addition to the governor and governess.[176] There was, however, an increase in response to expanding patient numbers, for in 1818 the staffing establishment for upwards of ninety patients consisted of the keeper and matron, with three male and two female 'assistants' and a porter who acted on occasions as an assistant keeper, in addition to a cook and three house maids.[177] Ratios were comparable at Liverpool; in 1812–13, there were two male keepers and two 'nurses', as well as cook, kitchen maid, housemaid, and three laundry maids.[178] The Newcastle Lunatic Hospital operated with minimal paid staff, assisted by convalescent patients. Sir George Paul in 1810 observed only one 'male officer'.[179] Before radical changes in the mid-1820s there had been only a male keeper, a 'matron', and two 'girls' to look after almost one hundred patients.[180]

The surgeon and private asylum proprietor William Ricketts criticized the lack of staff at St Luke's in 1816, suggesting that there were 'not half the servants employed that there ought to be'.[181] It was by then operating on the principle of one keeper for each gallery, with an assistant provided where necessary to cope with refractory or dirty patients.[182] In 1807, Thomas Dunston stated the staffing establishment to be six men and ten women servants, which partly reflected the higher proportion of female patients in the hospital.[183] In 1815, he advised the select committee that there were three male keepers, with two assistants, and four female keepers 'besides the matron and assistant matron'.[184] In effect, the staff-patient ratios were no more favourable than those at York and Manchester. It was also evident that the servants were quite dependent on the support of suitable patients. As Dr Sutherland explained in 1815, convalescent patients were 'exceedingly serviceable', for they 'frequently give assistance to the keepers, which renders a greater number of keepers unnecessary'.[185] After 1815, the numbers of paid staff at St Luke's increased slightly despite falling patient numbers, perhaps in response to the committee's investigations. By 1819 there were seven men and ten women servants.[186]

Staffing levels at the newer lunatic hospitals tended to be more generous. At the Exeter Asylum in 1812, with patient numbers around forty, there was a head keeper and two male 'under keepers', as well as the matron and five female servants who included three keepers, a cook and a washerwoman.[187] By the time that the Lincoln Asylum opened in 1820, clearer standards had been established in the wake of select committee reports and the practices of the post-1808 county asylums. A minimum of one keeper per gallery had become the established norm.[188] The number of keepers at Lincoln was gradually increased as patient numbers grew. In 1828, with forty-eight patients, there were three male keepers and two 'nurses' in addition to the matron.[189]

The quality of the servants was to some extent determined by the remuneration offered. Payment levels were not particularly high, reflecting a perception that the work was relatively menial. Wages were normally paid as an annual salary, inclusive of full board, with all servants expected to reside in the hospital. At Bethlem in the 1770s, basketmen were receiving £10 and maidservants £8, exactly the same as was being paid at St Luke's.[190] At both hospitals, however, staff were periodically rewarded with 'gratuities', amounting annually to £4 at St Luke's. In 1789 the position there was regularized, with gratuities abolished and wages doubled to £20 for males and £16 for females.[191] By 1808, male keepers were receiving £21 per annum and females £18, whilst the head male keeper received £26 and his female counter-part £25. Recruitment was, nevertheless, proving problematic. Thomas Dunston, in July 1809, advised the general committee that 'in consequence of the low Wages given to the Servants at the Hospital he finds it very difficult to procure proper persons to do the Business of the House'. His protestations secured an increase to £25 for the men and £20 for the 'Gallery Maids', levels comparable with the salaries being established within the new county lunatic asylums.[192]

In the provinces payment rates were lower, although generally exceeding those paid in private madhouses.[193] At the Manchester Lunatic Hospital in 1773, a male servant received £10 per annum and a female 'upper servant' £7.[194] As in London, there were gradual increases over the following decades. At Exeter in 1803, male keepers were paid £15 and females £6, raised to £7 in 1804.[195] At the Leicester Asylum, in 1812, the male keepers were each receiving £18 and the females £10.[196] At Liverpool there were marked differences between men and women, with keepers on £20 per annum and female staff receiving only £6.[197] At York Asylum in 1810, male keepers' wages ranged incrementally from £12 up to £20, with the head keeper paid £21. Two female keepers received ten guineas, and the head female keeper twelve guineas.[198] By the time the Lincoln Asylum opened in 1820, a standardized system of payment was developing with an accepted rate for the job. The first 'man-servant' at Lincoln was paid £20 per annum, and an assistant keeper was appointed in 1823 at £10 per annum. These wages, however, were clearly not attracting staff of sufficient calibre, and at the end of 1829 the salaries of male keepers at Lincoln were raised to £25, matching what was being paid at the new county asylums.[199]

Despite low wages and the demanding nature of the work, some staff remained in their jobs for many years and turnover was generally low. At York, James Backhouse worked at the asylum for twenty-six years before retiring as head keeper in 1810. Of the keepers in 1814, Henry Dawson had been there for over five years, Benjamin Batty for eight years, and Sarah Cuthbert for twelve years.[200] Edward Wakefield noted in 1814 that the 'humane, intelligent' head keeper of the Exeter Asylum had worked there for eleven years.[201] A notable example of longevity was Elizabeth Gibbons, a gallery maid at St Luke's. In 1816, in view of her 'long and faithful Services', amounting to seventeen years, she was allowed to continue with lesser duties at a reduced salary as a result of having become 'aged and infirm'. She stayed until her death three years later, and the hospital paid for her funeral.[202] Evidence from St Luke's for the period from 1808 to 1819 shows that several keepers, both male and female, remained in post for a number of years, though some remained for no more than a few months.[203]

The responsibilities entrusted to the subordinate staff of the lunatic hospitals were considerable. It was they who represented the face of the institution to the patients themselves. However, the evidence suggests that they were not usually of a sufficient calibre to match optimistic expectations. The issues were not dissimilar to those determining the quality of their managers. They were untrained, and their pay and conditions could hardly compensate for the gruelling and sometimes dangerous nature of the work. The pursuit of economy by governors and subscribers was one reason for the perpetuation of poor standards. More fundamental, however, was the perception that the staff were not agents of therapy and moral management but 'servants', with a role akin to that of people employed in domestic situations. Within the institution, servants or keepers were clearly at the bottom of the hierarchy, only above the patients themselves. It was inevitable that their shortcomings would periodically become apparent, although there were always the exceptions of those able to rise above their limitations. A keeper named Abraham at the Manchester Lunatic Hospital in 1801 was described by a patient as 'a man of grace and understanding', more suitable to be entrusted with the care of lunatics than 'any Doctor or Physician'.[204] It may well be that he was not unique.

CONCLUSIONS

Although formal control over the direction of the lunatic hospitals' affairs rested with the board of governors, as laid down in rules and constitutions, the reality was much more complex. Governors, who almost invariably had limited knowledge of the treatment of mental disorder, could not act alone. Effective direction was based ultimately on the forging of a partnership between men acting in a voluntary capacity and those who received a salary, and between men who were professionally qualified and those that were not. At each of the lunatic hospitals, whatever the original management arrangements, they were gradually adapted to meet the local circumstances and power balances between key individuals, professions and interest groups. Where these operated as checks and balances on one another, this could prove advantageous to the institution and prevent abuses of power. However, if the influence of particular individuals became paramount, as at St Luke's and the York and Leicester Asylums, there were almost always problems. Their ability to usurp the power of the governors and dominate the management of the lunatic hospital did at least ensure stability and consistency, but it also created risks that the best interests of patients, staff and subscribers could be compromised.

The physicians emerged as the single most influential group in the lunatic hospitals. As the apparent sole possessors of clinical expertise in a relatively uncharted area of medical practice, they were in the strongest position to take on the management responsibilities divested by the governors. It is clear that they accepted the leadership role in most places, particularly in the independent institutions not under the aegis of an infirmary board of governors. However, their other diverse commitments and interests would eventually restrict the amount of time and energy they could offer to management activities, and increasingly they needed to delegate. There was a significant group of medical men to whom it appeared convenient to pass on some of these responsibilities — the apothecaries. As the role of house apothecary was established, based on the example of the voluntary general hospitals, they emerged as the prototype of a new cadre of salaried public asylum managers.

The presence or otherwise of a house apothecary was a key factor in determining the nature and extent of power and authority exercised by unqualified lay managers. If there were a post of house apothecary, with managerial responsibilities, as at York and Exeter, the role of keeper or governor would be relatively limited in scope. If the apothecary was shared with a parent general hospital, as at Liverpool and Manchester, the keeper of the lunatic hospital could take on more of the practical management. At St Luke's, although there was a house apothecary, the high patient numbers necessitated his work being increasingly directed into the medical arena, leaving Thomas Dunston to take the lead on all management matters. Dunston was really the only lay manager to attain leadership and to exercise real power within his institution. In the provinces, though boards of governors made some attempts to create a management role for the governor of the lunatic hospital, in reality he was rarely more than a head keeper as the often-used alternative title of 'keeper' would suggest. In practice, the relatively low salaries paid were unlikely to attract candidates of a sufficient calibre to be effective in either managerial or therapeutic roles. The situation of the governor/keeper or matron was, in many ways, similar to that of the 'servants' whom they managed. At the same time, in the cases of both groups, the nature of their posts did allow for the exercise of considerable power over the patients and was always open to abuse.

Management arrangements demonstrated their greatest complexity at the York Asylum, the only provincial institution where patient numbers approached those of St Luke's. By the late 1790s, there were several posts with a managerial component — apothecary, steward, matron, and head keeper. Whether cause or consequence of this diffusion of roles, responsibilities and powers, most of the major decisions remained largely in the hands of Dr Alexander Hunter. The residual management and supervisory duties were shared between the others, in the context of a board of governors who were unwilling or unable to carry out their responsibilities. The resulting confusion of roles and absence of clear lines of accountability were significant factors in that asylum's descent into gross mismanagement.[205] Whilst the exposure of events at York suggested a singularly remarkable management system, it was perhaps only the most blatant example of how an institution might come to exhibit many of the hallmarks of the era of 'Old Corruption.'[206]

4   The physician's domain

The 'urban renaissance' that transformed towns and cities during the eighteenth century witnessed a remarkable flowering of civic institutions and culture, in which the professions have been identified as playing a particularly active part, and none more so than the medical professions.[1] Nevertheless, as Irvine Loudon, Joan Lane and others have shown, the three main groups of physicians, surgeons and apothecaries remained distinct and separated by hierarchical delineations. Any practical trends toward the equalization of status and the emergence of general practice were for the future. Physicians remained at the apex, both within the voluntary hospitals and in the wider community.[2] At a time when the social boundaries between ranks in urban society were relatively fluid, the physicians were increasingly able to forge a gentlemanly identity. That identity, based on their prominent public role and the connections developed in that role, and in private practice among the affluent and privileged, would be significantly reinforced by a conspicuous contribution to the developing socio-cultural infrastructure of the town.

The voluntary hospital was one of the key manifestations of the new urban fabric. The physician's participation in its foundation and operation demonstrated his sense of charity and public duty, with all the attendant status and prestige that followed. In the same way that the development of a hospital for lunatics could be construed to represent an additional degree of enlightenment among its projectors and subscribers, there was perhaps nowhere better for an ambitious physician to gain personal credit by demonstrating an unselfish concern for the most deprived, distressed and distasteful people. There were, of course, other potential opportunities of a more material nature, which more than counter-acted the effects of any lingering stigma that might attach to the role of 'mad-doctor'. The relatively poor state of knowledge of insanity and the difficulties in achieving successful treatment outcomes offered a serious professional challenge to the conscientious practitioner. The perceived expertise gained, and the associated reputation, might also lay the basis for a lucrative private practice.[3]

As was demonstrated in the previous chapter, physicians almost invariably emerged as the key figures in the direction of the lunatic hospitals and their affairs. The present chapter will survey the careers and activities of some of the most prominent of these physicians, namely William Battie, Alexander Hunter, Thomas Arnold, James Currie, John Ferriar, and Samuel Foart Simmons. It will initially consider briefly their individual backgrounds and the steps taken by them to become physicians and mad-doctors, before seeking to locate them within their wider medico-social context. Whilst each of these men had his individual characteristics and idiosyncracies, there were some notable commonalities. In several instances there was a clear Scottish connection, either by background or by medical training at Edinburgh University.[4] There was also a preponderance of dissent in their religious and cultural affiliations, William Battie being the notable exception. The most evident common feature, however, was in their professional development and activity. For each man, involvement in the treatment and management of insanity was only one aspect of a wider medical practice. That was no coincidence, in view of the prevalent acceptance that insanity had, at minimum, an intimate relationship with physical diseases, if it was not actually itself a physical disease.

MAD-DOCTORS IN THE MAKING

Dr William Battie (1701–76) was one of the first physicians to be identified as a specialist mad-doctor. The son of a parish vicar, he was born in Devon and educated at Eton and King's College, Cambridge, where he eventually gained his M.D. in 1737.[5] He practiced as a general physician for a few years at Uxbridge, before moving into London.[6] His great success there brought massive earnings in excess of £1000 per year. In addition to a substantial town house in Great Russell Street, Battie also acquired a fine villa on the Thames at Twickenham.[7] He became a particularly prominent and influential member of the College of Physicians, eventually holding the office of president in 1764–65. Battie gained something of a reputation for eccentricity and buffoonery. He demonstrated unusual sartorial tendencies, and social behaviours not normally associated with a gentleman-physician.[8] However, he could also convey sufficient gravitas when the occasion demanded, as in the debates of the College of Physicians, in his private consultations with members of the aristocracy, or in his attendance in 1763 as an expert witness before the House Of Commons Committee on the State of Private Madhouses.[9]

Battie's developing interest in insanity became apparent soon after his move to London. In 1742 he was elected a governor of Bethlem Hospital, having subscribed £50 for the privilege.[10] His knowledge of the operation of Bethlem, and of its shortcomings, gave him the credentials for appointment in 1750 as the first physician to St Luke's Hospital.[11] His formal post at St Luke's furnished him with the basis to develop an extensive private practice in the treatment and management of insanity, as well as the credibility to publish his main work, A Treatise on Madness, in 1758. Battie retired from St Luke's in 1764, with a characteristic flourish and words that have become incorporated into psychiatric historiography:

> Improvement in Medical Knowledge being one of the principal objects of Hospital Practice for which men growing old in confirmed Habits and Opinions are not so well qualified I cannot at present answer your good intentions better by retiring from that part of the Mad Business in time and resigning the Care of your Patients to some Younger Physician.[12]

Battie nevertheless continued for several more years as a governor of St Luke's and also of Bethlem Hospital, in addition to his private practice. He died in June 1776, following a paralytic stroke, at the age of 75. The considerable fortune he had amassed during his career has been estimated at anything from £100,000 to twice that amount.[13] Among his bequests was a rather modest £100 to St Luke's Hospital.[14]

The flamboyant Dr Alexander Hunter (1733–1809) was born in Edinburgh, the eldest son of a druggist.[15] He was educated at the city's grammar school and then at Edinburgh University. In furtherance of his medical studies, he spent several months in London and then in France before returning to Edinburgh and gaining his M.D. in 1753. Hunter opted to pursue a professional career in England and began practice at Gainsborough in Lincolnshire, before moving on to Beverly. He was invited to York in 1763 to take over from a recently deceased leading physician, and he became one of the physicians to the York County Hospital and later (in 1788) to the York Dispensary. Hunter developed wide medical interests, reflected in writings on the benefits of spa waters and on consumption. Much of his private work was as a general physician, and he built up a successful practice among the gentry and merchant classes of the city and county. He had probably never intended to become an insanity specialist. It was, however, as a mad-doctor that Hunter ultimately gained much of his professional reputation, in consequence of his long and often controversial association with the York Lunatic Asylum.

Dr Thomas Arnold (1742–1816) was the only man discussed here who intentionally set out to become an insanity specialist. A native of Leicester, his father was the successful proprietor of a private madhouse established in the early 1740s.[16] The younger Arnold was sent to Edinburgh University to study medicine, specifically with a view to taking over the family business.[17] Having gained his M.D., Arnold returned to Leicester in December 1766. In addition to his proprietorship of the madhouse, however, he also developed a private practice as a general physician and was appointed joint physician to the new Leicester Infirmary in 1771, along with Dr James Vaughan who was to become his implacable enemy.[18] With the eventual opening of the public lunatic asylum under his reluctant leadership in 1794,

Arnold took responsibility for its oversight in addition to the direction of his madhouse, his general private practice, and a continuing role as physician to the infirmary. He was assisted in all these ventures by his two sons, both of whom had followed him into qualification as physicians.[19] At the age of seventy-three, and under severe pressure from his critics, Arnold resigned as physician to the infirmary and the asylum in September 1815 and withdrew himself from public activities.[20] His death followed only a year later.[21]

Dr James Currie (1756–1805) might never have become a doctor at all. He was born in Annandale, the son of a Church of Scotland minister.[22] Educated locally and then at Dumfries Grammar School, he left Scotland at the age of only fifteen to go to Virginia to undertake an apprenticeship with a firm of merchants. He spent six highly eventful years in America during the period of political and commercial turmoil surrounding the war of independence. Soon after his arrival Currie caught a fever from which he almost died, the first of a series of serious illnesses that dogged him throughout his life.[23] After various hair-raising adventures he escaped to the West Indies before eventually returning to Britain for the sake of his health in May 1777.[24] It was whilst in America that his interest in a medical career was kindled, having stayed for a period with a relative, the eponymous Dr James Currie, the leading physician in Richmond, Virginia.[25] He commenced his studies at Edinburgh University in late 1777, and gained his M.D. in 1780.[26] At Edinburgh he had studied under William Cullen, and his contemporaries included Thomas Percival and John Aikin, with whom he retained lasting associations.

Despite an early intention to establish a practice in Jamaica or Virginia, Currie was persuaded to move to England and settled in Liverpool in October 1780.[27] After initial difficulties in establishing himself, he was elected as a physician to the Liverpool Dispensary in April 1781.[28] An advantageous marriage in January 1783 improved his financial and social standing, and in 1786 he became one of the physicians to the Liverpool Infirmary.[29] He gradually developed an extensive practice as a general physician, with a particular interest in the treatment of fevers.[30] Currie's growing interest in insanity was apparent in a letter written to his friend Dr George Bell in 1781:[31]

> There is a part of the philosophy of medicine that has as yet been little attended to; I mean that which treats of the diseases of the mind, of the influence of affections primarily, mental, on the corporeal functions, and particularly of the passions and emotions....If I ever do anything to be remembered, it must be on some such subject...the mind of man is, in my eyes, a noble field for speculation.[32]

Currie's successful promotion, in 1789, of the plan for a lunatic hospital occurred within the context of his role at the infirmary.[33] It proved to be one of his more significant achievements. However, his career was blighted by his recurrent debilitating health problems. He had to leave Liverpool for Clifton and then Bath in 1804, formally retiring from the infirmary in March 1805.[34] Currie died a few months later of chronic heart disease, at the age of only 49.[35]

Dr John Ferriar (1761–1815) also had to overcome adverse circumstances. He was born near Jedburgh, in the Scottish borders, the son of a Presbyterian minister. His father died when he was only three, however, and he was brought up and educated at Alnwick in Northumberland, going on to study medicine at Edinburgh University where he gained his M.D. in 1781.[36] Ferriar began practice at Stockton-on-Tees, and moved on to Manchester in 1785. In October 1789 he was appointed assistant physician to the Manchester Infirmary, and a few months later became one of its honorary physicians, with a role that also encompassed the lunatic hospital. He became the leading general physician in Manchester, with an extensive practice. Ferriar's diverse medical interests were indicated by his main publication, the first volume of which appeared in 1792.[37] The treatment of mental disorder had evidently become a significant area of his practice, as the *Medical Histories* demonstrate.[38] He regarded insanity as being closely aligned with physical disorders, which accorded well with his role as physician both to the lunatic hospital and the main infirmary.[39] John Ferriar died in Manchester at the relatively young age of 53, in February 1815.

Dr Samuel Foart Simmons (1750–1813), who was to attain prominence both as a mad-doctor and as a medical journalist, was the son of the town clerk of Sandwich in Kent. He was educated at a seminary in France, before going on to study medicine at Edinburgh and then at Leiden, where he obtained his degree of Doctor of Physic in 1776. He traveled extensively in Europe before returning to London, where he was admitted as a licentiate to the College of Physicians in 1778.[40] Simmons' medical interests were broad, evidenced by publications on subjects such as anatomy, gonorrhoea and consumption.[41] His first formal appointment, in 1780, was as physician to the Westminster General Dispensary. Being a Protestant Dissenter, the more prestigious hospital posts in London were hard to access, which may have been a factor inclining Simmons toward the insanity specialism.[42] He was elected physician to St Luke's Hospital following the death in October 1781 of Dr Thomas Brooke, who had taken over after Battie retired in 1764.[43]

Simmons' attention to his duties was assiduous, which the St Luke's governors recognized both by public statement and by financial acknowledgement.[44] He eventually resigned in early 1811, citing his age and state of health.[45] Simmons had been able to use his prominent role at St Luke's to enable him to become one of the foremost mad-doctors of his day. He has perhaps become best known for his involvement in the treatment of King George III's episodes of insanity.[46] He was first called upon in February 1804, after the king had expressed strong antipathy to being attended again by the Willis's. Within a few months of the monarch's recovery, however, he became equally resentful of the attendance of 'that horrible doctor' Simmons and his 'shabby' men.[47] Although Simmons was summoned again in 1810 and 1811, the queen also held a deep antipathy towards him and he was allowed no more than indirect access and was forced to act only as a consultant along with Drs Thomas Monro and John Willis.[48] Samuel Foart Simmons did not survive long after his retirement from St Luke's and his royal consultations. He died on 23 April 1813 at his house in Poland Street, London.

IDENTITY AND PRINCIPLE

> In large and opulent towns, the distinction between the provinces of physic and surgery should be steadily maintained. This distinction is sanctioned both by reason and experience. It is founded on the nature and objects of the professions; on the education and acquirements requisite for their most beneficial and honourable exercise; and tends to promote the complete cultivation and advancement of each.[49]
> — Thomas Percival, *Medical Ethics*, 1803

The late eighteenth and early nineteenth centuries witnessed the beginnings of erosion of the professional boundaries between the three main branches of the medical professions. The rise of general practice both reflected and accentuated the process. The increasing overlap between surgeons and apothecaries was particularly marked.[50] However, whilst physicians were not unaffected by the developments, they were able largely to remain aloof from them. There was little sign of any acknowledgement on the part of prominent physicians that their relative status might be waning, if indeed it was.[51] It may well be the case that the lowering of the tri-partite barriers was something of a provincial, small town phenomenon, where there were not sufficient prospective customers to support several medical practitioners, as compared to a large town or city with a general hospital as well as a numerous and affluent clientele. In those centres sufficiently prominent also to boast a lunatic hospital, there were invariably several practicing physicians who, whilst they might be in direct personal competition for custom and prestige, were also acutely conscious of their mutual interests in projecting themselves collectively as 'gentlemen of the faculty'.

A perception of gentility was at the heart of the physician's identity. It distinguished him from the surgeon, with the manual connotations of that profession, and from the apothecary, whose dispensing activities could be construed as being merely an aspect of 'trade'. The attainment of gentility was central to the medical education ethos at Edinburgh University, geared toward the physician's participation in the social and cultural elite of the town in which he practiced. Membership of the profession in itself provided a status as 'gentleman', with expectations of certain standards of behaviour and comportment. In provincial towns the physician's social visibility was most important, manifested by a suitable house, a carriage, a polished demeanour, and other norms of gentlemanly conduct.[52] The construction and maintenance of professional dignity were at the core of the public *persona*. This was well illustrated by Thomas Arnold on his return to Leicester from Edinburgh. Arnold was acutely conscious of the importance of 'settling in the World in the dignified Character of a Physician', which meant forming the right social connections and paying the necessary calls on appropriate people.[53] He welcomed the opportunity to join publicly with the established senior physician Dr James Vaughan in an 'external shew of the Doctoral Dignity'.[54]

The upholding of the practitioner's status and dignity was contingent on the community's acknowledgement of his professional ability, both as an individual and as a member of the general body of physicians. He will have held the superior medical qualification, having obtained his M.D. at a prestigious university. An honorary post as physician to a voluntary hospital provided recognition that he had achieved the requisite level of knowledge, and that he was gaining further valuable experience enabling him to enhance his skills. By providing those skills *gratis* to the community, the physician was making a clear and open display of gentlemanly conduct.[55] Another important means of practically demonstrating professional knowledge, and enhancing prestige, was publication. Battie, Hunter, Arnold, Currie, Ferriar and Simmons all published works on medical matters. These activities proved to be vital elements in the construction of a successful professional career, not least because the achievement of an accomplished and gentlemanly image brought considerable material advantages to a physician, by the attraction of a prestigious and affluent custom to his private practice.

To construe unremunerated work as physician to a voluntary hospital as being motivated primarily by considerations of personal gain, however, would be to do a disservice to some conscientious individuals. The principles of duty and service were propounded in the teaching of William Cullen and John Gregory at Edinburgh,[56] and were key elements in the practice of men such as Currie or Ferriar. Thomas Percival's profoundly influential pioneering work on medical ethics emanated from the approaches that he and his colleague Ferriar had been trying to adopt at the Manchester Infirmary and Lunatic Hospital.[57] Indeed, Percival stated that his first chapter had been written in 1792 'at the request of the physicians and surgeons of the Manchester Infirmary'.[58] His first and most fundamental principle concentrated on the medical man's duty to 'minister to the sick', in the context of a consciousness of 'the importance of the office'. He had to reflect that 'the ease, health, and the lives of those committed to their charge depend on their skill, attention, and fidelity.' He should conduct himself in a way that upholds an appropriate professional relationship with the patient — 'so to unite tenderness with steadiness, and condescension with authority, as to inspire the minds of their patients with gratitude, respect, and confidence.'[59]

Percival showed a keen awareness that a patient was far more than a set of symptoms to be managed and dealt with; he was a whole person who had to be approached accordingly:

> The feelings and emotions of the patients, under critical circumstances, require to be known and to be attended to, no less than the symptoms of their diseases…Even the prejudices of the sick are not be contemned, or opposed with harshness. For though silenced by authority, they will operate secretly and forcibly on the mind, creating fear, anxiety, and watchfulness.[60]

Percival also had quite profound insights to share specifically in regard to the insane, pointing out the painful nature of the physician's task 'when he is called upon to minister to such humiliating object of distress'. The potential reward was great when he could 'render himself instrumental, under providence, in the restoration of reason, and in the renewal of the lost image of God.'[61] If sensitivity to individual patients' needs was to inform the physician's practice, however, it had to be set against a background of the maintenance of the honour and integrity of the profession. Thus, the employment of 'quack medicines' had to be actively discouraged as 'disgraceful to the profession', and any dispensation of a 'secret nostrum' was equally to be censured.[62]

The expression of principles of duty and responsibility, as well as compassion and concern, are to be found in several of the writings of lunatic hospital physicians. For James Currie, the responsibility of a physician was much wider than considerations solely of disease, but was part of what members of the privileged classes owed to the 'labouring poor':

> They demand our constant attention. To inform their minds, to repress their vices, to assist their labours, to invigorate their activity, and to improve their comforts:—these are the noblest offices of enlightened minds in superior stations; offices which are of the very essence of virtue and patriotism….

This was also a religious imperative, for it would 'obtain the favour of the Eternal Being, who is the Great Father to us all.' From this premise of duty to the poor, Currie went on to expound the particular claims of those who were 'sinking under disease', and then more specifically insanity.[63]

Alexander Hunter expressed his perceptions of his responsibilities, as a physician and as a gentleman, in a number of different contexts. In the preface to one of his more successful publications, on the benefits of spa waters, he proclaimed that his sole motive in producing it was nothing other than 'a sincere desire to contribute to the ease and satisfaction of the infirm'.[64] His rather quirky book of aphorisms, *Men and Manners*, comprised brief *dicta* on many aspects of social relationships, including those that should subsist between doctor and patient. Hunter contended that it was the 'duty in a moral sense' of the medical man to take a 'warm interest' in his patients' recovery.[65] He suggested that a 'conscientious physician' was even likely to suffer disturbed sleep as a result of anxiety for his patients.[66] He went on to lament that a physician's life was 'not to be envied', for unlike other professions 'he has not a moment that he can call his own'.[67]

Hunter's commitment and compassion for his patients was, however, to some degree conditional. His controversial policies on the differential charges made to poor patients according to whether or not they were parish paupers were based on a conception, albeit sincerely held, that the non-pauper in 'low circumstances' was the most worthy of charitable assistance. Hunter was unapologetic in his resistance to any idea of reducing the charges for 'incurable mad paupers' and those who made up the ranks of the 'lowest and meanest of the poor'.[68] His motives have been, somewhat unjustly, characterized by his contemporary and subsequent critics as based largely or even purely on self-interest.[69] It could be interpreted that his espousal of higher charges for wealthy private patients was with the primary intent of providing the means for the asylum to offer affordable care to the deserving elements of the poor.[70] Hunter himself had little doubt as to the validity of his position. Reflecting on the history of the asylum in 1792, he insisted that he had always attended to the 'public good'. More specifically, he claimed to have consistently 'paid a diligent attention to the miserable inhabitants' of the asylum, including the paupers.[71] In upholding his position or his interests, Hunter was invariably forthright and often pugnacious. He was certainly not averse to the sorts of outspoken exchanges to which medical men were seemingly prone in defence of perceived matters of principle.

DISPUTATION AND CONFLICT

> The quarrels of physicians, when they end in appeals to the public, generally hurt all the contending parties; but what is of much more consequence they discredit the profession, and expose the whole faculty to ridicule and contempt. — John Gregory, *Observations on the Duties and Offices of a Physician*, 1770[72]

Gregory's strictures reflected a widespread tendency for physicians to indulge in the cut and thrust of disputatious controversy. Professional pride, expressed through an upholding of principle, tended to lie behind the fundamental disagreements that periodically arose among them. Personal vanity and self-interest could also be detected in the adoption of stubborn positions in a public argument. Indeed, many medical men appeared to relish engaging in disputes which at times could descend into the most rancorous, bitter, and even violent quarrels.[73] The complex issues surrounding the management of insanity evidently provoked some heated controversy, as witnessed by the much-discussed debate in print between William Battie and John Monro.[74] That particular argument remained relatively civilized, within gentlemanly bounds, and Battie and Monro were later able to work together reasonably amicably.[75] In other instances, particularly where material interests were directly affected, the conflicts could become more serious.

Major differences of opinion between medical men erupted around the Newcastle Lunatic Hospital in 1766–67. In 1765, the governors had resolved to replace the converted house with a new building.[76] Dr John Hall[77], the physician who had taken a leading role in the hospital's foundation, argued the case for another storey to be added to the building, to accommodate ten paying patients. As echoed in later controversies at York, Hall contended that the profits made by the charity could be used to subsidize the accommodation of more poor patients. He denied any personal interest, insisting that his intention was 'entirely calculated to serve the publick'. The governors, however, rejected Hall's argument and maintained that the lunatic hospital should provide specifically for the poor, advising him to open a private establishment to cater for the wealthier patients.[78]

Hall, clearly piqued at the governors' refusal to adopt his 'favourite plan', reluctantly took their advice, spurred on by moves by four of the infirmary's surgeons to establish a private madhouse.[79] He grudgingly entered into a partnership with them and in June 1766 they opened 'St Luke's House for Lunatics', explicitly for people 'whose Circumstances prevent their being admitted into the PUBLIC HOSPITAL'.[80] The joint venture was always doomed, with professional and private jealousies festering from the outset. Hall high-handedly insisted that he was to act as physician to all the patients in the house. Within a few weeks the relatives of a patient previously under the care of the surgeon Richard Lambert[81] refused to pay the physician's fees, precipitating an unseemly row between Lambert and Hall. The inevitable acrimonious break-up of the partnership followed, with Hall insisting that he would not be reduced to 'A CYPHER'.[82] He bought out the surgeons, who went on to open their own madhouse in opposition to St Luke's House, with adjoining rival advertisements appearing in the regional press for several months.[83]

The medical disputes surrounding St Luke's House were wider than just between Hall and the surgeons. Considerable mutual antipathy was also apparent between him and two of the city's other prominent physicians, Adam Askew and John Rotheram.[84] Hall was prepared to concede a certain amount of respect for Dr Askew's 'age and great reputation as a Physician'. However, Askew reciprocated with 'ill treatment and wanton ill-natured opposition' to St Luke's House and sought to 'ruin its credit'.[85] Dr

Rotheram had openly attacked St Luke's House in a parody circulated soon after its opening, seeking to 'render it ridiculous and contemptible'.[86] There was clearly no love lost between Hall and Rotheram. A further exchange took place between the two men in published pamphlets, with insinuations and insults freely traded.[87]

Hall's public position throughout the dispute was ostensibly based on a conception of professional honour. He maintained consistently that, in advocating provision for private patients within the lunatic hospital, he had been acting in a disinterested way, his goal being public benefit even at the sacrifice of his own interests. Once his intentions had been thwarted, he considered himself perfectly entitled to establish a private facility. Indeed, he claimed to be acting for the public good in relieving the pressure on the lunatic hospital.[88] In the dispute with the surgeons, he again justified his actions on the grounds of offended honour. As physician to the lunatic hospital, and by definition the city's leading authority on the treatment of the insane, he expected the proper rewards of the venture, including the right to sole oversight of the patients in St Luke's House, and payment accordingly.[89] By this code, the opposition of other physicians could be construed as merely malicious, originating from resentment at their exclusion from some lucrative work. Hall's sense of professional and gentlemanly dignity, however, did not extend far enough to prevent him from publicly aspersing fellow 'Gentlemen of the Faculty'.[90]

The bitter quarrels that developed in Leicester between Dr Thomas Arnold and Dr James Vaughan, and in which most of the city's medical community became embroiled, were also founded on a combination of professional rivalry and conflicting personal interests. Arnold had clearly anticipated that the relationship between himself, as a newly qualified young physician returning to Leicester, and the man who dominated the local medical market-place was potentially fraught with difficulty, accounting for why he was so careful to make the correct approaches. On the 'sage Advice' of a friend, one of his first actions in December 1766 was to present himself to Vaughan. The 'kind & gracious reception' with which he initially met seemed to bode well.[91] Arnold sought to consolidate the association. Having married in early 1767, at the beginning of April he and his young bride entertained Vaughan and family for tea, after which they all went together to the theatre. Arnold was conscious, however, of the possible fragility of their relationship, as he confided to the apothecary Richard Pulteney:

> I suppose Dr Sutton has told you on what <u>seeming</u> Terms we all are at present. I say <u>seeming</u>; — not because I have yet seen any particular Reason to doubt whether we are all sincere; but a Thing of this Kind you know is so uncommon among ye Faculty in the Country, that one is apt to fear it may last no longer than Views of Interest make it necessary to continue it.[92]

Arnold's apprehensions were to prove well founded. The rivalry and hostility that developed between the two men, and the ramifications, became increasingly poisonous elements in Leicester's medical community.

When the Leicester Infirmary opened in 1771, Arnold and Vaughan had been appointed as joint physicians. However, Arnold resigned his office in 1776, apparently in the wake of the resignation of the matron and several nurses after allegations of financial irregularities. This was almost certainly an episode in his simmering conflict with Vaughan, who remained as the infirmary's sole physician.[93] Arnold evidently then kept aloof from infirmary affairs, until his interests became directly threatened. When the governors proposed the establishment of a lunatic hospital, under Vaughan's guidance, Arnold rose to the challenge. After successfully fomenting Vaughan's resignation in June 1784, following the decision to abandon its opening, Arnold was duly re-elected as a physician to the infirmary, along with Drs Bree and Mackvie. These two were staunch in supporting Arnold against Vaughan, as Bree pointedly made clear to the public in acknowledging his own election: 'Convinc'd that my learned Friend, Dr. ARNOLD, will co-operate in promoting the Objects of this Institution, I rejoice in the Connection, and reflect upon the Secession of your last able Physician with less Regret.'[94] Vaughan, however, was not one to leave without a fight. Having joined the board of governors, he and his supporters lost no opportunity to make life difficult for Arnold, even to the detriment of the infirmary itself.[95]

The motivations of the protagonists were complex. It was certainly Vaughan who was the initial promoter and prime mover of the lunatic hospital, and it was almost equally certain that Arnold was responsible for blocking the project. Vaughan appeared initially motivated by a genuine intent to promote charitable provision for the insane poor.[96] Nevertheless, he must have been aware that a public institution in Leicester would materially affect the custom of Arnold's madhouse. For his part, Arnold undoubtedly derived commercial benefit from the indefinite postponement in 1784 of the lunatic hospital's opening. However, his extensive provision of charitable facilities for the poor, pauper and non-pauper, within his private asylum would suggest that he was driven by factors other than merely the maximization of personal gain.[97]

The quarrels even embroiled the men's respective offspring. The domination by the Arnold family of both the infirmary and of Leicester's provisions for the insane brought ongoing critical attack. In 1811 one of James Vaughan's sons, Rev. Edward Vaughan, an active infirmary governor who was intent on clipping the Arnolds' wings, sought a rule change to allow for a third physician, but his move was defeated.[98] Gradually, however, the Vaughan family gained some measure of consolation, if not actual victory. James Vaughan's most eminent son was none other than Sir Henry Halford, royal physician and future President of the Royal College of Physicians.[99] In September 1815, when the asylum was experiencing severe difficulties and Arnold's management was being seriously questioned, Sir Henry was drafted in to assist the infirmary governors' special committee of enquiry, whose membership also included Rev. Edward Vaughan and another brother, the barrister Serjeant Vaughan. Arnold immediately resigned as physician to the infirmary and the asylum, though his son Dr William Arnold continued in office.[100]

The depth of the enmity that developed between Vaughan and Arnold appears to have originated in sensitivities over conflicting professional and commercial interests. There were undoubtedly also fundamental social differences. Vaughan was one of a long line of eminent physicians, and was from a strictly Church of England background. Arnold's father, on the other hand, had been a baker who went on to become a madhouse keeper, and raised his son as a Baptist.[101] Someone who had known both men personally later recollected their differing characters. Dr Vaughan was 'a man of genius and quick perception; his practice bold and decisive', whereas Dr Arnold was 'the opposite; cautious, deliberate, and sure'.[102] Vaughan was evidently also quick-tempered, and became involved in violent confrontations on more than one occasion, though apparently with other medical colleagues rather than with Arnold himself.[103] Indeed, throughout the whole sorry saga, the gentlemanly conduct that might have been expected between medical men was abandoned.

Socio-political differences were rarely far from the surface in disputes between doctors. This was certainly the case in Manchester in the 1790s, when the physicians and surgeons of the infirmary battled over a range of issues.[104] John Ferriar was deeply involved along with Thomas Percival, both of whom were dissenters and adopted a radical Whig position on political and social questions. Their ongoing arguments with Tory Anglican elements within the infirmary and outside were primarily around matters of policy and practice in dealing with the city's growing public health crisis. Political positions were inevitably complicated by considerations of professional role and personal interest, creating a volatile cocktail of overlapping concerns. The disputes did not ostensibly include the care of the insane or the position of the lunatic hospital. However, they may well have influenced the decision to formally divide the Manchester Lunatic Hospital into 'hospital' and 'asylum' in 1791[105], and the subsequent debates in 1801 as to whether the lunatic hospital should be moved out of the city and the building converted into a fever hospital.[106] The latter issue certainly appears to have aroused a good deal of heated argument between the opposing parties.

Quarrels of a lesser degree arose among the physicians in Liverpool, emanating from the standard inter-mixture of concern for prestige, personal and professional, and pecuniary interest. Liverpool's medical arrangements were similar to those at Manchester, with its physicians taking joint responsibility for the lunatic asylum as part of their role at the Liverpool Infirmary. However, there was a further complexity after the establishment of the city's dispensary, creating additional voluntary posts for ambitious physicians. Competition developed between the physicians of the two institutions for spheres of influence, with the patients of the lunatic asylum becoming one of the main focuses. The initial arrangement had been that the paying patients were attended by the infirmary physicians, and the paupers by the dispensary physicians. The latter were clearly aggrieved at their exclusion from the more prestigious and lucrative work, and in early 1810 persuaded the governors to extend to them the right to attend on private patients, if wished by their relatives. The infirmary physicians led by Dr Joseph Brandreth, however, were fiercely opposed to sacrificing their pre-eminence and secured a reversal of the decision, as confirmed in the revised rules of 1813, making explicit their higher status.[107] However, the matter did not end there, for the infirmary's medical officers subsequently succeeded in having their dispensary colleagues excluded entirely from any attendance on the asylum's patients, leaving them in sole control. Grievances inevitably continued to fester, and contributed to the poisoned atmosphere between medical men that under-lay the scandals that erupted around the Liverpool Asylum in 1825.[108]

These various fraternal disputes among physicians engaged in the treatment of the insane were relatively restrained in relation to those that emerged at the Lincoln Lunatic Asylum in the 1830s, which are outside the scope of this volume.[109] The warning signs of trouble ahead were evident enough, however, some years earlier. The arrangement whereby the three physicians of the Lincoln County Hospital acted for the asylum on a monthly rotating basis was fraught with problems.[110] It proved to be the case that at least two of them, Dr Alfred Cookson and Dr Edward Parker Charlesworth, were particularly proud, stubborn, and strong-willed men who believed themselves actuated by matters of high principle.[111] Neither was averse to a public quarrel or to the use of language that bordered on the libellous.

Charlesworth, from the mid-1820s onwards, sought to bring about significant reforms in the way the asylum was operating, and was successful in convincing the governors to accept various progressive measures, notably structural alterations to improve patient classification and reductions in the use of mechanical restraint.[112] He published a book in 1828 which laid out, in a matter-of-fact manner, his vision of the asylum's operation.[113] Cookson, the senior of the two men in both years and status, was clearly jealous of the influence being gained by his junior. He regarded Charlesworth as a dangerous radical and his reforms as a threat to the stability of the institution. Each man acquired their group of supporters among the governors and the city's elite, and the arguments became thoroughly factionalised. From late 1828 into 1829 a newspaper controversy developed about the asylum and aspects of its management. The exchanges became increasingly vituperative and intemperate and there was little doubt in Lincoln that two of the main protagonists were Cookson and Charlesworth, both of whom were using pseudonyms.[114]

The Lincoln quarrels became focused on the role of the asylum's director, Thomas Fisher. Fisher, a surgeon-apothecary and himself a rather flamboyant character, was evidently not in accord with Charlesworth's reforming ideas and was equivocal in putting them into practice. Charlesworth sought to have him ousted, citing serious neglects of duty as well as various abuses towards both patients and the institution itself. However, despite Fisher provocatively referring to Charlesworth at a special board of governors' meeting in October 1829, as 'a *demon spirit* with the hand of an *assassin*' and a 'wretch', he was exonerated. Matters did not rest there, with both men continuing a newspaper war for several weeks, for which Fisher received only a reprimand from the governors.[115] Hostilities resumed in May 1830 when Fisher openly insulted Charlesworth within the hearing of the Dean of Lincoln Cathedral, a vice-president of the asylum governors. Special board meetings were held, at which Fisher was dismissed and then reinstated.[116] Unsurprisingly, Cookson took up a position actively in support of Fisher, openly calling for the removal of Charlesworth rather than the director.[117]

Matters came to a head at an over-heated special meeting of the board of governors on 13 October 1830, attended by no less than 180 people. The meeting, chaired by the Earl of Yarborough, lasted fully ten hours, with numerous speakers arguing for and against the dismissal of Fisher. Cookson and Charlesworth took the opportunity to trade verbal blows before an audience. Cookson lamented the deleterious effects on the institution of Charlesworth's 'extravagant management' and 'fantastical plans', complaining that his own contribution to the asylum's progress had been ignored. Charlesworth, on the other hand, defended his position in restrained terms and declined receiving a vote of thanks from the meeting, as he had only been doing his duty and acting on 'public grounds'.[118] Despite the efforts of Cookson and others, however, the case against Fisher was overwhelming and he was dismissed.[119] As for the Cookson — Charlesworth quarrel, it rumbled on until Alfred Cookson resigned in October 1832. By that time, however, he had passed on his mantle to his nephew Dr William Cookson, who would prove every bit as combative a few years later in his bitter confrontations with Charlesworth over the abolition of mechanical restraint.[120]

The longevity and the ferocity of the Lincoln controversies may have been exceptional. However, the apparently high incidence of quarrels and disputes among physicians with an interest in the treatment of insanity seems not to have been purely coincidental. Strong individual personalities, with firm convictions as to the correctness of their perspectives, were evidently impelled towards the advocacy or defence of entrenched positions. When personal financial interests or perceptions of public prestige were brought into the equation, the depth of the argument and the rancour engendered were even further magnified. With these combinations of circumstances, the standards and mores of gentlemanly conduct could be among the first casualties.

RENAISSANCE MEN

> A physician of spirit, who would wish to appear with dignity in his profession, must be acquainted with various branches of knowledge, which are rather ornamental than essential to the main ends of his art; although he will be able to make the separation in his own mind, between the liberal accomplishments that distinguish the gentleman and scholar, and that knowledge which is indispensably requisite to his practicing with any degree of credit or success. — John Gregory, *Observations on the Duties and Offices of a Physician*, 1770[121]

The cultivation of an image as an enlightened professional gentleman was central to the *persona* of the successful physician in the age of the 'urban renaissance'. There were various components that contributed towards the creation and maintenance of the image. An almost essential element was an active interest in the liberal arts, demonstrated by participation in the city's cultural institutions, even to the extent of the adoption of a leadership role in the promotion and management of those institutions. An interest in, and a knowledge of, areas of intellectual pursuit outside of medicine was particularly desirable.[122] If that interest was demonstrated and reinforced through the medium of publication, as a consequence adding magnanimously to the fund of public knowledge, there was likely to be a significant addition to reputation and prestige. In addition to participation in the cultural life of the city, the successful physician might also become involved in its civic and political activities, perhaps promoting reforms consistent with those aspects of his professional principles that were aimed toward the betterment of the health of the community.

William Battie, with his eccentricity of manner and of dress, was perhaps less interested than some of his other physician contemporaries in projecting a genteel and enlightened image. He had, though, experienced a quite wide-ranging education, prior to his entry into medicine. He had studied law both at Cambridge and for a period at the Middle Temple, though pecuniary constraints led him to abandon any ambition to practice. He was also an accomplished Latin and Greek scholar, having published edited versions of classical texts, including Aristotle's *Rhetoric* in 1728 and Isocrates' *Orations* in 1729.[123] In 1741 Battie was elected a Fellow of the Royal Society, though he subsequently resigned in 1752.[124] He also showed interest in some more practical projects, such as house-building and canal transportation.[125] The prominence that Battie achieved in the College of

Physicians, reinforced by his medical and related publications, brought him a degree of prestige that perhaps obviated any need to further display liberal gentility by other means.

Battie's later successor Samuel Foart Simmons demonstrated an extensive range of intellectual interests both within medicine and other fields. On completing his medical studies he had traveled in continental Europe. In Switzerland he had an audience with Voltaire and exchanged ideas with various people, including Baron de Haller to whom he sent books.[126] He became a fellow of various academies, including those of Nantes and Madrid, as well as the Societe Royale de Medecine at Paris. In Britain he accumulated memberships of various intellectual bodies, being elected a Fellow of the Royal Society in 1779 (on the recommendation of William Cullen), and a member of the Society of Antiquaries in 1791.[127] He also received honorary membership of the Medical Society of Edinburgh and of the Manchester Literary and Philosophical Society.[128] Simmons was a voluminous writer, particularly on medically-related subjects, one of his best known works being a biography of William Hunter.[129]

Much of Simmons' considerable energies were channeled into journalistic and editorial activities in the medical field. In 1779 he authored and published the first *Medical Register*, to be followed by another edition in 1780, and a third and much fuller edition in 1783. A publication that was both valuable to contemporaries and to medical historians, the *Register* utilized data obtained from correspondents around the country to provide detailed information on individual practitioners, as well as listing hospitals and other medical facilities in every locality.[130] In 1781 Simmons became editor of the *London Medical Journal*, the first medical periodical to achieve any significant longevity. It initially appeared monthly, and then quarterly; later re-named *Medical Facts and Observations*, it continued until 1800.[131] Simmons was quite indefatigable in his entrepreneurial activities. He established the Society for the Improvement of Medical Knowledge in 1782, a breakaway from the Medical Society of London, a body primarily comprised of religious dissenters, of which he had himself been the president in 1780.[132]

Alexander Hunter actively pursued an image as an enlightened gentleman-physician, ultimately becoming at least as well known for his wider activities as for his medical pursuits. As Michael Brown has shown, his publications on subjects connected with agriculture, botany and chemistry enabled him successfully to project a learned and genteel identity.[133] John Nichols awarded him the posthumous accolade of having been 'possessed of an active and liberal mind'.[134] Hunter had embarked on this aspect of his career even before his arrival in York, with the anonymous publication in 1761 of *A Treatise on the Nature and Virtues of the Buxton Water*; he published a longer version under his own name in 1768.[135] Aimed largely at a non-medical audience, the book laid the basis of his credentials as a knowledgeable man of science as well as of letters. Hunter's greatest literary successes, however, in both commercial and critical terms, were in botany and natural history. He regarded his much-enlarged revision of John Evelyn's *Silva* as his most important work. The first edition appeared in 1776, to be followed by four subsequent editions.[136] Its two handsome volumes, with numerous engraved plates, attracted a prestigious readership with subscribers among the aristocracy and gentry. It also attracted the interest of the intellectual elite; men such as Boswell, Priestley, and John Hunter appeared on the subscription lists. Alexander Hunter was himself gaining entry into that elite, recognized by his membership of the Royal Society in 1775, and later (in 1790) of the Royal Society of Edinburgh.[137] He followed up *Silva* with an annotated and illustrated edition of Evelyn's *Terra* in 1778.[138]

Some of Hunter's later publications were clearly aimed at a less specialist readership, providing homespun information and advice for a wider middle-class audience. In 1804, he published a volume dealing with the health aspects of cookery, which went into several editions.[139] Similar commercial success, indicated by a series of editions with enlargements, was achieved shortly afterwards with what was probably Hunter's most idiosyncratic piece of work, *Men and Manners*.[140] It comprised over a thousand brief maxims and aphorisms, containing advice and exhortation on many aspects of how a respectable person ought to conduct his life, concerning questions of social and class relations, politics, religion, health, domestic economy, and so on. Although medically related issues were not central, there were enough of them included to indicate Hunter's professional orientations. A few examples provide some illustration of the scope that he covered:

> Nothing is so endearing as being courteous to our inferiors.[141]

> If you have trusted your constitution in the hands of an empiric, why not act consistently, and send your watch to be mended by a blacksmith.[142]

> Whoever considers the nature of human society, must know, that, from necessity, there must be a subordination. Equality is theoretical nonsense.[143]

> If you are a medical man, take a warm interest in the recovery of your patients; it is your duty in a moral sense, and your interest in a political one.[144]

If nothing else, *Men and Manners* provides a perspective on aspects of Hunter's own character, and his priorities and prejudices. It lends a context for the tenaciousness with which he fought out the battles over the direction of the York Asylum's management.

It was in relation to agricultural matters, however, that Hunter achieved most prominence. In an era of agricultural improvement, he was able to establish himself in the vanguard of Yorkshire's progressive farming experimenters. In 1770 he founded the York Agricultural Society. Over the next two years he was responsible for collecting, editing, and contributing to four volumes of *Georgical Essays*, which comprised articles on agricultural, botanical, and natural historical subjects. The work proved a considerable success, with a second edition published in one volume in 1777, and a third in 1803.[145] Hunter's contribution to the dissemination of progressive agricultural practice was acknowledged well beyond the Yorkshire boundaries. He became one of Arthur Young's main collaborators, and in the 1790s he was officially rewarded with honorary membership of the newly established Board of Agriculture.[146] Increasingly, Hunter was projecting himself as a progressive intellectual gentleman, a promoter of the public good, whose professional occupation happened to be that of physician.

James Currie was another whose reputation rested more on activities outside of his practice as a physician. His wider intellectual and cultural interests had become apparent during his period as a student in Edinburgh, where he became an active member of several societies, both medical and philosophical, gaining a reputation as an eloquent public speaker. From his arrival in Liverpool he immersed himself in intellectual activities. He joined a literary society that met weekly. For some time the meetings were held at Currie's lodgings, and he was elected the president. Meetings continued for several years, until they were suspended after the outbreak of the French Revolution.[147] He co-founded the Liverpool Athenaeum and its library in 1797, and was its president by 1801.[148] He was elected an honorary member of the Manchester Literary and Philosophical Society, probably as a result of his association with Thomas Percival, with whom he maintained a regular correspondence on both literary and medical matters.[149] Both men were part of the intellectual corresponding network of dissenting physicians that Francis Lobo and Robert Kilpatrick have described, which also included William Cullen, John Aikin, John Coakley Lettsom, and Samuel Foart Simmons.[150] It was from Simmons that Currie first heard the news of his admission to the Royal Society in 1792.[151]

Currie aspired to be a serious literary contributor. In 1790 he wrote a series of essays for the *Liverpool Weekly Herald* under the anonymous cloak of 'The Recluse'. He also wrote book reviews for the *Analytical Review* and the *Critical Review*.[152] The pinnacle of this aspect of his career was his biography and collected edition of the works of Robert Burns, a project that he undertook some time after the poet's death in 1796. The four volumes were first published in 1800, with several editions to follow later. One of Currie's aims, in which he succeeded, had been to raise funds for Burns' family.[153] With the Burns biography Currie had firmly established himself as an enlightened man of letters. Of all his publications, however, the most commercially successful was a political polemic in June 1793, in which he launched a scathing attack on the government of William Pitt. Under the pseudonym of Jasper Wilson, Currie laid out the case against any declaration of war against revolutionary France.[154] The pamphlet made a considerable impression on public opinion and sold widely both in Britain and abroad. An edition was printed in America, and it was also translated into French and German.[155] Once the true identity of Jasper Wilson became known, in a political climate of patriotic ferment, Currie's private practice suffered for a period. [156]

Currie's radical perspective was also represented in his medical pursuits. He developed a particular interest in the treatment of fevers, which formed a key part of his *Medical Reports, on the Effects of Water, Cold and Warm*.[157] Like his colleagues Percival and Ferriar in Manchester, Currie became concerned with the health of the poorer classes, and the prevalence of epidemic fevers. He campaigned actively for a fever hospital for Liverpool, despite strong opposition that delayed fruition of the project until the eventual opening of a House of Recovery in the city in 1806.[158] His advocacy of the need for a lunatic hospital and the efforts he directed toward achieving his goal originated from the same current.

Currie was not one to be deterred by disapproval, gaining a reputation as a crusader on a range of humanitarian issues. He campaigned for improvement of the appalling and unhealthy conditions under which French prisoners-of-war were being held in Liverpool Gaol in 1799.[159] He was quite prepared to court unpopularity where fundamental matters of principle and humanity were at stake. He became a prominent activist in the movement for the abolition of the slave trade, risking the wrath of a wealthy and powerful element of Liverpool's merchant and commercial society.[160] Currie's interest in the subject had probably been kindled during his return passage from America, when he stopped at several West Indian islands *en route* and spent time in Antigua, providing the opportunity to witness at first hand some of the realities of slavery and the slave trade.[161] He corresponded regularly with William Wilberforce, providing him with practical information whilst expounding a position that was considered and gradualist.[162] At the same time he could be passionate and zealous, shown in a poem entitled *The African*, published in the London press in 1788. Jointly composed with the literary critic William Roscoe, it explored the trauma of a man being captured and torn from his homeland and his freedom.[163]

Despite the strength of his feelings on the subject of African slavery, one of Currie's particular qualities was his ability to appreciate the genuine dilemmas faced by his opponents, as he showed in a letter to Thomas Percival in 1788:

> The situation of a person of sense and feeling in society here, is at present very distressing. Men of any enlargement of mind, who have been concerned in the slave-trade, begin to reflect on their situation; and the struggle between interest and principle, between a lucrative traffic and

a sense of character, is productive of such embarassment and contra-
diction, as fills one with sorrow.[164]

This ability to condemn the practice, whilst seeking to understand the complex motives of the individual, was a major reason why Currie succeeded
in limiting the damage to his professional practice. Essentially, though
adhering to a radical political agenda, Currie was a committed moderate.
Writing to Percival on the urgent need for repeal of the Test and Corporation Acts, which discriminated against religious dissenters' participation in
public bodies, he affirmed that 'I detest oppression in every form'. At the
same time, he was convinced that the radical cause could only be advanced
by respectable behaviour, asserting that 'I am especially anxious that our
proceedings should be directed by candour and moderation.'[165] For Currie,
gentlemanly conduct was an essential pre-requisite in the proper advance-
ment of a principle. He was, in many ways, the archetype of the liberal
physician.

John Ferriar's intellectual and campaigning activities outside his profession also contributed to a position of prominence in cultural and political
circles in his adopted city. Like Currie and Thomas Percival, Ferriar was a
Nonconformist who adhered to all the associated liberal causes, including
the pursuit of parliamentary reform and anti-slavery.[166] Ferriar's preoccupation with public health issues developed from his indefatigable work among
the Manchester Infirmary's home patients, where he witnessed at first hand
the appalling conditions in which many working class people in the city
were living. He wrote several influential papers, highlighting the evils of
cellar dwellings, unregulated lodging-houses, ill-ventilated mills, and the
lack of adequate food and clothing. With the active support of Percival, he
campaigned for sanitary reforms aimed at tackling typhus and other fever
epidemics. Both men addressed large public meetings, ultimately achieving the creation of a Board of Health in 1796. Ferriar was prepared, like
Currie in Liverpool, to take up issues that might challenge the economic
interests of the wealthy middle classes who could form a significant part
of his customer base. He attacked the unhealthy conditions in the cotton
mills, and some of the practices imposed on the operatives such as the shift
arrangements. Again working with Percival, he called for shorter working
hours for the factory children.[167]

Ferriar became a well-known figure in Manchester liberal intellectual circles. He joined the Manchester Literary and Philosophical Society
shortly after his arrival in the city in 1785, reading his first paper in 1786 on
the subject of popular illusions. Over the following years he wrote several
papers for the society, comprising not only literary and poetical subjects,
but also philosophy, history, archaeology, and topography. He continued
to pursue scholarly activities, alongside his professional work and political campaigning. He retained a long-standing interest in the writings of
Lawrence Sterne, particularly *Tristram Shandy*, which eventually culmi-

nated in his most significant non-medical book, *Illustrations of Sterne*, first published in 1798.[168] An expanded second edition was published in two volumes in 1812, reflecting the celebrity that Ferriar's work had achieved in polite circles beyond Manchester.[169]

Thomas Arnold perhaps did not achieve an external reputation comparable to a Currie or a Hunter, mainly becoming known outside Leicester for his books on insanity. He became both a Fellow of the Royal College of Physicians and of the Royal Medical Society of Edinburgh. In 1800 he helped to found the Leicester Medical Society. His publications were all medically related. As well as the two substantial volumes of *Observations on the Nature on the Nature, Kinds, Causes, and Prevention of Insanity*, published in 1782–86, he produced another important work on mental disorder, *Observations on the Management of the Insane*, in 1809.[170] His work as a general physician was reflected in the publication of *A Case of Hydrophobia Successfully Treated* in 1793.[171] Arnold played an active part in most aspects of Leicester's social, cultural, and political life. He became the first president of the Leicester Literary Society. He adopted the role of patron of the arts, as well as being a book collector.[172] He maintained a lifelong interest in botany and natural history, and was a member of the Linnaean Society.[173] Having been brought up as a Baptist, Arnold's nonconformist background contributed to his consistent political liberalism, even though he had his children baptized as Anglicans. He was active in the movement for the repeal of the Test and Corporation Acts.[174] His published obituary confirmed him to have been 'an unshaken friend of civil and religious liberty', as well as 'the anxious promoter of every design which tended to ameliorate distress'. To his many supporters, Arnold was 'an enlightened ornament of his native town'.[175]

PUBLIC SERVICE, PRIVATE GAIN

Whatever the pretensions of many physicians toward gentlemanly status, they still had to earn a living. Indeed, there was scope to make a great deal of money within a medical market-place that was becoming increasingly diverse and sophisticated. The status gained by unpaid attachment to a hospital, dispensary, or other medical charity would go some way toward restoring any potential damage to character and prestige associated with involvement in commercial activities. A degree of respectability was also conferred by an extensive private practice among the privileged classes, based on individual consultation and emanating from personal reputation. For insanity specialists, or mad-doctors, there was the additional barrier to overcome of the stigma attached to the nature of their work.[176] Their most lucrative option was proprietorship of a private madhouse, but this carried the risk of incurring the particular distaste attached to what was a rather questionable aspect of 'trade'. The opportunities to generate a substantial income, however, could go a long way towards compensating for the effects of any deleterious public perceptions.

Private practice was to a degree encouraged as a consequence of the financial structures that emerged at the provincial public lunatic hospitals. Their viability was dependent on the payments received either by the patients' relatives or (if paupers) by their parish. Once the principle had been accepted at the Manchester Lunatic Hospital that admission could be extended to people beyond the ranks of the poor, and that a clear alternative to private madhouses was being offered, the voluntary institutions had plainly entered the market-place. With scales of charges according to ability to pay, it became accepted as reasonable for the medical officers to receive fees for attendance on people of 'superior Condition'.[177] In the rules of 1791, these fees were made explicit. A payment of one guinea was to be made to the attending physician on the admission of every patient charged at 8s. per week or more. A further sum, ranging from one to ten guineas (according to means), was to be paid upon their death, discharge, or after a period of two years' confinement in the hospital.[178] Although the potential earnings were not especially great, the voluntary principle had been clearly breached. The public service aspect of the physician's role was, however, still largely upheld by the continuance of free attendance on paupers and other poor patients.

Similar opportunities became available to the physicians at most of the lunatic hospitals, with the evident exception of the Leicester Asylum,[179] as their governors implemented arrangements similar to those at Manchester. Although Dr John Hall had failed in 1765 to convince the Newcastle Lunatic Hospital's governors to cater for private patients in their new building, the later expansion of the hospital did include some provision. Hall's successor Dr Wood became entitled to receive one guinea per month from the 'superior patients', as well as an initial entrance fee.[180] At the Liverpool Lunatic Asylum, the arrangements were similar to Manchester, with the 'Friends' of patients paying weekly charges above 8s. required to pay a guinea to the physician on admission, to be followed by a 'reasonable Acknowledgement' for his attendance on discharge, death, or after two years' residence.[181] At Exeter, a sophisticated and potentially lucrative structure was developed. Initially the physician received fees on a sliding scale for those patients paying over 10s.6d per week.[182] By 1824, there were two attendant physicians and fees were payable for patients charged over 15s per week, at rates ranging from one to five guineas, on admission and on discharge and also at six monthly intervals during their stay in the asylum. They additionally received 'more liberal Gratuities' from affluent patients whose cases had required 'long and assiduous attention'.[183]

It was at York that the physician was able to engineer the most favourable circumstances. Dr Alexander Hunter cited the Manchester precedent in contending for similar payment arrangements at the York Asylum.[184] Once the asylum began to accept private patients in 1784, with a scale of charges according to means and to standards of accommodation provided, Hunter could legitimately argue that his interests would be injured if he had to attend for free on people whom he might, in other circumstances, have treated as private patients. His contention that he should, therefore, be entitled to the 'reasonable emoluments' of his profession was easily conceded by the governors in 1785.[185] Any idea that payments to the physician were not compatible with service to a public hospital carried little apparent weight either with Hunter or the governors. Their agreement in 1787 to grant him an annual salary of £200, even if a short-lived experiment, showed how far the compromise of principle could be taken.[186] Hunter's opponents were given ample fuel for their attacks on his perceived subversion of the asylum's original charitable intent, even accusing him of operating it as a virtual private madhouse.[187] For his part he could demonstrate that he was not solely actuated by motives of personal gain, for it was acknowledged that he continued to provide 'liberal, disinterested, and charitable' attendance to all the 'necessitous objects' of the charity, including the paupers whose presence in the asylum he appeared to resent.[188] However, his charitable contribution notwithstanding, Hunter earned a very substantial amount of money from his private work in the asylum, as Godfrey Higgins later showed.[189]

Although the situation at St Luke's was somewhat different to the provincial lunatic hospitals, it also presented gainful opportunities to the medical officers. At first, there were no weekly charges for any of the patients. Once provision was made for incurables, however, charges of 5s. per week were instituted for them. Curable patients who were 'proper objects' of charity continued to be accepted without payment, funded from the hospital's considerable and accumulating wealth. There was never any provision for fee-paying private patients. Nevertheless, the governors brought in arrangements in 1789 whereby the physician (Foart Simmons) and the surgeon were rewarded with regular payment of an annual 'gratuity' for their attendance. The figure was set at £100 per year for the physician and £50 for the surgeon.[190] Although rescinded after Simmons' retirement in 1811, the arrangement was reinstated in early 1816 to the benefit of his successor Dr Alexander Sutherland.[191]

The most profitable aspect of medical attendance at St Luke's, though, was not the direct earnings from 'gratuities', but the lucrative private practice as a mad-doctor that could be built up on the basis of the acquired professional reputation. William Battie was able to develop an extensive practice, providing individual consultation to members of the wealthy classes, including the aristocracy. His later customers included the Earl of Orford and the M.P. and diplomat Sir Charles Hanbury Williams. He also attended on people whom he had placed in various madhouses in and around London, receiving substantial fees for so doing.[192] His most profitable ventures, however, were the two madhouses in Clerkenwell of which he was proprietor, one in Islington Road and one in Wood's Close, though he evidently sought to conceal his ownership of the houses.[193] According to Roy Porter, Battie was able to divert into his own care those affluent patients who had been referred to St Luke's but who would not have met the eligibility criteria.[194] The vast wealth he accumulated has been generally attributed to income obtained from his madhouses. The value of Battie's will occasioned considerable comment, not least from Horace Walpole, who in the context of describing his own 'melancholy ideas' and 'shattered nerves' was moved to exclaim in August 1776: 'What a distracted nation! I do not wonder that Dr Battie died worth £100,000. Will anybody be worth a shilling but mad-doctors?'[195]

Battie's successors at St Luke's were also able to do well for themselves. Samuel Foart Simmons was accumulating considerable wealth from the lunacy trade, even before the governors commenced paying him a salary. A consummate medical entrepreneur, he developed a range of private activities, which included acting as an expert witness in high profile court cases, such as the trial of the millenarian cleric Richard Brothers for treasonable practices in 1795.[196] By 1788, Simmons was visiting 'several houses of private confinement' in the London area, and had one 'under his own special direction'.[197] His proprietorship of Fisher House, the 'Islington Mad-House', led him to be pilloried in print by Brothers, who was confined there from 1795 until 1806.[198] His main motive, Brothers alleged, was to keep people confined for personal gain.[199] Dr Alexander Sutherland, who succeeded Simmons at St Luke's in 1811, appears to have acquired Fisher House from him. By 1815, Sutherland owned the madhouse, containing sixteen patients, as well as the larger Blacklands House in Chelsea with thirty patients.[200]

Despite the risk of adverse publicity, proprietorship of a madhouse was not uncommon among insanity specialists.[201] Dr John Hall at Newcastle was the first provincial lunatic hospital physician to enter into it when he opened St Luke's House in 1766. Although Hall alleged that he had reluctantly started the venture at the behest of the lunatic hospital governors, commercial considerations evidently soon became paramount. The initial publicity followed the usual pattern for private madhouses, declaring it 'a proper Place for the Reception of Persons of Fortune suitable to their Station', which would provide for the 'Convenience and real Welfare of Mankind', in a healthy setting on the edge of the city's Town Moor, and with the benefits of a 'spacious and very delightful Garden in Front.'[202] Following the break-up of Hall's partnership with the surgeons in 1767, he continued the house on his own, offering to receive patients at the comparatively low rates of £20 per year for board, or 8s. per week, with an additional weekly charge of half a guinea for attendance on those receiving active medical treatment. Hall was anxious, though, to show that he was not profiteering, waiving the additional charges for incurables and offering reduced rates to people in poor circumstances.[203] His promise was that the 'Greatest Care' would be taken of 'all Patients intrusted to him.'[204]

Alexander Hunter was evidently not satisfied with his earnings from private patients in the York Asylum. He had even made a case similar to Hall's, employing the argument that suitable recompense for his attendance on private patients in the York Asylum would discourage him from feeling impelled to open a private madhouse.[205] Notwithstanding the endeavours of the governors to meet his requirements, Hunter nevertheless went ahead and opened his own house in 1790, despite an awareness that this was in conflict with the early intention of the York Asylum to 'lessen the number of private madhouses'.[206] Hunter's advertisements stressed the exclusivity of his 'House of Retirement, for Persons of Condition only', which received only 'a few Persons' who laboured under a 'recent or continued Derangement of Mind'. Claiming that the house would avoid all the 'Inconveniences' complained of in private houses of confinement, the proprietors promised 'Neatness, Cleanliness, and gentle Usage'. Patients were to be waited on by their own attendants and could dine in their own 'apartments' if they so chose.[207] Hunter presumably wanted to ensure a clientele of sufficient respectability, accommodated in suitably salubrious surroundings, in order to maintain his gentlemanly image as far as was consistent with being owner of a madhouse.

Thomas Arnold's circumstances were quite different to those of Hall and Hunter. His proprietorship of a private madhouse pre-dated his tenure as physician to the Leicester Lunatic Asylum by many years. He was also seeing individual patients, in the wake of his growing reputation as a specialist mad-doctor. His clientele included prestigious figures like the Birmingham physician Dr John Ash, who consulted him in 1783 in relation to a prolonged episode of depression.[208] The reputation Arnold gained from his private work was the reason for his being invited to manage the asylum in 1792, rather than the more normal reverse situation. Having taken over the madhouse in Bond Street from his father in 1767, Arnold had developed the business considerably.[209] Early in the nineteenth century he relocated it to Belle Grove, the large suburban house to which he had moved with his family in 1791.[210] The considerable success Arnold achieved, in therapeutic and particularly in commercial terms, had given him the wherewithal to be able to establish his 'hospital for lunatics', making available free and subsidized places for members of the poorer classes.[211] That ostensibly magnanimous demonstration, combined with his important contributions to the infirmary and the lunatic asylum, exemplified how a physician could reconcile the diverse elements of both private practice and public service.

CONCLUSIONS

Physicians acquired and retained the key leadership role in the voluntary lunatic hospitals. Yet, with the exception of Thomas Arnold, none of the men considered in this chapter had actually planned to become an insanity specialist. Even where practice as a mad-doctor became the predominating element of their work, they ensured the retention of professional credibility and prestige by their continued involvement in the wider aspects of medical practice. There was a clear logic to this for, even with the development of the principles and techniques of 'moral management', the diagnosis and treatment of insanity remained rooted firmly within the medical sphere.[212] The successful physician, therefore, needed to maintain a rounded and eclectic professional perspective. Beyond that, it became important to establish a position in the town and community that was commensurate with the role of physician and the associated aspirations to be regarded as a gentleman.

The construction and exhibition of a gentlemanly identity was a paramount element of the physician's public presentation. Of our main subjects, only William Battie had the natural advantages of birth into the correct circles. Church of England, Eton and Cambridge gave him the right credentials for membership (and later leadership) of the College of Physicians and the development of a highly successful and profitable career. He could afford both to lead an eccentric life-style and to risk acquiring the stigma attached to mad-doctoring.[213] The relatively modest middle-class Scottish origins of Hunter, Currie and Ferriar, and particularly their educations at Edinburgh University, were significant in shaping their approaches to medical practice and to their engagement in activities in other arenas. Arnold and Foart Simmons emanated also from middle-class nonconformist backgrounds, which directed their medical education northwards. The Edinburgh experience, in the great era of William Cullen and John Gregory, was of profound influence on all of them (excepting Battie), as on so many other of their contemporaries. It was there that they not only learnt the practices and the art of physic. The duties and the responsibilities of the liberal gentleman-physician were instilled into them, as well as an appreciation of the literary, scientific, philosophical and socio-political knowledge that they would need to develop a successful career wherever they chose to settle.[214]

An unpaid attachment to a general hospital or a lunatic hospital was a prime exemplar of the physician's acceptance of an obligation to serve the public. It demonstrated philanthropy, duty, and the unselfish dissemination of the fruits of his acquired professional skills to people less fortunate. This voluntary activity formed one part of his engagement in the wider public sphere. In almost every case, the physicians' cultural activities or participation in public affairs became at least as significant as their medical practice. They were able to achieve prominent social positions in their respective cities or towns, even to the point of acquiring a leadership role. There was an evident consciousness of being in a position of influence, allied to a perception of duty to make constructive use of that position for the benefit of the wider community. Currie and Ferriar exercised their influence by involvement in radical political activity and in campaigning for improvements in the conditions of the poor as a means of countering disease, whilst Hunter made his contribution through the promotion of agricultural improvement. In every case, they sought to advance knowledge by means of literary contributions, whether in medicine, science, politics, literature, or in more than one of these fields. The ostensibly selfless exercise of communal and social responsibility proved to be the essence of the liberal gentleman-physician. There were, of course, great incidental benefits to be gained. The prestige and public regard acquired, not to mention the connections developed among members of the local elites, proved most advantageous in building up private practices both as general physicians and as insanity specialists.

Even in the larger towns and cities physicians remained relatively few in number in the late eighteenth and early nineteenth centuries. Notwithstanding similarities in education, career development and cultural orientation, they tended to be fiercely individualistic. A strong upholding of professional dignity and honour was a common characteristic, which could unite them against challenges from outside. However, it also fed the obstinate pride and vanity that became evident in the rancorous quarrels that appear to have been endemic anywhere that two or more physicians were in practice. Differences of principle provided the ostensible rationale for arguments that were often fuelled by more basic considerations of material self-interest. The prolonged trans-generational enmities that developed between the Arnolds and the Vaughans in Leicester were only the most graphic example of a volatile admixture of professional self-righteousness, offended dignity, and threatened commercial interests.

Comportment as a gentleman required an income sufficient to permit the physician to have sufficient leisure time to pursue non-medical interests. In order to achieve this level of prosperity, there was no alternative to active participation in the medical market place. This meant the development of a private practice among those wealthy enough to pay for his services. As William Battie and his contemporary John Monro demonstrated, there were lucrative opportunities in private consultation for the successful insanity specialist.[215] The real money, though, was to be made in owning and operating a private madhouse. However, the whole question of madhouse keeping highlighted the paradoxical and complex position of the physician mad-doctor. With the increasing criticism of madhouses and some of the dubious practices that had received public exposure, there was a risk that even the most respectable proprietors could be tainted by the associated stigma. The dilemma to be faced was that the activity that would contribute most to the financial security that a gentleman needed could also potentially threaten the image of gentility that he had so carefully constructed.

5 'Proper objects'

Social historians engaged in considering the history and development of provision for mentally disordered people have, in recent years, rightly sought to divert some of the emphasis previously placed on institutions and on the prominent individuals who ostensibly shaped events, to focus more on the people on the receiving end of their ministrations. In particular there have been several major studies of the patient populations of nineteenth century county lunatic asylums.[1] These studies have utilized the voluminous material which asylum superintendents were obliged to keep after 1845. Record-keeping was, however, considerably less sophisticated in the period before the state intervened actively in institutional provision, which in itself places considerable limitations on the availability of useful data regarding the patient population. The problems are even further accentuated by the vagaries of survival or otherwise of the documents which might provide evidence.[2] In order, therefore, to construct a representation of those who populated the lunatic hospitals it is necessary to assemble and interpret evidence from disparate sources.

The most comprehensive analysis of institutionalized insane patients in the eighteenth century has been provided by Jonathan Andrews within his extensive study of Bethlem Hospital.[3] His consideration of elements such as the social and economic background of the patients, the areas from whence they came, and their anticipated prognosis in terms of the expectation or otherwise of 'cure' provide some possible bases for comparison with successor lunatic hospitals. One of Andrews' key sources of evidence consisted of the petitions for admission to Bethlem. These provided important information regarding the circumstances that had precipitated or led up to admission, which were likely often to include contemporary perceptions of the 'causes' of the mental disorder. Unfortunately, comparable documents do not appear to have survived either for St Luke's or for the provincial lunatic hospitals.

Committal to an institution for the insane in eighteenth-century England, whether a public lunatic hospital or a private madhouse, was not undertaken lightly or casually. Even with the growth that occurred in the last quarter of the century, places were relatively few in number, reflecting the overwhelming tendency to maintain mentally disordered people within family and community.[4] It would only be when certain factors came together, in the severity of the individual's presentation and the capacity of others to deal with it, that committal was the consequence. Those factors might comprise behaviours or patterns of thinking that posed a risk of harm to the sufferer or to those around him, or inter-personal dynamics within the family which both affected the patient's condition and impaired their ability to cope. The emergent therapeutic orthodoxy, stressed by Battie and others, that separation and removal of the lunatic were a pre-requisite of curative treatment, served to legitimate the option of committal.[5] Nevertheless, with hospitals, asylums, and madhouses catering probably for only a small minority of sufferers of mental disorder, it followed that the people who entered those institutions were likely to consist of the most potentially dangerous to themselves or others, the most distressed, the most disinhibited, the most socially unacceptable, and the hardest to manage.

This chapter sets out to construct a picture of the patient population of the lunatic hospitals. It initially examines the growth in their numbers through the period, before a consideration of the main social factors that influenced who those patients were. The procedures and, more importantly, the criteria for admission are described, for these both reflected and determined some of the key qualifications for entry. Curability was strongly emphasized in accepting people into St Luke's Hospital, as at Bethlem before it, but appears to have been a less significant determinant for reception into the provincial institutions. The geographical factors that had been apparent in the patterns of location of the lunatic hospitals were similarly important in influencing where their patients emanated from. As conceptions of what constituted a 'proper object' widened beyond the 'poor', social class considerations proved increasingly significant in influencing the composition of the inmate groups, as well as being important determinants of the ways in which the lunatic hospitals developed and functioned. The chapter concludes with some descriptive, impressionistic contemporary perceptions of the characteristics and behavioural presentations of the patients themselves.

A GROWING PATIENT POPULATION

Although committal remained an option of final resort, there is little doubt that the threshold was shifting in the latter part of the eighteenth century. Reliable figures are not available on the confinement of the insane in private madhouses, but it is clear that the number of houses was steadily increasing both in London and the provinces, as were the numbers of people that individual houses could accommodate. In particular, capacity was expanding to meet a growing demand to accommodate pauper lunatics referred and paid for by their parishes.[6] To some extent this was a consequence of the accelerating population growth characteristic of the period, but which alone was not sufficient to provide an explanation.[7] There has been some inconclusive historical debate as to whether the incidence of insanity was on the increase as a response to the social upheavals related to economic change and the emergence of an urban-industrial society.[8] The factors that almost certainly did contribute to the rising numbers of committals included socio-demographic changes, particularly in the north and the midlands, allied to gradual shifts in perceptions of what was tolerable in the community and a growing acceptance that there could be positive benefits from confinement in a specialist institution.

The expanding provision within the private sector was more than matched by the charitable institutions. The first St Luke's Hospital, having opened initially for twenty-five patients in August 1751, contained forty-seven a year later, and fifty in 1753[9] (see Table 5.1). Following admission of the first group of incurable patients in 1754, they were recorded separately from the curables, who continued to be the predominant group in the hospital.[10] By the end of 1755, there was capacity for twenty incurables in addition to the fifty curable patients. Maximum patient numbers continued at seventy until early 1765, when an additional building for twenty curable

Table 5.1 St Luke's Hospital — patient numbers, 1751–1821

Year	Numbers
1751	25
1755	58
1760	67
1765	97
1770	100
1775	110
1780	110
1785	103
1790	183
1795	267
1800	305
1805	301
1810	298
1815	295
1820	227
1825	273
1830	235

Source: St Luke's Hospital, General Court Books.

and ten incurable patients came into use; there were ninety-seven in the house in February.[11] Accommodation for ten more patients had been provided by February 1772.[12] After that, the hospital largely remained full to its capacity of 110 for more than a decade, until its replacement at the beginning of 1787.[13]

It was the pressure of growing demand for places, both for curable and incurable patients, that provided the impetus for the projection and building of the second St Luke's in Old Street. The new hospital opened with those transferred from Windmill Hill, plus a few additional patients.[14] Expansion was gradual, however, for it was several years before the maximum capacity of 300 was reached. In February 1789 there were 170 patients, increasing to 218 in 1791.[15] By 1794 the numbers stood at 252, reaching a pinnacle of 305 in January 1800. St Luke's was now the largest lunatic hospital or asylum in the country, providing for more patients than Bethlem.[16] Numbers remained close to 300 for several years, until 1815.[17] However, over the following five years there was a fairly dramatic fall, from 295 in February 1815 down to 227 in February 1820.[18] The main cause of this appears to have been the opening after 1811 of the various new county lunatic asylums established under the Act of 1808, which deflected some patients who might otherwise have been referred to St Luke's.[19] This decline, though, proved to be only temporary for numbers then rose sharply again, reaching 284 in early 1821.[20] It seems, nevertheless, that the hospital continued to function at below capacity, with 270 patients recorded in 1827, followed by another fall to 235 by 1830.[21]

One very notable factor in the pattern of admissions to St Luke's was the disparity between the genders. This was particularly significant in the first half-century of its operation. By the end of 1760, 510 females had been admitted and only 225 males, amounting respectively to sixty-seven per cent and thirty-three per cent of the total. This clear preponderance of women continued to 1800. In the decade 1790–1800, 1403 females (sixty-two per cent) were admitted and 913 males (thirty-eight per cent).[22] From then onwards the number of male admissions steadily increased. Thomas Dunston observed to the 1807 select committee that the proportion of females to males admitted was 3:2.[23] Within a few years the balance was more even, though female admissions did continue to exceed those of males. St Luke's appears to have been unique in this high incidence of female admissions, and there is no ready explanation other than Dunston's suggestion that female patients displayed higher rates of cure.[24] A tendency toward more female admissions had not been apparent at Bethlem Hospital earlier in the eighteenth century.[25] Similarly, the St Luke's phenomenon was not reflected in the provincial lunatic hospitals. Porter's view generally held true that the numbers of males admitted to institutions for the insane exceeded those of females.[26]

Of the provincial institutions, only the York Lunatic Asylum came anywhere near St Luke's in its extent. It also had commenced on a fairly mod-

Table 5.2 York Lunatic Asylum — patient numbers, 1777–1828

Year	Numbers
1777	10
1780	28
1784	43
1790	75
1794	83
1800	112
1805	142
1808	188
1813	199
1814	103
1820	108
1821	130
1828	144

Sources: Gray, A History of the York Lunatic Asylum, p.24; Report of the Committee of Inquiry into the Rules and Management of the York Lunatic Asylum, p.48; The Rules and Regulations of the York Lunatic Asylum, With a List of Governors, &c.&c., York: Thomas Wilson and Sons, 1820, p.4; University of York, Borthwick Institute, RET 8/1/1/1, Annual Reports, 1821, 1828.

est scale, in 1777. The building was designed to accommodate fifty-four patients but only ten were admitted initially, followed a few months later by another twenty.[27] The story thenceforth was one of steady growth in patient numbers, accompanied by periodic additions to the building (see Table 5.2). A new section with twenty-four rooms was completed in 1788, and an extensive detached building was added in 1795.[28] The increase in numbers was rapid over the next twenty years, peaking at 199 in 1813. A high proportion of these additional patients were pauper lunatics, though there had also been a significant increase in private patients.[29] In contrast to St Luke's, in the years from 1777 to 1820 male admissions to York consistently exceeded those of females, by an average of about fifty-five per cent to forty-five per cent.[30]

The York Asylum's infrastructure was severely stretched to cope with this growth, and the stresses engendered undoubtedly contributed to the developing crisis in its affairs. The ensuing collapse in patient numbers was related largely to the disastrous fire of December 1813, which destroyed the detached building housing female patients. Only four people died, but numbers had to be drastically pruned by early discharges, restrictions on admissions, and transfers to other asylums.[31] By the end of 1814, there were just over one hundred patients in the asylum. Even though a replacement new building for forty females was opened in 1817, the reforms that followed the scandals ensured that the severe overcrowding of 1812–13 would not be repeated and that numbers were kept to a level that provided for adequate space, comfort, and security for patients.[32]

The Manchester Lunatic Hospital also experienced a significant growth in its patient population, emerging as the leader among those attached to a general hospital, and the third largest overall numerically. It opened with only four patients in 1766, and contained thirteen by the middle of the following year[33] (see Table 5.3). By 1787 the lunatic hospital had expanded to a point where it actually contained more people than the main infirmary. Considerable extensions had been made to the building, in 1773 and 1781, to be followed by another in 1789.[34] By the early nineteenth century, the lunatic hospital and asylum could accommodate one hundred patients, and numbers hovered between eighty and one hundred over the next twenty years. There was a steady decline in the 1820s, so that by 1830 there were only forty-five patients. Like at St Luke's this appears to have been to a large extent associated with the establishment of the county asylums, in particular that at Lancaster which had opened in 1816.[35] In the lunatic hospital's early years the numbers of males and females admitted had been virtually identical.[36] However, figures for the years 1812–14 show that by then, and again in contrast to St Luke's, twice as many males were being admitted as females.[37]

The Newcastle Lunatic Hospital conformed to the expansionary trend. For its first few years it was providing for more patients than Manchester. The converted house that comprised the original lunatic hospital opened in

Table 5.3 Manchester Lunatic Hospital — patient numbers, 1767–1818

Year	Numbers
1767	13
1773	32
1784	47
1789	60
1801	64
1804	85
1805	98
1808	86
1813	97
1814	88
1818	90+

Sources: Manchester Infirmary Archives, Annual Reports, 1766-1814; Warneford Hospital Archives, W.P.5, xv, letter 7 April 1818 from Mr Taylor, Manchester Infirmary.

Table 5.4 Liverpool Lunatic Asylum — patient numbers, 1794–1831

Year	Numbers
1794	5
1796	36
1798	51
1802	55
1808	64
1812	69
1815	53
1820	45
1827	49
1831	59

Sources: Liverpool Record Office, 614 INF 5/2, Annual Reports, 1793-1831; Staffs CRO, Q/AIc, Box 1, letter 11 March 1812, Squires to Aylesbury.

1764, and within six months it was full to its capacity of nineteen patients. This remained the position until the new hospital replaced it in 1767, providing for in excess of thirty patients.[38] Clearly some subsequent expansion did take place but, unfortunately, no reliable figures for patient numbers are available for the intervening years before 1810 when Sir George Paul visited. He put the numbers at approximately sixty, tallying with a published report of 1817, according to which there were fifty-nine people in the hospital.[39] Ten years later, following some extensive renovations and improvements to the building, the capacity had been raised to eighty.[40] By this time, though, it was questionable whether the house at Newcastle still properly constituted a public lunatic hospital.

Of the other lunatic hospitals established during the latter part of the eighteenth century, only the Liverpool Asylum was operated on a substantial scale (see Table 5.4). The building was designed to accommodate between sixty and seventy patients.[41] After a slow beginning, numbers grew steadily, reaching a maximum of sixty-nine in 1812. Thereafter there was a marked decline which, as at Manchester, was largely the effect of the opening of the Lancashire County Asylum in 1816. Indeed, sixteen Liverpool pauper lunatics were removed in 1815 to the workhouse, apparently preparatory to transfer to the county asylum.[42] From then onwards, pauper lunatics were being regularly transferred to Lancaster after initial admission to Liverpool.[43] With the opening of the new Liverpool Lunatic Asylum in 1831, patient numbers again began to rise, no doubt in response to 'the superiority of accommodation afforded there for every class of its inmates'.[44]

The Leicester Lunatic Asylum, which opened shortly after Liverpool, began on a small scale and never really progressed beyond that. The building had been designed for twenty patients, but it opened at the end of 1794 for ten.[45] By June 1796 there were twelve patients in the house, rising to fourteen by 1803. Numbers remained at that level for several years, before falling to just eight in 1814, when the building was in a deteriorated state.[46] After renovations and reforms, there was a moderate increase in patient numbers, which rose to fifteen in 1821 and then to a maximum of still only eighteen by 1830.[47] The other lunatic hospital that opened in the 1790s, at Hereford in 1799, was also designed for twenty people, but by 1801 it had effectively ceased to be a charitable facility.[48]

Developments at the Exeter Lunatic Asylum followed more conventional expansionary patterns. The original Bowhill House accommodated fourteen patients when it opened in 1800. Extensive additions to the building were made in 1803, which increased the capacity to forty-eight. There were thirty-nine in the house in 1807, and by 1812 the numbers in the asylum were averaging forty-two.[49] Following further building work, the asylum's capacity had risen to fifty-four by 1824.[50] The Lincoln Lunatic Asylum also commenced on a relatively modest scale. In March 1825, five years after it had opened, there were thirty patients in the asylum, and at the end of 1830 it contained forty.[51] However, its major expansion was to come during the following decade, with numbers climbing to 109 by 1840.[52] The Oxford (Radcliffe) Lunatic Asylum, which opened in July 1826, contained thirteen patients a year later. Some expansion in numbers began to take place after 1828.[53]

By any standards, the growth in the number of patients in the voluntary lunatic hospitals in the second half of the eighteenth century had been extremely significant. From the small beginnings at St Luke's in 1751, the combined figures had reached about 630 in 1800. These numbers constituted about a fifth of the estimated population in voluntary hospitals as a whole.[54] After 1800 the situation became somewhat more complex. The number of patients in the lunatic hospitals had actually fallen to about 580 by 1820 before they rose again to around 680 in 1830.[55] Certain factors had served to curtail the rate of growth. The circumstances at York, particularly the disastrous fire, had led to a halving of its patient capacity between 1813 and 1815.[56] Most significantly, however, public efforts in the field of lunacy had been largely re-directed following Wynn's Act of 1808, with its provision for rate-supported county asylums. The Act's facilitation of joint action between counties and voluntary subscribers bore fruit in the asylums built in Nottinghamshire, Staffordshire, Cornwall, and Gloucestershire. By 1830, the voluntary elements of these asylums were providing between them for about seventy charitable patients and a similar number of private patients.[57] It can be argued, consequently, that there had continued to be a real overall growth in patient numbers in the voluntary sector.

ADMISSION — PROCEDURES AND CRITERIA

The legislative basis for committal in the eighteenth century was far from clear, even though addressed within various acts of parliament. The first specific provision appeared within the Vagrancy Act of 1714, which laid down that two or more justices of the peace could authorize the apprehension and confinement by parish officials of lunatics who were 'furiously mad and dangerous'. The Act was amended and amplified by that of 1744, which gave parishes the added responsibility of payment for the 'curing' of pauper lunatics, in addition to 'removing, keeping, and maintaining' them in a secure place.[58] There was no explicit provision for medical certification before the Act for Regulating Madhouses of 1774, which required the completion by a physician, surgeon, or apothecary of a certificate of insanity.[59] However, this related only to non-pauper patients committed to private madhouses; there was no legislation requiring medical certification for admission to a public lunatic hospital. It was left to the governors of the respective institutions to determine their own arrangements and processes for securing admission, as well as the criteria to be met. The County Asylums Act of 1808, as amended in 1811, 1815, and 1819, provided for medical certification of paupers admitted to county asylums. The law regarding committal to county asylums and to private madhouses was further clarified in 1828, though once again voluntary lunatic hospitals were not directly included.[60]

The governors of St Luke's were, from the outset, careful to ensure that proper admission procedures were in place. They took the precedents offered by practices at Bethlem Hospital and adapted them in order to demonstrate the probity and openness of the new hospital's approach.[61] The basic requirement for admission was for two certificates, one to be completed by the minister and churchwardens or the overseers of the poor of the person's place of residence, and the other by a physician, surgeon or apothecary who had visited the patient. The signed certificates had to be presented to a justice of the peace and an affidavit sworn. These certificates, accompanied by a petition, were then to be submitted to the hospital's secretary. The petitioner was required to attend at the hospital on the following Friday morning. If the application was approved by the house committee, arrangements would be made for the patient to come for examination, subject to there being a vacancy. Once he or she was accepted for admission, there was a further requirement that two 'substantial Housekeepers' who resided within the 'Bills of Mortality' (i.e. London) had to provide security in the form of a bond for £100, to ensure the patient's removal when discharged. The 'securities', who could not be governors, were expected to attend at eleven o'clock a.m. precisely on the day of admission.[62]

Procedures at the provincial lunatic hospitals were generally rather less demanding, especially for pauper lunatics. At the Newcastle Lunatic

Hospital there was no requirement for a medical certificate. The only certification was from the parish officers, attesting to the person's poverty, accompanied by a petition containing their personal circumstances and brief details regarding the nature and degree of their insanity. If deemed potentially suitable, when a vacancy occurred the patient would be brought by his 'friends' for examination by the committee. Some security would be required from the parish, to guarantee the payment of the weekly charges, and to provide for clothing and for burial, should it become necessary.[63]

Although the trustees of the Manchester Infirmary stated that they had modeled their rules for the admission of lunatic patients on those of the 'London Hospitals', the early arrangements bore more resemblance to those at Newcastle. A petition was required either from two relatives or from the parish officers, giving details of the person's mental disorder and the reasons why admission was needed. No medical recommendation was called for. Two 'substantial House-keepers' had to provide a bond to cover the weekly payments and any delays in removal of the patient after discharge. In addition, the overseers of the poor had to submit a certificate as to legal settlement. In the case of patients of 'superior condition', no certificate of any sort was required. The final decision regarding eligibility for admission of patients of all classes would be made following examination by one of the infirmary physicians.[64] Eventually, by about 1816, the rules were revised to provide for medical certification. This could come either from one of the infirmary physicians or, in the cases of patients referred from places outside Manchester, from a local practitioner.[65] Presumably the trustees were seeking to match the higher standards of scrutiny being implemented in the new county asylums. At the other two lunatic hospitals connected to infirmaries, at Leicester and Liverpool, there were requirements from the outset for a certificate of insanity completed by a medical practitioner, to accompany the petition for admission. As elsewhere, bonds of security were required from either the relatives or the overseers of the poor.[66]

The governors of the York Asylum chose initially to adopt the high standards inherent in the St Luke's model, by requiring a petition accompanied by two certificates — one from the minister and churchwardens, and the other from a physician, surgeon, or apothecary.[67] However, Dr Hunter's increasing preoccupation with attracting private patients to the asylum brought some dilution of the requirements, with the agreement that patients of the 'higher classes', or those paying more than eight shillings per week, were allowed the 'privilege' of admission without any certificates.[68] The reforms that were introduced in the asylum after 1815 brought a reversion to the general requirement for medical certification as a condition of admission.[69]

The decisions taken as to admission by the hospital's weekly board or house committee were usually on the basis of advice from the attending physician, informed by the background information that had been received from the petitioner, in answer to a number of questions regarding their circumstances and the nature of their condition. In the early days the expectations were fairly basic. At Newcastle, in the 1760s, there were only two questions regarding the person's mental health — 'How long distracted, and whether ever so before', and 'Whether melancholy, or raving, or had attempted to do any Mischief.'[70] The Manchester Infirmary governors, in 1766, advised relatives or overseers of the poor that the petition for admission should specify:

> the Age, Sex, and Condition of the Patient, how long ill, whether he or she has any, or what lucid Intervals, whether any means have been used for his or her Recovery, and with what Success, whether he or she has been afflicted with Fits, Epileptic orothers, or has any Venereal Taint.[71]

The information required at the York Asylum was much less prescriptive. The medical man providing the certificate was merely asked to describe the patient's 'present state of mind', with particular regard as to whether he or she was 'furious, flighty, or melancholy'.[72] At St Luke's also, despite the declared intent to promote good practices, there does not appear to have been a specific set of questions. By 1790, the certifying medical officer was being requested to send to Dr Simmons 'a State of such Patient's Case, and an Account of the Methods (if any) used to obtain a Cure'.[73]

The content of the information sought, and the questions asked, gradually became more sophisticated. At the post-reform York Asylum, some key questions were asked at the application stage, including how long the patient had been 'affected with derangement', whether there had been 'considerable violence' or the person was 'tractable', and what was the state of their bodily health? Once he or she had been accepted for admission, further particulars were sought from 'friends' and medical attendants. Nineteen questions were asked in all, covering all aspects of the history of the disorder — previous episodes; changes in symptomatology; attempts to injure self, clothing, or other people; 'impropriety' and 'false notion'; 'exciting' causes; family history of disorder; habits and interests; religious adherence; physical ailments. Those providing the information were assured that their answers would serve as an aid to successful treatment.[74]

Criteria for admission centred around the determination of whether the person was a 'proper object'. There were two main elements to achieving this status —mental disorder, and financial or social circumstances. The governors of St Luke's, borrowing from Bethlem, put it quite succinctly in declaring that to gain admission to the hospital the patient had to be 'Poor and Mad', requirements that were periodically reiterated.[75] There was generally little definition as to the nature or degree of insanity that would merit admission. At York it was resolved at the outset that the charity would receive 'all persons labouring under an unsound mind', without concern as to potential curability.[76] In regard to the pre-requisite of poverty, this was only adhered to consistently at St Luke's and, possibly, the Leicester Asylum. At all the other lunatic hospitals, arrangements were implemented to accept private fee-paying patients.[77]

There were much clearer definitions as to what factors would preclude admission. These were stated explicitly at St Luke's, where there were several exclusions — people who had been 'a Lunatick more than twelve Kalendar Months'; those who had been 'discharged uncured' from another lunatic hospital; anyone 'troubled with Epileptick or Convulsive Fits'; someone who was 'deemed an Ideot'; persons 'infected with the Venereal Disease'; and, any woman 'with Child'.[78] From the opening of the hospital, these exclusion criteria were adhered to strictly by the House Committee, which vetted admissions on the basis of Battie's guidance.[79] Within the first few years of operation several patients were refused admission as not being a 'proper object', usually because they had been ill for more than a year, though occasionally for other reasons, such as the predominance of physical illness or evidence that they were not really 'poor'.[80] In many other cases, people who had been admitted were subsequently discharged, frequently because they were found by Battie to be idiots rather than lunatics, and sometimes because he 'hath not discovered any symptoms of Lunacy'.[81] A similar pattern of exclusions continued under Battie's successors.[82]

Other lunatic hospitals adopted comparable exclusion criteria. At York, they were initially copied verbatim from those at St Luke's.[83] By 1787, however, the governors had made some important changes. They lifted the prohibitions on people who had previously been discharged from elsewhere as incurable, and on the admission of pregnant women, provided that security was given that the child would not become a burden on the parish in which the asylum was located.[84] The governors of the Hereford Infirmary, in its brief existence as a charitable institution, adopted a reverse position for their lunatic asylum. Its only specified exclusions were pregnant women, and patients who had been discharged as incurable from a public hospital.[85] At the Exeter Asylum, a similar position to that of York had been adopted by 1812, 'women with child' being allowed admission subject to security against their becoming a burden upon the parish.[86]

As the lunatic hospitals developed, admission arrangements had steadily become more sophisticated. Medical certification, though not a formal legal requirement in voluntary institutions, was increasingly accepted as a standard of good practice, providing both some protection for the patient and legitimization for the admitting hospital. The requirement to submit prescribed information regarding the person's history and onset of their disorder also reflected a more professional approach to diagnosis and treatment. However, although admission criteria were becoming less rigid, the charitable ideal that the patient should qualify as a 'proper object' remained a central principle in the lunatic hospitals' operation

CONSIDERATIONS OF CURABILITY

The concept of curability as an achievable goal was fundamental to the developing therapeutics of the management of insanity in the eighteenth-century.[87] It became increasingly central to the admissions policies adopted at Bethlem Hospital.[88] The pursuit of cure was at the heart of William Battie's approach to treatment, and was embraced by the governors of St Luke's. They intended that it would be a curative institution, and this premise under-pinned the clauses initially adopted whereby people were excluded from admission if their disorder had lasted for more than twelve months, or if they had previously been discharged uncured from another lunatic hospital. The initial plan adopted by the governors was that people deemed incurable would not be admitted. Furthermore, if a patient's stay in the hospital became protracted, due to a lack of response to treatment, he or she would be discharged at the end of a year.[89]

The house committee upheld these policies quite strictly. When someone remained uncured at the end of their designated twelve months, the opinion of Battie (or one of his successors) would be taken. If he reported no prospect of recovery, notice would be issued to the securities to have the patient removed. For example, in the case of Mary Magson in September 1752, Battie advised that she was 'still a Lunatick and not better than when first admitted'. In November of the same year he apprised the committee regarding Sarah Hicks that 'from the present Circumstances of her Case he hath not Sufficient reason to expect a Speedy Recovery'. Their discharges were consequently ordered.[90] However, there was some limited scope for flexibility. In cases where the person was showing evidence of improvement, indicating the likelihood of recovery, the physician would gain the agreement of the committee for an extension of their stay for a few weeks, with the situation being kept under close review. In the case of Thomas Chambers in June 1754, for example, he was still deemed by Battie to be a lunatic after a year in the hospital; however, 'he has greatly recovered his Senses and is at present very nearly in a State of Sanity'. He was therefore granted an additional month in the hospital, but Battie then reported him to be no better and he was discharged.[91]

The curability policy at St Luke's inevitably came under a degree of strain. Practical considerations were given extra impetus by a developing charitable perspective that incurable lunatics were a group of people for whom there ought to be some provision.[92] Bethlem had been accepting incurable patients for some time, and from 1734 was providing specific accommodation for them, as did Guy's Hospital.[93] In 1754 the St Luke's governors decided to follow suit. Initially, ten beds were allocated to patients who had been or would in future be discharged uncured, with payments to be levied at the rate of five shillings per week. The first six incurable patients were admitted at the end of June 1754.[94] This proved to be the beginning of a steadily increasing provision, which became a significant part of the hospital's operation. Admissions of incurable patients were recorded in separate books, and their annual statistics were calculated and published separately from the figures for curable patients.

Additional provision for ten more incurable patients was made in 1755, and again in 1765. When the new St Luke's opened in 1787, thirty incurable patients were transferred out of the total of 110.[95] In the new hospital the division between curable and incurable was strictly maintained. The proportion of incurables was allowed to rise steadily until 1800, when there were 120 incurables among the total of 305 patients (approximately forty per cent).[96] This presumably reflected the patterns of demand. By 1810, incurable numbers were being held at one hundred, to allow for more curable admissions. With the falling demand for places for curables in St Luke's later in the decade, and the drop in overall numbers to only 227 in 1820, the proportion of incurables had risen to forty-four per cent.[97] Had they so chosen, the governors could have more than filled the hospital with incurable patients, as the numbers on the waiting list for a place stood at 600 in 1810, and nearly 700 in 1815.[98]

It would appear that it was only at St Luke's that there was this sharp distinction between curable and incurable patients. Certainly, most lunatic hospitals' governors sought to present their curative credentials in annual reports highlighting the proportions of patients who were discharged recovered, or at least improved. However, admissions policies were fairly open, with both the potentially curable and those considered incurable being accepted. At Newcastle it was made explicit from the outset that the lunatic hospital was intended for 'incurables, as well as those whose Complaints may admit of Relief'.[99] The policy was evidently maintained, for more than fifty years later it was declared that it was not only 'an Hospital for the Cure of the Insane', but also 'an Asylum for the *Incurable*'.[100] As previously mentioned, at York a resolution was passed fairly early in its history that the charity would receive any insane patient 'whether curable or not'.[101] In July 1788, the York Asylum governors did place some restrictions, by reserving a third of the cells for incurables, and limiting their numbers accordingly. A few weeks later, they specified the number of rooms reserved for incurables as twenty-five.[102] At Exeter, it was agreed in 1804 and reinforced in 1812 that incurables could be admitted.[103] Elsewhere, the lack of mention of preferential status for curable patients or of exclusion of the incurable, tends to suggest that curability was not a primary consideration.

CONSIDERATIONS OF GEOGRAPHY

The location of the lunatic hospitals in London or regional provincial centres reflected the anticipated demand for their services. Whilst St Luke's was established with a view to accepting patients from throughout the country, the provincial lunatic hospitals were intended to cater primarily for people living within their city and its hinterland. Where data is available, it largely confirms a strong regional emphasis in admission patterns. Studies undertaken of admissions to county asylums in the nineteenth century have highlighted a similar tendency. The most recent, completed by Melling and Forsythe in relation to the Devon County Asylum (opened in 1845), stresses the importance of distance as an influence on the incidence of admissions to the asylum. Although patients were admitted from across the county, there was a markedly greater concentration of people from parishes nearer the asylum.[104] An earlier study by Philo, citing the example of the Bedfordshire Asylum, drew similar conclusions about the significance of distance.[105] Interestingly, he pointed out that a comparable phenomenon had been apparent in the earlier subscription lunatic hospitals. He argued that it was not only a matter of convenience, but was considered to be in the patient's best interests to be placed in an institution in proximity to his home area. The significant exception that Philo noted, however, was in relation to people of the higher social classes, where the motivations might be more toward being placed at a greater distance from their families.[106]

Bethlem Hospital had never functioned solely as a resource for London and its surrounds, but drew from a national catchment.[107] St Luke's was to follow suit, with referrals accepted from all over England, though subject to the important constraint (similar to Bethlem) that the securities for the patients had to come from within the London area.[108] Consequently, the majority of people admitted tended to be from London and the adjoining counties. Nevertheless, admissions from more distant places continued. Despite this, however, the perception in the northern cities, as expressed in the proposals and appeals for the building of their lunatic hospitals, was that it was extremely difficult for insane patients inhabiting places distant from London to gain admission to St Luke's or Bethlem, quite apart from any questions of distance or accessibility.[109] This provided one of the key motivations for establishing local facilities.

It is possible to analyze the places of origin of patients admitted to St Luke's on the basis of the very comprehensive admission books that have survived, both for curable patients and for those admitted or re-admitted as incurables. The information regarding curable patients is summarized in Table 5.5.[110] The figures show that, for the first sixty years of the hospital's operation, a majority of patients came from parishes in London and from the adjoining metropolitan parts of Middlesex, Surrey and Kent. Until 1800 the conurbation provided a remarkably consistent proportion of admissions, at around fifty-seven per cent. However, there was a perceptible shift over the next twenty years, the proportion falling to fifty per cent in the decade 1801–10, and then down to an average of forty-seven per cent in the following decade. Indeed, the figures for individual years reveal an even more marked decline, for in 1820 itself admissions from metropolitan London, at ninety-seven, amounted to only forty per cent.[111]

Table 5.5 St Luke's Hospital — curable admissions by placy of origin, 1751–1820

Years	London area %		Home counties %		Out counties %	
1751–60	429	58.6	198	27	105	14.3
1761–70	553	57	258	26.7	158	16.3
1771–70	653	57.2	294	25.7	195	17.1
1781--90	786	56.9	390	28.3	204	14.8
1791–1800	1332	57.6	620	26.8	361	15.6
1801–10	1406	50.3	852	30.5	537	19.2
1811–20	1242	47.6	865	33.2	501	19.2
Total	6401	53.6	3477	29.1	2061	17.3

Source: St Luke's Hospital, Curable Patients Books.
Note: 'London Area' includes the City, Westminster, and metropolitan parts of Middlesex, Surrey, and Kent; 'Home Counties' comprise other parts of Middlesex, Surrey, and Kent, in addition to Essex, Hertfordshire, Berkshire, Buckinghamshire, and Sussex; 'Out Counties' comprise all other areas.

The numbers of patients originating from outside London were consistently significant. These have been separated into those emanating from the 'home counties' and those from further afield.[112] Admissions from the home counties remained fairly constant until 1800, at around twenty-seven per cent, thereafter increasing to thirty-three per cent in the years 1811–1820 as those from London itself decreased in proportion.[113] Taken together, admissions from London and the home counties were consistently in excess of eighty per cent, confirming that St Luke's primarily served the south-east of England. Similar general patterns were apparent in the admissions of incurable patients, as evidenced in Table 5.6, although the smaller numbers involved could produce occasional anomalies.[114]

The regional concentration notwithstanding, there was a constant stream of admissions to St Luke's from other parts of England, and occasionally from Wales, with certain counties being particularly prominent. An analysis of curable admissions between 1751 and 1820 shows Hampshire to be the most significant external county of origin, accounting for 355 patients (approximately three per cent of the overall total), followed by Oxfordshire (214), Northamptonshire (187), Wiltshire (141), Gloucestershire (134), Warwickshire (130), Suffolk (122), and Cambridgeshire (100). Other regular sources of referrals included Somerset, Bedfordshire, Huntingdonshire, and Lincolnshire. These were all counties in which no lunatic hospital had been established.[115] Clearly this was a significant determinant, because counties like Lancashire, Yorkshire, Norfolk, Northumberland and Durham, and Devon (after 1800), where charitable institutions had been opened, were responsible for comparatively few admissions to St Luke's. Nevertheless, the considerable geographical spread of people admitted demonstrates conclusively that St Luke's did still continue to function as a

Table 5.6 St Luke's Hospital — incurable admissions by place of origin, 1754–1820

Years	London area %		Home counties %		Out counties %	
1754–60	32	59.2	12	22.2	10	18.6
1761–70	17	56.7	9	30	4	13.3
1771–80	9	60	2	13.3	4	26.6
1781–90	36	56.2	19	29.7	9	14
1791–1800	72	59	27	22.1	23	18.8
1801–10	24	51.1	16	34	7	14.9
1811–20	46	47.9	29	30.2	21	21.9
Total	236	55.1	114	26.6	78	18.2

Source: St Luke's Hospital, Incurable Patients Book.

national hospital, despite its particular focus on London and the south-east of England.[116]

The provincial lunatic hospitals, as their projectors intended, provided for a more localized constituency. The Newcastle Lunatic Hospital was established specifically to cater for people from the counties of Northumberland, Durham, and of Newcastle-upon-Tyne itself.[117] No records are available to show conclusively whether this policy was adhered to. There is, however, valuable surviving evidence for the Manchester Lunatic Hospital, the York Lunatic Asylum and the Exeter Lunatic Asylum. The admission records for these institutions show that, although they upheld a local focus, they were catering for an area considerably wider than the towns in which they were situated.

The only admissions book that has survived for the Manchester Lunatic Hospital covers the period from February 1773 to July 1777.[118] As is shown in Table 5.7, 151 patients were admitted during that time. Of those, 23 (fifteen per cent) came from Manchester itself. A substantial majority, though, came from the surrounding area, particularly from various parts of Lancashire. Of the other towns or parishes of the county, Wigan accounted for the most admissions, with seven, followed by Bolton and Prestwich, each with five, then Liverpool with four, and Blackburn, Burnley, and Leyland with three apiece. Much of Cheshire could also be considered to fall inside the Manchester hinterland. Within the county, the parish of Budworth accounted for four admissions, with Stockport, Mottram, Macclesfield, and Sandbach each responsible for two. The number of admissions from Yorkshire is particularly significant, as it could not be considered to lie as directly within Manchester's orbit. Most of the Yorkshire patients emanated from the western side of the county, within reasonable reach of Manchester, with seven from Sheffield, four from Halifax, three from Elland, and two from Leeds. The opening of the York Asylum in 1777 would

Table 5.7 *Manchester Lunatic Hospital — Admissions by place of origin, 1773–77*

Place	Numbers	%
Manchester	23	15.2
Other Lancashire	57	37.7
Cheshire	25	16.6
Yorkshire	21	13.9
Other:	(25)	16.6
North Staffordshire	5	
Derbyshire	5	
Nottinghamshire	4	
North Wales	4	
Westmoreland	3	
Miscellaneous	3	
Unspecified	1	
Total	151	

Source: Manchester Royal Infirmary Archives, Lunatic Hospital Admissions Register,1 773–77.

doubtless have diverted most subsequent Yorkshire referrals. Amongst the 'other' category, most noteworthy were three admissions from Mansfield in Nottinghamshire, two from Kendal in Westmoreland, and single admissions from Bath and from Boston in Lincolnshire. Notwithstanding these individual exceptions, it is clear that the Manchester Lunatic Hospital, like its parent infirmary, was functioning as a regional facility, reflecting the domiciles of its subscribers.[119]

A similar pattern of admissions is evident for the York Lunatic Asylum, for which much fuller admissions records are available, summarized in Table 5.8.[120] The asylum began with a policy of providing primarily for insane patients from York itself and the wider county. However, in an appeal of 1777 it was stated that 'this Asylum is confined to no district, but extends its arms to receive poor and afflicted lunatics from every part of his majesty's dominions'.[121] It seems likely that Dr Hunter had been responsible for the insertion of the phrase, for he ensured that it was repeated and amplified in several subsequent publications.[122] This was related to his single-minded policy of seeking to deter the admission of paupers, whilst encouraging charitable patients and private patients whose payments could subsidize their care. Nevertheless, the figures show that people from the city of York and the rest of Yorkshire accounted consistently for around ninety per cent of admissions. The main urban centres like Leeds, Sheffield and Hull provided the largest numbers, but patients were admitted from

Table 5.8 York Lunatic Asylum — admissions by place of origin, 1777–1824

Years	York %		Other Yorks %		Lincs %		Notts %		Other %	
1777–80	24	23.8	69	68.3	4	4.0	3	3.0	1	0.9
1781–90	124	25.3	322	65.7	23	4.7	11	2.2	10	2.0
1791–1800	79	12.9	477	77.8	31	5.0	9	1.5	17	2.8
1801–10	69	7.8	729	82.0	57	6.4	17	1.9	17	1.9
1811–20	44	7.6	498	83.7	32	5.4	4	0.7	16	2.6
1821–24	11	5.7	158	81.9	0		5	2.6	19	9.8

Source: University of York, Borthwick Institute, BOO 6/2/1/1-3, York Lunatic Asylum, Admissions Books.

towns and villages all over Yorkshire. Of those coming from elsewhere, the most significant numbers were from the adjoining counties of Lincolnshire and, to a lesser extent, Nottinghamshire.[123] The remainder of the external patients came mainly from Derbyshire, Cumberland, Westmoreland and Durham, with only a few emanating from southern areas. It is clear that the York Asylum was essentially operating as a county and regional facility.

The Exeter Lunatic Asylum also catered for the city, the county of Devon, and a wider hinterland. An early report had suggested that people could be admitted from 'any part of the kingdom', but it acknowledged that its 'local situation' meant that 'this Asylum is particularly calculated for the four Western Counties'.[124] The surviving admissions register for 1801–05 confirms a clear county and regional emphasis. (See Table 5.9). The pattern was remarkably similar to that at York and Manchester, with over eighty-five per cent of patients coming from Exeter and the rest of Devon. The remainder were from Somerset, Cornwall and Dorset.[125]

Although comparable evidence is not available for the origins of patients admitted to the other lunatic hospitals, it is likely that they also provided for regional catchments. The Liverpool Lunatic Asylum appears to have covered west Lancashire, Cheshire, and parts of North Wales, as well as

Table 5.9 Exeter Lunatic Asylum — admissions by place of origin, July 1801–July 1805

Place	Numbers	%
Exeter	14	15.2
Other Devon	66	71.7
Somerset	8	8.7
Cornwall	3	3.1
Dorset	1	1.0

Source: Devon CRO, 3992 / F / H21, Exeter Lunatic Asylum, Register of Admissions, 1801-5.

the city itself. Agreements were made to receive pauper lunatics from out-side Liverpool, at charges higher than those for the city's paupers.[126] The model of a lunatic hospital that provided for a regional clientele was evidently one that had impressed Sir George Onisephorus Paul, to judge from evidence given to the 1807 select committee. It was at the heart of his plans for a network of rate-assisted public asylums, to be based partly around the further development of the existing voluntary institutions. Each would be situated within a designated catchment region, with York, Exeter, Hereford, Leicester, and Liverpool among the proposed locations.[127] As Philo has demonstrated, through the mediation of the select committee the model established in the eighteenth century of regional catchments proved highly influential in the subsequent development of the county asylum system.[128]

CONSIDERATIONS OF RANK

Perceptions regarding rank were at the very heart of the functioning of English society in the eighteenth century. A finely graded social hierarchy had yet to give way to the more monolithic and all-embracing concepts of 'class'. The ongoing transformation of society, whereby commercial and industrial interests were making steady inroads into territory that had been within the sphere of control of landed and agricultural interests, may have begun to alter some of the established boundaries within the hierarchy. It had, however, certainly not eliminated them. The 'urban renaissance' that accompanied the dramatic expansion and growing sophistication of commercial activity was accompanied by a multiplication of the numbers, and a growing diversification of the nature and occupations, of people comprised within the middle orders of society. With their increasing economic power, these middling groups were becoming intent on securing their social position, especially within the towns and localities where they could wield some influence. In these conditions, conceptions of rank could even become more solidified. Whilst people within the range of middling ranks might seek to permeate the boundaries above them, or at least to imitate the customs and mores of their perceived social betters, there was a marked tendency to try to protect the integrity of the boundaries that still lay below them.[129]

Issues of social rank became increasingly significant in the development of the lunatic hospitals. Like the voluntary general hospitals, their subscribers and governors were drawn not only from the aristocracy, gentry, and clergy of the region but also from the commercial, manufacturing, and professional classes.[130] The question of for whom the lunatic hospital should be providing, or who was a 'proper object', became potentially a matter of controversy between the different interests. There was little disagreement that it should cater for 'the poor', but at York at least there were great difficulties in agreeing as to who rightfully deserved to be included under that heading. Within most of the lunatic hospitals the poor became divided into paupers and those who were above the rank of pauper, but dependent on charitable support.

Once the view was taken at Manchester, and accepted elsewhere, that one of the lunatic hospital's functions was to offer patients and their families an alternative to exploitation or abuse by private madhouse proprietors, the admission of patients from across the middling ranks became an accepted part of their charitable function. It was then a relatively short step to bring in a commercial element by admitting people who were more affluent, based on the rationale that their payments would bring additional income to the charity, so enabling it to support more of the 'proper objects'. Having taken this step, the governors then had to ensure that the facilities and accommodation of the hospital were suitably adapted to meet the needs and expectations of the different ranks of people for whom they were now providing.[131]

With its secure funding base, questions of whether to admit people who had some financial means never became a serious issue at St Luke's Hospital. However, there was a degree of discernment in its admissions policies for, although it catered exclusively for the 'poor and mad', preference was clearly given to non-paupers. From the hospital's inception, a charge of £1.12s for bedding was made to the parish of any pauper admitted. This was strictly enforced, and a failure of the parish to pay would result in a refusal of admission.[132] The charges were periodically raised, and in early 1809 they stood at £6.[133] In the first twenty-five years of the hospital's operation, pauper admissions accounted for only 280 out of 2280, or slightly over twelve per cent. (See Table 5.10). The opening of the new hospital, with its greater capacity, facilitated an increase in both the number and the proportion of pauper admissions. By 1807, according to Thomas Dunston, sixty paupers were being admitted annually out of an average of 263 people.[134] The figures from the admission books confirm this upward trend, with paupers constituting over twenty per cent of admissions between 1810 and 1820.[135] These were all people deemed 'curable', for paupers were actu-

Table 5.10 Pauper admissions to St Luke's Hospital, 1751–1820

Period	Admissions	Paupers	%
1751–60	732	97	13.2
1761–70	969	113	11.7
1771–80	1142	145	12.7
1781–90	1380	207	15.0
1791–1800	2313	424	15.5
1801–10	2795	544	19.5
1811–20	2608	558	21.4
TOTAL	11939	2088	17.5

Source: St Luke's Hospital, Curable Patients Books

ally excluded from admission on to the incurable list. Consideration had been given in 1814 to allowing pauper incurables to be admitted, but the idea was rejected.[136]

The Newcastle Lunatic Hospital appears initially to have provided exclusively for paupers, with certificates of poverty required from the parish officers prior to admission. Although some private patients were later being admitted, a published report of 1817 referred to the relief provided by the hospital 'to all the Poor-Houses around'.[137] At Liverpool the acceptance of people from the city's poor house was set forward by James Currie as one of the main reasons for establishing the asylum. Following its opening, agreement was made with the parish officers for the removal there of the lunatics, and favourable rates of five shillings per week were negotiated to pay for their board.[138] The Manchester Infirmary governors had in 1775 offered rates of five shillings for paupers from all the parishes and townships in the area.[139] In both cities there was a clear acceptance of responsibility for pauper lunatics.

There had, however, to be some limits to pauper admissions, especially if adequate provision was to be made for charitable and private patients. At Liverpool, in 1812, it was agreed to restrict the number of pauper patients to thirty-two, or half the asylum's capacity, at the same time as charges for paupers from outside the city were raised as high as 15s per week.[140] Similar considerations appear to have prevailed at Exeter, where the asylum's main protagonist and projector Rev. James Manning advised the secretary of Stafford Infirmary, whose governors were contemplating the establishment of an asylum, that the presence of too many paupers had acted as a deterrent to the referral of other patients. Charges for them were now set at the high rate of 15s per week, which Manning, in an argument reminiscent of Alexander Hunter twenty years earlier, rationalized by suggesting that parishes composed of 'opulent farmers' could afford to pay.[141] In 1820, Manning expressed the view that those members of the poorer classes above the rank of pauper were the 'greatest objects of charity'.[142] This was an idea that became increasingly prevalent as the nineteenth century progressed, and which provided the rationale for the Oxford Lunatic Asylum not accepting paupers at all.[143]

The attitude toward pauper lunatics inherent in the position taken at Exeter reflected a perception of their position as being at the very bottom of the status hierarchy. An evident contempt lay behind the disparaging views articulated by Hunter regarding 'incurable mad paupers', who constituted the 'lowest and meanest of the poor'.[144] His perceptions were evidently supported by the majority of the York Asylum governors, even though an influential minority were outraged. The protagonists at York appeared almost to be contending for the very soul of the institution, although the ostensible argument was about which sections of the poor were entitled to the relief afforded by the charity. Reverends William Mason and William Burgh and their supporters asserted that the asylum had been intended for the poor, and among those paupers were as needy as any. Hunter, however, was in no doubt that it was those 'in low Circumstances, or of a middling Rank in Life' who ought to obtain the most benefit, and his views carried the day. Later commentators considered that his arguments, and the position adopted by the governors, betrayed nothing other than a deep prejudice against paupers.[145] Nevertheless, despite all the heat that had been generated, the numbers of paupers in the York Asylum did continue to rise steadily, standing at eighty (or forty per cent of the total numbers) in 1814.[146]

Although York was the focus of controversy surrounding the acceptance of private patients, the practice had been initiated at the Manchester Lunatic Hospital. Its infirmary trustees proceeded with their intent to protect 'Persons of middling Fortunes' from the 'Impositions' of madhouse keepers, and the argument was subsequently adopted and acted upon at York.[147] The policy was translated into practicalities by establishing scales of payment rates. At Manchester, these ranged initially from five shillings for 'poor Lunaticks' to a maximum of one guinea for those in 'affluent Circumstances', the actual amount determined by 'what is judged to be the Ability of the Patients'.[148] A more sophisticated scale was established at York, determined according to 'class'. In 1785, seven classes were delineated, extended to eight by 1788. Class one, the poorest charity patients, paid a maximum of six shillings per week. The charges then ascended by two shillings for each class, with people in class eight paying 20s and upwards.[149] When Sir George Paul visited in 1810, a few months after Hunter's death, he found a slightly modified arrangement of charges, but the principles similar.[150]

These elaborate payment scales at York, however, did not represent the actual classification of the patients. According to Hunter in 1788, the sixty-six patients were arranged into only three divisions. The 'first division' consisted of twenty patients of 'better condition', whose payments provided a profit that could be used to subsidize the payments of others. The 'second division' of twenty-six people, which included the paupers, were all being charged eight shillings per week. The twenty charitable patients, whose charges might be as low as four shillings per week, comprised the 'third division'. These arrangements were to continue for several years.[151] By 1810, the three divisions had been re-constituted as classes, with the first class now the charity patients, and the third class the private patients.[152] Within four years, however, the arrangements had become more complex, reflecting the creeping privatization that was taking place. There were officially five classes. The first class, containing 107 people, now included the paupers. The second, third, and fourth classes, totaling forty-five people, were entirely made up of private patients, paying upwards of 9s. The fifth class was the most exclusive group, the sixteen 'Physician's private Patients', for whom Dr Best paid 14s per week to the asylum and received unspecified fees from the patients or their families. The twenty-eight charitable patients were not formally included within any of the classes.[153] By this time, however, the whole system at York had been exposed as deeply flawed and corrupt.

The differentiation of patients by rank at Newcastle remained relatively crude in comparison. According to Paul in 1810, there were three classes. The great majority, fifty people, were the paupers who constituted the first class, paying between 6s and 8s shillings per week. There were eight in the second class paying 10s or 12s, whom he described as 'not paupers: these live something better than paupers', and only three people in 'superior circumstances' in the third class, who each paid £40 per annum.[154] Elsewhere, gradations of payment were established which corresponded more to the York model. At Liverpool in 1812, payments were on five points of a sliding scale, from 8s–31s and upwards.[155] At the Exeter Asylum, the early plan had been for three classes, although there were four when it opened. Subsequently the system was developed to comprise first six and then seven classes. The charges ranged from 5s per week for the first class, or charitable patients, to three guineas for the seventh class, the wealthiest private patients. Paupers, for whom their parishes paid 15s, were included within the third class.[156]

Alexander Hunter had developed the case for 'the indigent' to be 'relieved at the expense of the affluent' to a point where it was, in effect, an expression of charitable virtue for the admission of wealthy patients to be actively encouraged.[157] James Currie at Liverpool was convinced by Hunter's argument, and employed it in his proposals for the city's asylum.[158] Sir George Paul was equally persuaded of the merits of such an arrangement and incorporated it into his local schemes in Gloucester and, more significantly, in his proposals for a national asylum system.[159] Once the principle had been accepted that people from across the social scale could be admitted to a lunatic hospital, adaptations had to be made to the buildings to make suitable provision for the different ranks of patients. At Manchester, when new accommodation was opened in 1783, separate 'apartments' were provided for 'poor Persons' and for those of 'superior Fortunes'. In language redolent of a prospectus for an exclusive private madhouse, the latter were offered accommodation suitable to 'their Condition in Life', where they were to receive 'the greatest Privacy, the best Advice, the most tender Treatment, and every Comfort and Assistance that can be afforded to them in their unhappy Situation.'[160] The York Asylum also began to provide separate and more luxurious accommodation for the patients in 'affluent circumstances'. They could be offered a second room, so as to accommodate a personal servant, for whom an additional charge of six shillings per week was payable. They were also provided with separate dining areas and better food.[161]

At the Exeter Asylum, where the governors could use the experience gained elsewhere, the matter was taken into account in their original plans. The projectors in 1795 sought to provide 'larger and more convenient Apartments' for the 'more opulent' patients, and to ensure 'every Attention given them in the Articles of Conveniency, Comfort and Secrecy'. Private patients were to be allowed the luxury of their own 'confidential Servant'. It became possible to put these aspirations into practice with the opening of the new building in 1804, in which the rooms were 'neatly fitted up in a manner suited to their Ranks in Life.'[162] Similar considerations were applied to the next new building opened in 1824.[163]

The classification of patients by rank became formalized at the two main lunatic hospitals with infirmary connections, by dividing them into two separate entities. This occurred first at Manchester by 1791, where it was re-named the Manchester Lunatic Hospital and Asylum. The 'asylum', comprising the better accommodation, provided for the private patients, while the 'lunatic hospital' continued to house the poorer patients.[164] The Liverpool Infirmary governors eventually followed suit, and had made a similar distinction by 1810; it was contained in the new infirmary rules of 1813. The building was re-named, and again there was an internal division of the 'different Classes' of patients, with the 'better Apartments' making up the 'Asylum'. The section of the building housing the poor was re-designated as the 'Lunatic Hospital'.[165]

The social composition of the provincial lunatic hospitals' patient population had become varied and complex. It was also clearly unusual for public charitable organizations, and has to be accounted for by the particular problems associated with the perception and management of insanity. The measures taken to allow for the nuances of rank, and to respond to the associated expectations, did materially affect the nature and character of the institutions. The social experiment, if such it was, had evidently been considered a success. The arrangements were to be perpetuated, and even developed further, in several of the new lunatic asylums that followed the legislation of 1808.[166]

'UNHAPPY SUFFERERS'

The people who entered the lunatic hospitals were a diverse and disparate group. Their previous circumstances, and place in the social structure of family and community, were important influences on their presentation inside the institution and on how officers and staff responded to them. The most significant determinant, however, was the nature and manifestation of the condition from which the person was suffering. The hospital's population ranged from those with acute and florid disorders, which might abate after a few days, to those whom Hunter dismissed as 'idiots, bedridden, diseased and incurable mad paupers'.[167] Inmates exhibited all manner of behaviours, which might not be significantly checked by the treatments or methods of control available in the late eighteenth century. The techniques of 'classification' that were to become refined in the nineteenth century were still in their infancy, and any given group of patients was likely to provide a representation of the various typologies of madness that made up what Dr Thomas Arnold characterized as 'these most pitiable and degraded of mankind'.[168]

It was the 'great terror and concern' aroused by the violent lunatic that was most likely to propel him or her toward confinement.[169] Within the institution, violence and dangerousness were seen to represent the worst features of the madman. A minister at York, James Scott, graphically characterized 'the wild ravings of outrageous frenzy, gnashing his teeth, tearing his hair, threatening destruction to those who approach him'.[170] Dr Thomas Arnold considered that some patients were 'incapable of refraining from outrage and mischief', and he compared many to 'violent and dangerous wild beasts'.[171] Thomas Dunston told Samuel Tuke, visiting St Luke's in 1812, that 'we have many patients who come to us in a very violent state'. Dunston prevented Tuke from seeing some of the worst cases, claiming that 'I have men in this place who would tear to pieces every means of precaution or safety'.[172] In published case histories John Ferriar and James Currie described patients in their lunatic hospitals who were raving and 'furious' for days and even weeks on end, and who required drastic treatment interventions.[173] People like these posed considerable management problems both for the medical officers and for the more junior staff.

Much of the violent behaviour was directed toward fellow inmates. The York Asylum investigations revealed numerous cases, including particularly severe incidents in 1813–14 when two men were killed by other patients, one having been attacked by the three with whom he shared a sleeping room.[174] Whilst these were the most serious instances lower level violence was apparently endemic, with fighting being frequent among both male and female patients.[175] The problems were clearly exacerbated by the conditions in which people were being held. S.W. Nicoll, one of the York reform campaigners, described a small room that had contained thirteen people for some months, and was 'filled with clamorous maniacs, who were reciprocally stimulating each others fury'.[176] These events occurred in a context both of very poor supervision and regular physical abuse by staff toward patients. However, even a well managed regime could not prevent violent excesses, for a male patient was killed by another in the privy at the end of 1817, well after major reforms had been imposed on the York Asylum.[177]

Staff were also exposed to risk of serious injury from attacks by violent inmates. Thomas Dunston reported in 1815 that there had been 'a great many' patients in St Luke's who were 'outrageous' and presented considerable danger to the keepers.[178] In 1808, Jane Hughes, who had worked in the hospital for fifteen years, was badly injured by a blow from a patient and was unable to continue in post.[179] In another incident in 1814, a male keeper named William Ayres received 'a very dangerous hurt from one of the male Patients'.[180] The keeper of the Manchester Lunatic Hospital was actually stabbed to death in early 1774, a widely reported incident that was used to support the argument for proposed legislation on the regulation of madhouses.[181] Visitors to lunatic hospitals noted the air of menace and threat, even when there was not actual violence. Based on his visits to the York Asylum, Samuel Tuke suggested that the attendants in large public institutions had to use repressive measures to control 'such a formidable body of malcontents'. The stronger patients would intimidate others and steal their food.[182] John Thomas, the St Luke's apothecary, commented in 1827 that when he and the physician went round the hospital, they were 'obliged to get from some of the patients as quickly as possible' due to the 'excitement' produced by their visit.[183] Thomas Dunston had previously commented on the disturbances that followed governors' visits.[184]

Arrangements had to be made to contain people prone to violence. Separate cells would be provided for the most serious cases, usually away from the other patients, as Paul discovered when visiting the Newcastle Lunatic Hospital in 1810.[185] At the Lincoln Asylum, where governors had the benefit of others' experience, the cells for violent patients were initially sited at the ends of each gallery, but were re-located in 1822 to 'the bottom of the garden'.[186] There as elsewhere mechanical restraint was widely employed as a method of containment. The lunacy reformer Edward Wakefield found several violent patients in chains at St Luke's in 1815. He commented particularly on a sailor, whom he considered 'one of the most dangerous animals I have ever seen'. The man had to be both leg-locked and hand-cuffed, for otherwise 'he flies at you, and would seize anybody within his reach with his teeth'.[187]

Restraint implements were also often required for another significant group of dangerous patients — those with suicidal intent. Despite precautions some did succeed in their efforts, like a man at the Manchester Lunatic Hospital in early 1774, who 'found the means to destroy himself' within a few hours of being admitted.[188] In July 1797, Elizabeth Shelton hung herself using a handkerchief tied to the top of a fire grate in the dining room. It occurred without warning for, according to the matron Mrs Bagshaw, three hours earlier she had appeared 'considerably better and more composed in appearance'.[189] In 1815, a St Luke's patient set her clothes on fire by laying in the burning cinders. A passer-by in Old Street raised the alarm, having seen her walk past a window in flames. Although a 'maid' extinguished the flames, the patient later died.[190] People with this level of determination could find ways to evade close supervision. In 1817, in the reformed York Asylum, a male patient used a sharpened metal button to cut into his body causing his intestines to protrude. The inquest concluded that no blame attached to the keepers.[191] Occasionally serious attempts were foiled. At Manchester in 1801, a private patient named Hugh Williams heroically saved the life of Matthew Jepson, 'a respectable tradesman from Sheffield', after he and another patient deliberately went and sat down in the fireplace. Williams described how Jepson had 'smiled at me, tho' his coat was in flames'.[192] A St Luke's patient, Catherine Rivers, set herself on fire in a gallery in February 1804; her life was only saved by a 'Gallery Maid' who 'at the hazard of her life' extinguished the flames, severely burning herself in the process.[193]

Based on his familiarity with the York Asylum, Rev. James Scott graphically described to his congregation in 1780 the type of patient 'ready, through excess of anguish, to lay violent hands on himself'. They were among 'some wretched souls' who were 'in that deep black melancholy', and who appeared as 'a group of miserable objects, silent and sullen, wrapt up in a profound trance, in a lethargic stupor, with their eyes open, and their senses shut.'[194] Profound depression characterized a significant proportion of lunatic hospital patients. John Ferriar detailed several in his Manchester case histories. A female of sixty, A.W., admitted on 30 August 1791, 'laboured under a total alienation of mind'. Her 'aspect' was 'extremely dejected', she constantly muttered to herself and 'often groaned and wept'.[195] Another female, L.H., aged forty-eight, had been admitted a few weeks earlier, 'in a very low desponding state, and fancied she had destroyed part of her family.'[196] Mrs T., a middle-aged married woman, who had attempted suicide, 'became melancholy without any sensible cause. She talked incoherently, was fretful, and frequently wept.'[197] Ferriar's melancholic patients were of both sexes and from right across the age range,[198] a picture likely to have been replicated elsewhere.

Although diagnoses like melancholia or mania appeared quite frequently in contemporary writings and reports, patients were more often described in terms of behavioural presentations. This was particularly so where undesirable traits like 'noisy' or 'dirty' required intervention. Dunston in 1816 spoke of some St Luke's patients who 'will bawl from Monday morning to Saturday night'.[199] According to a Manchester Infirmary report in 1818, ten of the ninety patients in the lunatic hospital were 'noisy and troublesome'.[200] The response to these behaviours tended to involve separation and restraint, as at St Luke's where some of the 'very noisy' patients were 'confined to a cell'.[201] These methods, though, could sometimes actually exacerbate the problems.

Dirty, or incontinent, patients were also liable to be placed in the refractory cells, normally on beds of straw. They were even referred to as 'Straw Patients' at the Manchester Lunatic Hospital, where they were 'kept out of view from the others on account of being unclean'.[202] Edward Wakefield observed people 'not aware of the necessities of nature', chained naked in their beds at St Luke's.[203] The exposures at the York Asylum produced much evidence regarding the presence of this type of patient. According to one of the prominent reformers, at any one time there were ten or twelve of each sex whose 'foul and offensive habits' required 'extraordinary attendance'.[204] Several rather graphic individual cases were described during the investigations.[205] These paled into insignificance, though, next to the descriptions of the women 'discovered' by Godfrey Higgins secreted in cells 'in a state of filth horrible beyond description'.[206] The York revelations showed, however, that when incontinent patients were placed in distinct and not very salubrious accommodation it could become difficult to determine cause and effect of their uncleanliness.

Incontinence might be consequent on various conditions, including the disinhibition associated with mania, the absence of awareness characteristic of some delusional disorders, or the lack of volition and the self-neglect that accompanied melancholia. It could also be part of the spectrum of deficiencies presented by the chronic, 'incurable' patients. These were the people described at Newcastle in 1817 as suffering 'unmanageable mental Derangement' arising from 'Fatuity, Palsy, or Epileptic Fits', Hunter's 'idiotic, bed-ridden, diseased' incurable mad paupers at York, or those described as 'in a state of idiotism' and in need of feeding at the Manchester Lunatic Hospital in 1818.[207] These least promising of patients, from a therapeutic perspective, formed a not insignificant minority of the lunatic hospital population, as also did those who appeared to be in a 'poor lost state', characterized in 1816 by Thomas Dunston of St Luke's.[208] Apathetic, isolated and preoccupied individuals were vividly portrayed by Samuel Tuke in a typical scene in the York Asylum:

> I could perceive no attachments, and very little observation of one another. In the midst of society, every one seemed in solitude; conversation or amusement was rarely to be observed — employment never. Each individual appeared to be pursuing his own busy cogitations; pacing with restless step from one end of the enclosure to the other, or lolling in slothful apathy upon the benches.[209]

These passive and introspective people were particularly vulnerable to exploitation and bullying. A lack of supervision at meal times might result in 'the strong often devouring the portion intended for the weaker patients'.[210] Those under restraint could be at a particular disadvantage. It was reported at St Luke's in 1827 that convalescent patients detailed to take food to those in chains ate it themselves, leaving 'the man who is confined' to 'go for two or three days without anything to eat.'[211]

Vulnerability to sexual abuse was also an occasional hazard. A married female at York Asylum, Dorothy Exilby admitted in July 1801, became pregnant by a male patient named Parkin from Hull, though she was nevertheless subsequently discharged as cured in February 1802.[212] Five years earlier Elizabeth West from Louth in Lincolnshire, a patient of 'exceedingly good character', became pregnant by one of the asylum's keepers, James Backhouse. He managed to retain his post and retired as head keeper after twenty-six years' service in 1810.[213] A St Luke's patient, described later by Dunston as 'a vicious kind of young woman', became pregnant by the keeper Edward Dowding, around 1810. The act evidently took place 'in the dusk of the evening, when he went up with the beer, behind the door', despite the presence in the room of two other patients who remained oblivious. Dowding was dismissed, whilst the patient went on to have subsequent admissions to Warburton's madhouse at Bethnal Green.[214]

There was, of course, a substantial body of patients who presented as perfectly quiet and settled most of the time. John Howard, visiting St Luke's in 1789, saw women who were 'calm and quiet, and at needle-work with the matron'.[215] Sir George Paul, in 1810, noted that most York Asylum patients were in a 'state of association' with one another. He was particularly impressed with a dinner scene of thirty private patients 'seated in perfect order', whilst the matron at the head of the table 'carved for, and served her company'. He was surprised to witness a 'more numerous class of paupers' dining together with 'a decorum nearly equal to that of a rational family'.[216] A German visitor to Manchester Lunatic Hospital in 1816 described a similarly tranquil picture. The males 'all behaved very quietly; some were sitting and amusing themselves at draughts; while others were playing on the flute, writing, and employed in various ways.' Most of the women were also 'very quiet', apart from one 'continually speaking with great vehemence'.[217] Orderliness was, indeed, most likely the prevailing norm in a lunatic hospital, for otherwise it was barely conceivable that the small numbers of keepers could maintain any semblance of control. Consistent well-ordered behaviour would usually be interpreted as a sign of recovery, with 'convalescent' patients treated accordingly, like the female convalescents at St Luke's in 1815 who were observed knitting and lace-making.[218] At Manchester in 1818, males and females 'in a Convalescent state' were allowed to mix together, and had the use of a private room and a garden to walk in.[219] Recovering patients would be called upon to assist hard-pressed keepers. In fact, the institutions' smooth functioning was often dependent on their active, unpaid participation.

Patients were certainly not, however, a body of universally compliant people who never registered dissent. There is little doubt that some of the reported destructive, threatening, or 'dirty' behaviour contained an element of protest. There was also some more articulate dissent that surfaced occasionally from people above the rank of pauper. Hugh Williams, admitted to Manchester Lunatic Hospital in March 1801, managed to achieve the publication of a short pamphlet highly critical both of his incarceration and his treatment. The title referred to his being in the fifty-fourth day of his 'confinement in bondage' in the lunatic hospital. He accused the doctors of having given orders 'not to let me see the word of God', whilst he praised the actions of his sympathetic 'turnkey', Abraham, described as a 'man of grace and understanding'. This was in sharp contrast to the physicians whose knowledge and motives Williams dismissed disparagingly:

> Lunacy is a disorder of the mind and Soul, and not of the Body; for a carnal physician knows nothing about it, nor never will; it's like a carnal minded man attempting to preach the Gospel of Christ to a carnal-minded Physician, to attempt to cure the Lunacy; they are only aiming for the loaves and fishes.

The keeper, he suggested, was far better equipped to care for a lunatic than one of the doctors.[220]

Godfrey Higgins, in his exposures of the York Asylum, cited a letter written by a 'man of rank', who complained that he had been 'most arbitrarily confined in the York medical inquisition'. The man suggested that those patients who had unaccountably died were 'fortunately released... from the most shocking cruelty of doctors and their keepers, and the most dangerous tyranny ever invented by the devil, doctors, or men'.[221] Similar sentiments were expressed by some patients in the Liverpool Asylum when its particular scandals arose in 1825. Several of them, who included military officers, gave lucid and eloquent testimony as to the abuse and violence to which they had been subjected by the keepers. One had kept a detailed journal of the events that had occurred. Their evidence, carefully marshaled and placed with sympathetic infirmary governors, provided the ammunition for the establishment of an enquiry.[222] Dr Thomas Renwick, one of the infirmary physicians subjected to most criticism, dismissed the problems as having been mainly created by one particularly plausible but insane patient who had succeeded in forming a 'cabal, with other lunatics' in order to 'harass and distress the Governor, Matron, and keepers'.[223] If this were indeed the case, a determined patient had succeeded in creating a considerable upheaval. Protest and dissent were, however, far from easy to manifest in a closed institution. Those patients who succeeded in making their point to a wider public were clearly people of unusual resource and ability, hardly typical of the inmates of a lunatic hospital.

CONCLUSIONS

During the second half of the eighteenth century there was a notable expansion in the numbers of people confined in specialist institutions for the insane. Although part of this increase was accommodated in the private madhouse sector, the voluntary lunatic hospitals were the key new element in the range of provision. Patient numbers grew most rapidly in the decades up to 1800, driven largely by the expansion of St Luke's, the York Asylum and the Manchester Lunatic Hospital. The leveling off that followed in the early decades of the nineteenth century was associated partly with the particular difficulties that arose at York, offset mainly by the emergence of the new institutions at Exeter and Lincoln. The legislation of 1808, and the subsequent development of county lunatic asylums, was influential in several ways. Some of the paupers admitted to the new asylums might otherwise have been placed in voluntary institutions, and this certainly affected admission numbers at St Luke's, Liverpool, and Manchester. On the other hand, several of the new post-1808 asylums constituted joint endeavours with voluntary subscribers, and their acceptance of charitable and private patients effectively added to the numbers of patients admitted into lunatic hospitals.

In the absence of a clear legislative framework, the governors of lunatic hospitals were able to establish their own criteria and arrangements for admission of 'proper objects'. The variations in systems and standards between different places were quite marked. Formal medical certification was not required prior to admission at either the Newcastle or Manchester Lunatic Hospitals. At the latter, however, the requirement for examination by one of the infirmary physicians probably ensured a more rigorous vetting than would often be provided by an outside practitioner. Elsewhere, particularly at St Luke's, York and Exeter, the arrangements established generally matched the standards set by law for admissions to private madhouses or, later, county asylums.[224] As physicians and governors gained experience in the assessment and treatment of insanity, their requirements for prior information developed accordingly. A steady process of professionalisation was reflected in the increasing sophistication of the questions asked of referrers, as the basis for informing admission decisions and treatment plans.

Although the pursuit of the curative ideal was central to the emerging literature on insanity and its treatment[225], it was only at St Luke's that curability was established as a central criterion for admission and discharge of individual patients. In the provincial lunatic hospitals, whilst their governors would seek to illustrate their successful achievement of high rates of cure, there was always an acceptance of responsibility to receive and retain people deemed to be incurable. Even at St Luke's it was not long before the problem was recognized and then addressed by the establishment of an ostensibly separate facility for incurable patients, with its own distinct admission arrangements and administrative systems. As the numbers of patients in the new hospital grew after 1790, the extent of provision for incurables became increasingly significant, whilst still not making great inroads into the long waiting list.

Geographical considerations became increasingly influential in determining both the pattern of establishment of lunatic hospitals and the localities from whence their patients were admitted. Although St Luke's continued to function throughout the period as a national hospital, accepting people from throughout England (and occasionally Wales), the large majority of admissions were from London and the south-eastern counties. The projectors of the northern institutions cited the inaccessibility of St Luke's and Bethlem among the primary reasons for their foundation. Admissions reflected a clear localized pattern, with the lunatic hospitals at Newcastle, Manchester, York, Liverpool and Exeter all providing primarily for their cities and counties and the region beyond. The outline of a national system of public institutions for the insane, based on a regional geography, was in place even before parliament intervened in 1807 and 1808.

Social class, and the associated financial considerations, became increasingly pertinent issues. Whilst St Luke's retained being 'poor' as one of the key admission qualifications, the criterion was not generally applied elsewhere for reasons that were apparently both philosophical and pragmatic. Certainly the governors of the provincial lunatic hospitals accepted that their main responsibility was to cater for the poor, whether parish pauper or otherwise. However, the distaste for private madhouses expressed at Manchester and York was sincere enough and there was a real desire to offer a superior alternative and even to compete actively for middle (and even higher) class custom. The potential financial benefits to the institution became increasingly apparent to the extent that, at York and Exeter in particular, the attraction of fee-paying private patients was promoted as a charitable necessity. People well above the rank of pauper therefore became a significant element in the lunatic hospitals' population.

A construction of images of the institutions' patients has to be based on various pieces of evidence, some of them impressionistic. What emerges is a picture of a very diverse group of people, emanating from varied social, economic, cultural and geographical backgrounds. Intellectually, they ranged from the idiotic and the fatuous to the highly intelligent and articulate. They could present with varying types and degrees of mental disorder, both 'curable' and 'incurable' in nature. These disorders manifested themselves in all manner of symptomatology, as well as in problematic, difficult and at times incomprehensible behaviours. Some patients were sullen, threatening and even violent, whilst others exhibited little more than passivity or vulnerability. Some were in a poor physical state, unable or unwilling to control basic bodily functions. The challenge to be addressed by governors, physicians, and staff was considerable if they were to effectively manage and contain such disparate groups of people, let alone to go on to help them toward recovery and a return to family and community.

6   Managing and curing the patients

The opening of St Luke's Hospital in 1751, with its high principles and declared therapeutic intent, represented a signal that profound shifts were occurring in approaches to the treatment and management of madness in England. As Roy Porter has clearly demonstrated, the half-century or so that followed was something of a heroic period in the history of psychiatry.[1] Practitioners, activated by a mission to relieve suffering and to achieve cures, set about confronting madness and attacking it on several fronts — medical, psychological, and institutional. These curative orientations were becoming increasingly influential, providing a real alternative to the less savoury aspects of practice present in some domestic and institutional settings around the country, and which tended to dominate historical discourse before Porter rescued the eighteenth century from perceptions that neglect and brutality were the norm.[2] The lunatic hospitals, steeped as they were in charitable ideals, were significant sites for the implementation of the new therapeutic approaches, even if achievement did not always match intent.

The decision by the subscribers to the proposed lunatic hospital at York to call it an 'asylum' was not insignificant. The word, already adopted in the titles of institutions for other needy groups of people, contained connotations of tranquility and refuge long before it acquired stigmatized meanings. Indeed, 'asylum' initially carried very similar inferences to 'retreat', the term adopted fifteen years later in naming York's second charitably funded institution for the insane. A lunatic hospital or asylum was intended as a place where treatment would take place in a conducive and caring environment. If actual cure or recovery could not be achieved, there still remained an intention to promote at least the relief of suffering and distress for both the patient and his family.

However, unlike the general hospital, the lunatic hospital also had to meet other expectations — safety and security. The patient was likely to require restraint, in its broadest sense, in order to protect others and himself from the unpredictable excesses associated with madness. This brought certain requirements for the material fabric, the equipment, and the management system, tending inevitably toward a custodial orientation.

The need for security and control provided an over-arching context for the therapeutic regime, and indeed tended to support those aspects of the heroic approach that were based on the analogy of confrontation between practitioner and the dark forces of madness.

Although aspects of the running of institutions, public and private, might be left to laymen without formal medical knowledge or training, the curative treatment of the patients was clearly perceived to be the province of the medical man and of the physician in particular. Medical treatment continued to be the accepted primary curative agent and this constituted a key justification for the development of the lunatic hospitals, particularly those that emerged from general hospitals. Many of the pharmacological techniques of treatment had been well established before 1750. The practitioners of the later eighteenth century, however, armed with their liberal medical education and in the context of the intellectual ferment of Enlightenment and 'urban renaissance', showed a great preparedness for experimentation and eclecticism. The range of drug treatments utilized was being widened, and other physical treatments were added to the treatment armoury, particularly involving water, but also making use of new contraptions like the circular swing chair.

The most significant element to emerge in the therapeutic armamentarium, though, was 'management' or, as it later became known, 'moral management'. Battie famously reiterated that 'management did much more than medicine'.[3] Although he and his rival John Monro were hardly in full agreement on some basic principles, this was one significant issue on which they occupied common ground; according to Monro, the cure of madness 'depends on *management* as much as *medicine*'.[4] In the course of the following half-century or so, the techniques of management were being refined and perfected, and aspects were implemented to greater or lesser extent in all institutions for the insane, including the lunatic hospitals. Management methods operated on the general and the specific level, comprising both the overall regime within the institution and the regimen prescribed for the individual patient. The most successful practitioners were those able to combine effectively the principles of management and the range of medical or physical interventions into one therapeutic system.[5]

THE DISEASE OF INSANITY

The growth that occurred in the second half of the eighteenth century in the number and size of specialist institutions was accompanied by an expanding literary output. Publications on the nature of mental disorder, its origins and 'causes', and the means by which it might be treated, reflected a growing academic, professional, and public interest in the whole subject. A number of practitioners went into print to advance their theories, with a view either to the improvement of treatment practices or the development of their private practices, or conceivably both. Several physicians directly associated with the lunatic hospitals were among those who published influential works, including William Battie, Thomas Arnold, and John Ferriar.

It became an established orthodoxy among those seeking to treat mentally disordered people that madness had its basis in physical disorder. The Chester surgeon George Nesse Hill was confirming what had long since been accepted when he entitled the first chapter of his 1814 book 'Insanity Has Always Corporeal Disease for its Foundation'.[6] Writers on insanity had been placing emphasis on the intimate linkage between bodily and mental illness since the early part of the eighteenth century, if not before.[7] James Currie asserted it to be beyond dispute that 'madness is a disease of the body'.[8] Other practitioners, like Joseph Mason Cox, did not quite go that far but maintained that madness 'is always accompanied by corporeal disease'.[9] There were some, nevertheless, who dissented from this position, like Andrew Harper, who argued that the mind could become deranged independently of bodily ailment,[10] though this perspective remained very much in the minority.

Most practicing mad-doctors, and physicians with an interest in mental disorder, continued to reiterate the connections between body and mind. Thomas Arnold, like others influenced by Locke, was a strong adherent and argued that 'certain states of the one infallibly produce, or are accompanied with, certain states of the other.'[11] James Currie put the interconnection forward as a primary rationale for locating the Liverpool Lunatic Asylum next door to the infirmary, under joint management and medical oversight.[12] His contemporary in Manchester, John Ferriar, clearly considered his practice with patients in the lunatic hospital as an aspect of his general work in treating sickness. He looked specifically at how 'conversions' could take place between one disease and another, and included within his analysis not only insanity and 'maniacal complaints' in general, but also particular conditions such as 'puerperal mania'.[13]

The acceptance of an intrinsic organic element to insanity did not prevent the identification of a wide range of causal factors, some physiological and some psychological or even social. Whilst bodily ailments might directly contribute to the onset of madness, external non-organic causes were seen to act on physical elements in precipitating the disorder, as William Battie carefully expounded.[14] His summary of causes was relatively modest in comparison to the highly detailed delineation of Thomas Arnold, who began his extensive survey with the caveat that 'In treating of causes of insanity we tread upon slippery ground' and that it was advisable to 'step with caution'.[15] He proceeded to exercise that caution over about 400 pages in which he divided a very large number of conceivable causes into 'remote' and 'proximate', and then into 'bodily' and 'mental' causes.[16]

Arnold's range of bodily causes included the involuntary effects of particular ailments, lesions, or circumstances. Thus, damage to the skull or a lack of nourishment could be material causes.[17] Environmental influences, like the sun's rays or the climate, were significant, insanity being observably more frequent in summer 'and especially during the heat of the dog-days, or after a long continuance of very hot, dry, and sultry weather.'[18] Mental disorder might also result from factors that a person could control, like the extremes of either excessive exertion or a 'defect of exercise'.[19] Arnold, like other observers, paid particular attention to intemperance, and especially to habitual excessive drinking.[20] His delineation of mental causes was equally detailed, and included categories such as 'intense application of the mind', and the sudden or violent exercise of the 'passions', of which he cited no fewer than 18, ranging from 'joy', through 'avarice', to 'religious fear'.[21] So comprehensive was Arnold's overall schema that even the most obscure potential causes were included.

Other practitioners also published their views on causative factors, though not in the intricate detail of Arnold. Among them was John Ferriar, who provided a brief summary, distinguishing particularly by gender. Those chiefly affecting men were 'hard drinking, accompanied with watching; pride; disappointment; the anguish arising from calumny; sudden terror; false opinions respecting religion; and anxiety in trade.' Due to the 'peculiar situation' of their sex, women's minds were 'sometimes deranged by the restraint or misdirection of passions, which were bestowed to constitute their happiness.' Ferriar did also note some physical precipitants. As well as direct 'conversions' from other diseases, there were factors such as the 'imprudent suppression of eruptions' and 'the irregularities of circulation produced in the puerperal state', as well as the effects of diseases like fevers and scrofula that could lead directly to insanity.[22] Ferriar's ascription of causation was probably not intended to be comprehensive. Other writers, like Haslam and Cox, tended to go into rather more detail, picking up on the sort of ideas that Arnold had put forward.[23]

The development of classifications of mental disorders was becoming, even by mid-century, a preoccupation of some practitioners.[24] In considering causality, Battie sought to divide madness into two main categories, 'original' and 'consequential'. Original madness, he suggested, was 'solely owing to a disorder of the nervous substance'. Its origins could be identified as essentially organic for, as he went on to say, 'we may with the greatest degree of probability affirm that Madness is Original, when it both ceases and appears afresh without any assignable cause.'[25] Consequential madness, on the other hand, was 'chiefly to be attributed to some remote and accidental cause' external to the person.[26] This was more than an academic differentiation, for Battie suggested that there were significant differences in prognosis. The physician could do little about original madness, for it was not susceptible to physic and indeed was 'never radically cured by human art'.[27] Consequential madness was a quite different proposition, however, for it was 'frequently manageable by human art'.[28]

Battie's delineation was relatively straightforward, in contrast to Thomas Arnold's highly elaborate classificatory system. Arnold developed a complex nosology, based on a division into 'ideal insanity' and 'notional insanity'. Ideal insanity referred to conditions where the person experienced auditory or visual hallucinations, or conversed with persons or things not present or that did not exist. Notional insanity comprised various manifestations of delusional misinterpretation of events or objects.[29] These two main categories were then further sub-divided, with ideal insanity broken down into four types and notional insanity into no fewer than nine.[30] Arnold described every one in detail, on the basis that each was a separate illness with its own distinctive symptomatology. His minutely differentiated system was far from easy to follow, not least because of the frequent overlap of symptoms between many of the thirteen types of insanity.[31]

In both his extensive analysis of causes and his ambitious classification, Arnold may well have been seeking to demonstrate his professional expertise, in order to promote his Leicester madhouse. Whatever the motives, the critical response was mixed. Dr Johnson's biographer, James Boswell, considered Arnold's *Observations* a 'very entertaining work'.[32] Arnold's influential teacher and mentor William Cullen was, however, rather less impressed. He suggested, somewhat condescendingly, that 'The ingenious Dr Arnold has been commendably employed in distinguishing the different species of insanity' and that 'his labours may hereafter prove useful'; however, Cullen concluded, 'at present I can make little application of his numerous distinctions'.[33] His verdict may have been somewhat harsh, for his pupil had at least made a genuine attempt to break new ground in delineating varieties of insanity. The problem about Arnold's system, like most classifications of mental disorder, was that whilst it might conceivably aid understanding of the different manifestations of the disorders, it could do little to assist actual treatment. It is even questionable whether it materially influenced practices in the modest surroundings of the Leicester Lunatic Asylum.

MEDICAL TREATMENT — 'A DOSE OF PHYSICK OR A VOMIT'[34]

The therapeutic principles that guided physicians seeking to treat the insane through medical means were essentially the same as those underpinning their general medical practice. Imbalances in the bodily constituents or in its actions had to be detected and diagnosed, before being redressed through the use of medicines or the application of other physical or surgical interventions. The restoration of a proper equilibrium within the constitution formed the essence of the therapeutics. To that end, treatment was largely directed toward the key elements of the blood, bodily temperature, sleep patterns, and the digestive system. The last was consistently the focus of most attention, with the various types of evacuative medicines consolidating their place as the mainstay of the treatment armoury. What was most striking, however, about treatment practices was the eclecticism and energy demonstrated by practitioners in their endeavours to achieve cures. Pragmatic action to deal with particular symptoms was augmented by a willingness to experiment with a range of interventions, to be discarded if they proved ineffective and replaced by others until beneficial change occurred in the individual patient's condition.

Drug Treatments

Dr Alexander Sutherland, the fourth physician to St Luke's, told the 1815 parliamentary select committee that 'I myself generally attack the cases of mental disorder through the medium of the stomach, I find it answer exceedingly well'.[35] He was reflecting long-accepted practices both at St Luke's and elsewhere. Two main categories of 'physic' dominated therapeutic practice – emetics and purgatives. Although opinions might differ on the circumstances which indicated their usage, or the extent to which they should be employed, there was little argument among mad-doctors as to their significance as effective means of treatment in combating both physical symptoms and actual manifestations of insanity.

Emetics, often referred to as 'vomits', were an apparently essential element of treatment in many cases. Whilst Battie did not specifically recommend their use, he acknowledged that they were widely employed and sometimes had their place.[36] John Monro of Bethlem was more forthright in their advocacy, maintaining that 'evacuation by vomiting is infinitely preferable to any other', insisting that he 'never saw or heard of the bad effects of vomits'.[37] Later writers were yet more positive. The private madhouse proprietor Joseph Mason Cox was convinced from his own experience that vomiting 'takes the precedence of every other curative mean'; emetics were needed in nearly every case. They acted, he suggested, by removing impurities from the stomach.[38] Similar ideas actuated Sutherland of St Luke's, who sometimes found it 'absolutely necessary to employ emetics', in the same way as he would to 'any other patient whose stomach required it'.[39]

John Ferriar had been more specific, arguing that in 'recent cases' of mania there is 'commonly much disorder in the functions of the stomach', and vomiting was the usual remedy. His published case histories provide the clearest examples of actual practice in a lunatic hospital. He cited M.P., a young woman admitted to Manchester in 1792 'in a state of furious agitation' and with 'totally confused' ideas. She 'could not be brought to attend to any object', and would not answer any questions. Ferriar 'ordered her a vomit of tartar emetic, in the usual manner'. It operated 'briskly' and 'had an instantaneous effect in restoring a degree of rationality.' Five days later she was reported as continuing to be 'rational', and was discharged 'cured' soon afterwards.[40] Ferriar was an eclectic practitioner, employing emetics alongside other treatments. He particularly used emetic tartar (antimony) in cases of recent onset of mania, in 'nauseating and vomiting doses', following up with purgatives and tonics.[41] He was candid enough to acknowledge, however, that his methods had little direct success in some of the cases and that other remedies had to be tried.[42]

Importantly, Ferriar realised that emetics were capable of having effects more significant than merely acting on the stomach. As well as 'clearing the first passages', vomiting might also directly produce 'a favourable change in the mental disease'.[43] The medicine could be effective in 'diverting patients from capricious resolutions'. He developed this psychologically based perspective further:

> The repetition of vomits, and the use of antimonial preparations, in nauseating doses are certainly proper in maniacal cases: the uneasy sensations which they excite, seem to recal (sic) the patient's attention to a regular train.[44]

Ferriar, however, expressed caution about the possible behavioural influences of emetics in some conditions. Although they were useful in maniacal cases, they might actually be harmful to melancholics, for the distressing associations could worsen the symptoms by 'furnishing an opportunity for some new fancies'.[45]

Like other physicians, Ferriar also made extensive use of purgatives, considering them 'undoubtedly useful in most cases of insanity, but only when moderately given.' He used 'the celebrated melampodium' in numerous cases, two or three times per week, in order to 'purge the patient gently'.[46] His purgative of choice, though, was calomel (chloride of mercury), despite unpleasant side effects such as a very sore mouth emanating from its mercury content. Ferriar did raise doubts about its efficacy, citing several cases where little benefit had been gained.[47] There were, though, other cases where he claimed at least partial success with calomel. In the case of J.B., for whom tartar emetic had been ineffective, calomel brought some abatement of his 'fury', rendering him 'brutal and stupid' before he gradually improved sufficiently to be 'completely cured' after five months in hospital.[48] On balance, Ferriar considered that calomel 'deserves to be farther tried in cases of insanity'. It was particularly effective, he thought, in mixed cases of mania and melancholy, if used in conjunction with emetic tartar.[49]

Notwithstanding the side effects, calomel remained the purgative medicine in widest usage. Cox, for example, considered it the most effective purge.[50] Others such as magnesia, hellebore, magnesium sulphate and castor oil were also employed in lunatic hospitals and asylums. In the case of a young woman Ferriar had treated initially with tartar emetic, he then 'kept her bowels freely open with magnesia' for fifteen days, and also ordered occasional purges at night with black hellebore. He used black hellebore, along with other treatments, in the case of T.R., a man who had remained for some time in a 'furious state'.[51] James Currie described the treatment of L.I., admitted to Liverpool Asylum in June 1796 in 'a state of furious insanity'; after being restrained his bowels were cleared by means of a 'saline purgative', before various other treatments were implemented.[52] Ferriar likewise recommended regular 'saline purgatives', particularly in gradually restoring the health of people with disorders precipitated by 'hard drinking'.[53]

The main rationale for the use of purges, as Cox explained, was that maniacs were 'frequently and almost uniformly costive'.[54] The medicine would both unblock the system and remove impurities. Experienced practitioners, however, counseled discretion in prescribing purgatives, as their excessive use could be harmful. Battie expressed reservations over the use of cathartic salts, suggesting that 'sharp purges' should only be employed with great caution, and not at all with patients who were in 'fits of fury'. Along with vomits, he contended that rougher purges should only be used in spring or autumn, 'as being neither extream (sic) of cold or heat', and that they should not be given for more than six or eight weeks at a time. As soon as the patient approached sanity they, 'and all other violent methods', should be discontinued.[55] Ferriar advised against the practice of 'brisk purging' in maniacs, for there were few instances in which the patient's 'robust, even luxuriant health, and undisturbed natural functions' would justify carrying it out to any great extent.[56] Thomas Arnold was also concerned that excessive evacuative measures, including purging, might be damaging. However, he recommended that the insane, if 'strong and healthful', should have their bowels 'kept in a constant state of moderate evacuation', and that some with 'very strong constitutions' needed 'a considerable purging'.[57]

Purgative and emetic medicines were employed in conjunction with general measures to promote a healthy digestive system. Attention to individual diet was, as far as practical, an important part of a lunatic hospital's therapeutic regime, and was under the clear direction of the physician. The intention would generally be to ensure an adequate food intake that was not over-stimulating. As Currie advised a correspondent, 'I restrict the diet to articles that are mild.'[58] He, Ferriar and others frequently had recourse to 'low diet' with a view to reducing over-activity and bringing the patient under control.[59] Sir George Paul noted in 1810 that, at the Newcastle Lunatic Hospital, medicine and diet were used by Dr Wood for 'reducing the habit' in order to render the patients manageable.[60] Arnold recommended a lower and stricter diet for patients who were 'remarkably strong, or of a gross habit of body'.[61] When employed as a means of control, however, dietary regulation was open to misuse. Alexander Sutherland at St Luke's accepted that diet ought to be 'occasionally regulated', but only in cases where actual 'bodily indisposition' was present; he considered that treatment relied 'generally too much on the system of lowering'.[62]

A common problem, however, was the inclination of some patients to refuse food, consequent either on the depth of their melancholia or delusional ideas regarding the food. Force-feeding was a likely response; Thomas

Dunston told the select committee in 1816 that he had forced unwilling St Luke's patients to take food 'many score times'.[63] In less serious cases, tonic medicines would be employed to promote improvements both in digestion and in the overall constitution. The most popular of these was Peruvian bark, which Currie employed in rebuilding the strength of his patient L.I.[64] Ferriar also made frequent use of bark, often together with wine which was employed quite frequently by mad-doctors to fortify the constitution.[65]

Various types of 'physic' were also used for purposes of sedation. Lack of sleep was symptomatic of both melancholia and mania, and its restoration could form an important part of the treatment and recovery processes. For Currie sleep disturbance was the 'leading symptom of the beginning disease', and its significance was self-evident:

> By procuring sleep that is sound, where it was fugitive and broken, the disease may in general be prevented: and by producing it, where the disease is formed, if it be not of long continuance, it may in general be cured.

Currie's drug of choice in combating 'watchfulness' was opium.[66] He had found in some cases of insanity that there were 'very extraordinary effects from such doses of opium as induced profound sleep', though he had to acknowledge that substantial doses of it had limited effect in the case of L.I..[67] Ferriar also used opium in several of his cases, either on its own or in combination, with mixed results. It seems that he was sometimes employing it for general calming purposes, rather than solely to aid sleep.[68] Battie had suggested forty years before that opium could relieve symptoms in certain circumstances, though he too noted its limitations as a narcotic.[69]

Another drug that came increasingly into vogue for mental disorder was digitalis. Developed from the foxglove, its diuretic effects and other medical benefits were expounded by the Birmingham physician William Withering in 1785. He described a case of a man 'in a state of furious insanity' where digitalis had proved effective.[70] Other practitioners took note and tried it out for themselves. Ferriar employed digitalis in several cases, 'even to nauseating doses', but to little evident effect. He commented dismissively that the drug had become 'fashionable', though acknowledged that others had found it useful 'for the removal of insanity'. He would only concede that it had been sometimes employed successfully 'in cases of melancholy'.[71] Currie considered digitalis a suitable drug for treating insanity. He tried it in L.I.'s case, after opium and a low diet had brought little real change. However, several courses of digitalis proved hardly more successful.[72] Other physicians were quite convinced of its benefits. Joseph Mason Cox, for example, after several years experience with digitalis, ranked it second only to emetics as a remedy.[73]

William Battie had generally adopted a cautious position on the use of medicines, questioning the efficacy of many in current usage to deal with mental symptoms.[74] His successors, both at St Luke's and elsewhere, tended to be more adventurous, showing a preparedness to move quickly from one drug to another and to prescribe several simultaneously. According to interpretation, specialist physicians either had little clear idea how to effectively and consistently prescribe to tackle insanity, or they were creatively pragmatic in their treatment approaches. Assuming the latter, they showed a similar eclecticism in their employment of interventionist physical treatments, either in conjunction with physic or as an alternative approach after it had proved ineffective.

Physical Treatments

Blood-letting in its various forms was central to eighteenth-century medical practice, but it was certainly not universally regarded as effective in the treatment of insanity. Battie suggested that bleeding was 'no more the adequate and constant cure of Madness than it is of fever'. A lancet applied to a 'feeble and convulsed Lunatic' might be no 'less destructive than a sword'.[75] Despite the risks, however, bleeding retained its place in both private and public practice. Its excessive use, on a regular seasonal and sometimes apparently undiscriminating basis, became one of the chief criticisms of practices at Bethlem.[76] Alexander Sutherland was keen to distance St Luke's from any such methods: 'Certainly not' was his dismissive response to the 1815 select committee when asked if 'periodical bleeding of a number of patients' was followed at the hospital.[77]

Thomas Arnold articulated the rationale for bleeding, claiming in 1786 that the increased activity of the small arteries and consequent 'turgescency' of the brain's vascular system 'seldom fail to accompany the beginning, and are never absent from the violent states' of the disorder. He argued that this causal link led to important 'practical considerations' and pointed towards 'a rational method of cure'. His conclusion was that, 'in almost every recent, and violent cases of Insanity', great advantage could be derived from 'topical evacuations from the head' and from other means that could 'divert the impetus of the blood from the vessels of the brain, and abate their preternatural activity.'[78] It is significant that, in his two earliest volumes, Arnold gave few other definitive opinions on treatment methods. In his later writings he had evidently moderated his position, concluding that over-use of bleeding was a 'dangerous error'. He still acknowledged that the insane, if 'strong and healthful', should have blood removed 'occasionally, in such quantities as the symptoms seem to demand'. However, although 'copious bleeding' might sometimes be beneficial, it was more commonly otherwise and ought only to be 'the result of much experience and judicious discrimination.'[79]

Arnold's more circumspect later position was reflected by other discerning practitioners. Currie told a correspondent in 1790 that, when symptoms were becoming evident, 'I sometimes bleed' according to the 'vigour and fulness of the patient'.[80] Ferriar recognized its beneficial effects in certain cases and circumstances, whilst conscious of the need for caution and discrimination. He suggested that general blood-letting was a 'valuable remedy' in 'young plethoric subjects' who were not completely unmanageable, but it was a dangerous practice for those in a 'frantic state'. Repeated bleeding was hazardous and risked bringing on debility. He had fewer reservations, though, about topical bleeding, either by cupping or the use of leeches, methods that were 'attended with no danger' and were an effective alternative to general bleeding.[81] In his second volume, Ferriar reiterated strong reservations against general blood-letting, because of the risk of precipitating the patient into an 'irrecoverable state'. He spoke of having 'seen maniacs bleed till they became melancholy, and melancholics, by repeated venaesection reduced to despair.' However, he did not completely discount the practice, referring to one case where a 'single, copious bleeding' had worked effectively for a woman 'of full habit' whose maniacal symptoms followed an episode of cholera.[82]

Topical bleeding was clearly not subject to the same constraints. Leeches were widely used, to judge from financial accounts for the Exeter and Leicester asylums.[83] The other significant topical treatments in common usage were what Ferriar referred to as 'drains', specifically blisters and setons.[84] Once again, Battie had acknowledged the availability of these treatments but was unenthusiastic about their efficacy.[85] Ferriar was more positive about the benefits. He rationalized their action by suggesting that melancholia and mania were 'sometimes produced by the suppression of habitual eruptions, or discharges' and might, therefore, be cured by 'restoring, or irritating them.' He cited two cases where application of a seton had contributed significantly to recovery. For L.H., a woman of forty-eight admitted to Manchester Lunatic Hospital in July 1791 in a 'very low, desponding state', various treatments had little effect until in September Ferriar ordered a seton to be put in the nape of her neck. After it began to 'suppurate' there was an immediate change, sustained by daily improvement until she was discharged 'perfectly well' in October. As for blisters, Ferriar considered that they 'generally answer very well' for patients not 'sufficiently tractable' to accept drains requiring more management.[86]

The physical treatments that became most central to therapeutics in the lunatic hospitals, and later in the county asylums, were those utilizing water. A cold bath had been installed at St Luke's by 1773; the master, Mr Mansfield was ordered to purchase a 'pair of steps' to enable patients to get into it.[87] This evidently was intended for purposes of therapy as well as cleanliness. In the new building cold baths were provided on both the men's and the women's sides. In 1793, George Dance junior, the surveyor, was instructed to provide an estimate for a cold bath lined with marble, on the east side of the hospital.[88] To judge from Sutherland's comments in 1815, they received plenty of use, for he admitted to 'often' employing cold bathing in the form of the 'bath of surprise'.[89] Baths intended for treatment purposes became standard equipment in all lunatic hospitals and asylums. The Exeter Asylum was equipped with a shower bath from the outset.[90] With the opening of the new building in 1804, all the latest contrivances were installed. There was a hot bath and two cold baths, in addition to a shower and a 'Vapor Bath'.[91]

After publication of his most important medical text, James Currie attained the status of an authority on the use of water in treatment of a range of conditions.[92] His explanation of its utility in 'maniacal diseases' was based on Erasmus Darwin's ideas regarding the close connection between insanity and convulsive disorders.[93] Currie expounded his theories and practices by the detailed presentation of the complex case of L.I. (thirty-two), admitted to the Liverpool Lunatic Asylum on 2 June 1796 in a state of 'furious insanity'. After initially being subjected to powerful restraint, followed by opiates to induce sleep, low diet, and vomits, his condition was 'as violent as ever' after two weeks. Digitalis and other medicines were then tried, with limited success. After six weeks, he was put on a course of tepid baths, which was then altered to a twice daily 'tepid affusion' lasting a minute or two at a time, with the water being gently poured over him. Despite sporadic 'lucid intervals', Currie was not satisfied and admitted himself 'perplexed'. Considering cold baths to be effective in convulsive disorders, he ordered a trial. When L.I.'s insanity returned 'with great violence' on July 21st, he was forcefully 'thrown headlong into the cold bath'. He emerged 'calm, and nearly rational', and remained so for 24 hours. However, this state was not maintained and the forceful process was repeated with apparent success, as reported on 30 July:

> on the morning of the 23rd, he was again thrown into the cold bath in the height of his fury, as before. As he came out, he was thrown in again, and this was repeated five different times, till he could not leave the bath without assistance. He became perfectly calm and rational in the bath, and has remained so ever since.

L.I. continued to have baths every other day, in addition to fortifying medicines. Having no further relapse, he was eventually discharged 'in perfect health of body and mind.'[94]

Across in Manchester, Ferriar had become equally convinced of the therapeutic value of baths, and was making use of them in the lunatic hospital before Currie. He did not take the same forthright approach, though, differentiating the type of bath according to the patient's presentation, with cold for melancholics and warm for those with mania. Ferriar believed that if a maniac was kept in a warm bath for an extended period, 'he will become entirely passive'. He illustrated with the case of T.R. (twenty-eight) admitted in 1791, who had remained in a 'furious state' despite various interventions. Warm baths were instituted for a half hour each morning. This was no easy task as it 'required six men to carry our patient into the bath'. However, the 'relaxing effect was so great' that only one person was needed to return him to bed afterwards, where he remained 'in a sort of comatose state'. T.R. became generally calmer and more rational. Regular baths were continued, along with the application of cold water sponges to his shaven head for 'a considerable time' each day. He gradually fell into a 'harmless, stupid state', before gradually regaining his reason. His recovery was aided with tonics, sedatives and emetics, and he was 'dismissed, cured' after several months in the hospital.[95] Ferriar cited another case where he had used the warm bath to calm someone with 'furious mania', as well as two cases where cold baths had provided relief for patients suffering from melancholia.[96] There was no advocacy of the forcible cold plunge baths recommended by Currie.

Currie was unapologetic about his more drastic approach, fully recognizing that the psychological aspects were key to the treatment's efficacy. In a paper given in London in 1790, he had argued that madness is 'best combated in the height of the phrenzy'. The 'plentiful affusion of cold water' was an 'infallible remedy' for a 'hysterical paroxysm'. It was legitimate to create 'powerful dread' or even 'terror' of the treatment. He claimed from experience that 'a tub of cold water kept in readiness, with the certainty of being plunged into it on the recurrence of the paroxysm' could be sufficient to cure the disorder 'without the remedy actually being tried'.[97] The approach that Currie recommended and 'so successfully practised' proved very influential, as Joseph Mason Cox acknowledged, in particular the mode of 'suddenly immersing the maniac in the very acme of his paroxysm'. As Cox added, however, the patient needed to be 'secured by a strait waistcoat' and strapped into a chair.[98]

Once particular therapies began to rely on the deterrence of fear, or required the use of physical coercion, they ceased to be purely medical treatments. The intent was increasingly to alter behaviour as well as to relieve symptoms, based on an assumption that the patient was, at least in part, able to exercise some control. Almost inadvertently, specialist physicians were expanding the whole territory of treatment, to a point where medically based techniques and 'management' were becoming closely linked and inter-dependent. The cold plunge bath, with its origins in medical theories, was perhaps the most striking example. Some of the drug treatments, such as vomits, could have similar additional ramifications. The treatment most overtly combining medical and behavioural management properties was the circular swing chair, perfected by Cox.[99] The extent of its dissemination in the lunatic hospitals is unclear, though 'one of Dr Cox's rotatory chairs' had certainly been installed at Exeter by 1815. Significantly, it was located in the same room as the cold bath.[100]

MANAGEMENT AND MORAL MANAGEMENT

By the time that William Battie stressed the significance of 'management' in relation to 'medicine', there was already some recognition that the success-ful treatment of insanity depended to a degree on the skilled use of interac-tive techniques. In the half-century after Battie wrote, the nature and range of those techniques were refined in both private and public practice. The growing confidence in the curability of madness was a product of practi-tioners' commitment to its achievement, utilizing whatever methods proved effective. Although medical approaches were becoming more diverse and sophisticated, the late eighteenth and early nineteenth centuries were par-ticularly characterized by the application of management techniques, and by a growing intellectual conception of how they operated. Moral manage-ment, or 'moral treatment', may have been most associated by historians with the emergence of the York Retreat in the 1790s but, as Roy Porter has demonstrated, the paradigm was already becoming established before then, not least by the work of lunatic hospital physicians like Battie and Ferriar.[101]

Among John Ferriar's most significant statements was the assertion that 'the management of hope and apprehension in the patients forms the most useful part of the discipline.'[102] He may have inadvertently encapsulated the essence of the two main strands of 'management'. On the one hand, 'hope' was promoted by those practices rooted in humane, conciliatory principles. Other principles, those related to discourses of custody and containment, tended more toward the generation of 'apprehension'. The strands, how-ever, were far from being mutually exclusive. Both were seen to have their place in the pursuit of the goal of 'cure'. Indeed, most practitioners accepted them to be essentially complementary.

Certain principles of patient management were present whatever the ori-entation of the institution's regime. Fundamental was the conception that, for treatment to be effective, the lunatic had to be separated from undesir-able outside influences. As Battie expressed it, madness required removal from 'all objects that act forcibly on the nerves, and excite too lively a perception of things, more especially from such objects as are the known causes of the disorder'.[103] Ferriar adopted a similar position, contending that 'lunatics recover more quickly when they are removed from home'. If they remained with their families, the 'concern and exclusive attention' of which they were the objects would lead the disease to gain 'additional strength'.[104] Arnold argued similarly, though from a slightly different premise. Cure should not be attempted in the person's own home because 'the familiarity of domestic scenes' and the presence and conversation of 'intimate friends' presented a 'serious impediment' to the process. Separation was needed because the sufferer would not 'easily submit to the refusal of indulgence by those from whom they think they have a right to expect or demand it', and also because he was likely to be aggravated by their presence.[105] Dr Wood at Newcastle was quite blunt on the issue in 1810, thinking it 'necessary to remove his patients out of the reach of all impressions on the senses from outward objects; and this, even to total seclusion from society.'[106]

The emphasis on removal and separation became an orthodoxy for practitioners.[107] The key associated requirement was for the patient to be confined in a specialist institution, 'under the Management of Strangers', as aptly expressed in the initial proposals for the establishment of St Luke's in 1750.[108] According to Thomas Arnold in 1782, a 'house adapted to the purpose' was required, which had an 'appropriate apparatus' and 'properly instructed' servants.[109] The Manchester Infirmary trustees in 1766 had also referred to the need for 'proper Servants', as well as an 'experienced Governor and Governess' and skilled medical attendance.[110] Location was an important consideration. Battie argued that ideally the place of confinement should be 'at some distance' from the patient's home.[111] Arnold, writing in 1809, also favoured removal to a distant place, preferably in a 'retired, pleasant, and rural situation'.[112] Presumably, he had in mind somewhere like his madhouse at Belle Grove, in the country outside Leicester, rather than the public lunatic hospital in the city centre.

The principle of separation was also developing within the institution, under the guise of classification. There appeared to be therapeutic advantages in dividing patients according to their diagnoses, mental states, and behavioural presentations. These divisions were added to the spatial separation routinely imposed in regard to gender and, in some circumstances, social class. Thomas Arnold suggested that, where mutually beneficial, patients should be classified and associated 'according to the nature of their several cases'. Those 'unfit for association with others' ought to be kept entirely separate.[113] For most of the period, classification arrangements remained relatively crude in practice. At the Manchester Lunatic Hospital, by 1791, it was decided to provide separate accommodation for people deemed convalescent, 'that they may not be incommoded or disturbed by the unhappy sufferers under more violent degrees of insanity.' The same criteria were later adopted at Liverpool.[114] In the Leicester Asylum, the intention was also, as far as possible, to separate convalescent patients from those who were noisy and disturbed and 'even from the sight of such patients as are violent, untractable, or shocking' in appearance or conduct. The 'violent and noisy' were to be kept at 'as great a distance as the convenience of the house shall admit' from the more 'peaceful and manageable'.[115] A similar basic classification was instituted at Hereford in 1799.[116]

Classification was perhaps more an aspiration than a reality. St Luke's, as the largest lunatic hospital, should have had the most practical scope, but Edward Wakefield in 1815 noted its lack of 'means of classification'. There was 'some degree' on the men's wing, with most of the 'idiots' kept apart in the basement, and also separate day rooms where convalescent females could engage in lace-work and sewing. Another visitor confirmed that there was a 'great want' of classification at St Luke's, as in all other public lunatic hospitals.[117] A year later, the private madhouse proprietor and surgeon William Ricketts was yet more dismissive, claiming that there was 'no attempt' at classification there; the 'furious and melancholy' were all together and there was no distinct provision for convalescent patients.[118] As late as 1827, the surgeon John Dunston admitted that there was only limited classification at St Luke's, in the form of separation of the 'noisy and offensive'.[119] It would appear that the methodology of classification only attained any real level of sophistication in some of the new county asylums developed after the Act of 1808.[120]

At the heart of the therapeutic process, as Porter has emphasized, was the individualized relationship developed between practitioner and patient. The doctor had to engage with the lunatic and use a range of stratagems in order to confront and dispel erroneous ideas and inappropriate behaviours. Techniques were developed whereby psychological control could be gained over the patient, using methods that might be either conciliatory or intimidatory. Perhaps best known amongst these was the use of 'the eye', or the piercing stare, to subdue him. Such methods, at times bordering on the theatrical, were perfected and expounded by men like William Pargeter, Francis Willis, and Joseph Mason Cox.[121] The influence of these ideas was clearly evident in the writings and practices of Ferriar, Percival, Currie, and Arnold. William Cullen, in his professorial role at Edinburgh University, would undoubtedly have had direct influence on the thinking of Arnold, Currie, and Ferriar. Cullen's treatment principles were based on intimidation, isolation, and restraint of the lunatic, and he argued that it was necessary to inspire him with 'awe and dread'.[122] The overall tenor of the Cullen approach, based on subjugation, was perhaps not completely in accord with the new therapeutics. Nevertheless, aspects were incorporated, even by Ferriar who emphasized that treatment practices had seen a replacement of brutality with humanity and the general implementation of milder and more conciliatory methods.[123] Notions regarding the importance of the assertion and maintenance of authority, control and discipline remained as integral elements in management methodology, along-side the more liberal and gentle approaches.

The centrality of order and control in the management both of the lunatic hospital and its patients was made explicit in institutional rules. The phraseology that became incorporated into most was that patients were to be treated with care and indulgence as far as 'compatible with steady and effectual government'.[124] At Leicester, there was a significant variation of the latter phrase to 'consistent with their good government'.[125] These considerations effectively reconciled therapeutic principles with the pursuit of an orderly house. The model was best exemplified in the Newcastle Lunatic Hospital, as described by Paul in 1810. Dr Wood considered that success in attempting to cure his patients depended on imposing the idea of 'great restraint' on their minds. They were kept in 'sufficient order' by 'a constantly enforced attention to certain rules of discipline'. He advised

Paul that: 'I rely very much on discipline in the management of lunatics. By discipline, I do not mean severity, but strictness.' He drew an interesting comparison between his system of 'moral management', operated for the last eighteen years, and the new educational principles being implemented in some schools.[126]

By the time that the ageing Thomas Arnold published his book on 'management', he had the benefit of extensive practical experience in his madhouses as well as in Leicester's lunatic hospital. It had a good deal to say regarding matters of authority and obedience. Arnold's initial statement of 'rules' to be observed by those undertaking the cure of the insane comprised several clear injunctions. He contended that sufficient control should be exercised to correct or prevent 'improprieties, eccentricities, inconveniences, and dangers', and was quite explicit about the implications:

> No pains should be spared to procure their ready and quiet, or at least their actual, submission to all due controul. Authority over them is absolutely necessary; to the attainment of which firmness and resolution will greatly contribute.[127]

Arnold advocated relationship-building and the development of 'esteem and confidence' to achieve these ends, but 'obedience to orders' was essential if treatment was to succeed.[128] In his elaboration of basic principles, Arnold repeatedly emphasized these aspects. It was of considerable importance for the keeper to bring about 'great tractableness and compliance'. This entailed achieving 'ascendancy' over the mind of the patient at an early stage. However, he distinguished that this should be obtained by 'determined authority, as over children' rather than by 'severity, as over brutes'.[129]

Arnold was not advocating particularly new ideas, but rather was re-stating them in a clear and succinct format. Battie, fifty years earlier, had placed discipline at the heart of his conception of the appropriate management regimen for treating the lunatic, insisting that 'Every unruly appetite must be checked, every fixed imagination must if possible be diverted.' However, he had surprisingly little to say about the actual techniques of management.[130] The Lancashire physician John Aikin, who was well acquainted with the Manchester Lunatic Hospital, suggested in 1771 that 'the attention or art' needed to be directed toward the acquisition of a 'proper government over the temper and passions'. This required 'constant observation', together with 'firmness', though Aikin stressed that there should be a 'total absence of terror'.[131] Ferriar, in the 1790s, adopted a similar perspective. Although arguing primarily for a conciliatory approach, he recognized the need for a 'system of discipline, mild, but exact'. That discipline, he suggested, should be directed toward enabling the patient to 'minister to himself' and to exercise the 'command of his intellectual operations'.[132] Here was the essence of moral management.

Arnold and Ferriar tended not to dwell on aspects of management that might be deemed intimidatory. There is little doubt, though, that they had their place. Cox was quite open in suggesting that maniacs particularly 'susceptible of fear' were more easily managed, and that this was a legitimate element of treatment.[133] The fear principle was consistently employed at St Luke's during Thomas Dunston's long tenure as master. He adhered to the fundamentals established by Battie for, according Samuel Tuke who visited in 1812, he had 'never seen much advantage from the use of medicine, and relies chiefly on management.' It was a particularly authoritarian form of management, for Dunston candidly told Tuke that he considered fear 'the most effectual principle by which to reduce the insane to orderly conduct.'[134] Other statements by Dunston illustrate the paradoxes inherent in the principles and methodologies of moral management. In 1807, he told the select committee that 'much is certainly to be done by management', and a key element was to 'animate all with a hope of recovery'.[135] In 1815, under strong questioning, he insisted that 'The most tender treatment is always the best and will do the most.'[136] However, Dunston also justified the extensive use of various methods of control and coercion, including strong measures for force-feeding reluctant patients. Like other proponents of management strategies, he saw no inconsistency. If a technique was shown to work, it was legitimate.

Lunatic hospital rules contained injunctions for patients to be treated with 'tenderness and indulgence', and with no 'unnecessary severity' used against them.[137] The implication was that management was at least as much about facilitation and encouragement as control and authority. Thomas Arnold included 'the Agency of Humane and Kind Treatment in Effecting Their Cure' in the main title of his 1809 book.[138] He placed a strong emphasis on developing a positive relationship with the patient, as an essential precursor of effective treatment. To achieve this, 'great pains' were to be taken to gain his 'respect and confidence', by convincing him that everything done was with a view to his welfare and based on 'real regard and good will'.[139] The practitioner's genuine concern would be demonstrated by attention to the patient's comfort, by carefully listening to his 'notions and complaints' and 'indulgently sympathizing' with his feelings.[140] The empathic approach was to be reinforced by soothing agitated or depressed minds by 'kind and gentle treatment' and 'insinuating attentions'.[141] However, a humane style of interaction was not to be adopted merely for its own sake. As Arnold made clear, it was the best means of securing obedience to 'all orders and directions', which would contribute significantly to the achievement of a cure.[142]

Arnold stressed that his 'Observations' were not merely theoretical ideas and principles, but had been put into practice in his madhouse for forty years. He claimed that the Leicester Lunatic Asylum had been conducted on the same basis, though he added the revealing caveat that this was 'as much as the difference between a public and a private asylum would allow.'[143] John Ferriar, with no private establishment of his own, was restricted to developing his methods in the lunatic hospital. He too placed greater emphasis on the gentle rather than the authoritarian elements of the 'management of the mind', with techniques based on a 'system of mildness and conciliation'. Whilst he acknowledged that this did not necessarily lead to a cure, it did 'soften the destiny' of the suffering patient, which was equally important.[144] Ferriar considered that the experience of confinement should not have to be made unpleasant, and that everything 'painful and terrible' ought to be excluded from the 'lunatic-house'. The goal of treatment should be recovery, and this was most effectively furthered by 'small favours, the shew of confidence, and apparent distinction' toward individual patients.[145]

The sorts of principles expounded by Ferriar, Arnold and others have tended to be more associated with the York Retreat, whose later reputation benefited greatly from Samuel Tuke's skills as a publicist. Central to the Retreat's therapeutic ideology and its moral management was the concept of the desire for esteem. Tuke argued that this operated more powerfully than the principle of fear (which also had its place). It had great influence over the conduct of the insane; when 'properly cultivated' it led many to overcome 'morbid propensities' and 'deviations' whereby they became less 'obnoxious' to those around them.[146] This perspective had, however, previously been anticipated by Ferriar. He had put forward a strikingly similar proposition in his characterization of the lunatic as having a 'high sense of honour' with which the practitioner could engage in trying to bring about beneficial change. Both approaches were, in effect, based on a similar positive reinforcement of socially appropriate attitudes and the promotion of personal responsibility.[147]

One area of moral management where the Retreat did proceed considerably further was in relation to diversionary activities. Tuke emphasized the importance of 'exercise and labour' in the 'moral treatment' of insanity. The essential intent was to shift the patient's trains of thoughts away from distressing or delusional preoccupations.[148] Similar methods were implemented in the best managed of the private madhouses.[149] Arnold outlined a programme of outdoor exercise, recreations and indoor amusements in which patients should be encouraged to participate.[150] However, although he may have been providing these activities at Belle Grove, there is little evidence of similar things happening in the restricted confines of the Leicester Asylum. The lunatic hospitals' urban sites usually militated against outdoor activities, beyond what was possible in enclosed yards. At Manchester, a large garden was available for some patients by 1783.[151] At Exeter Asylum, its suburban location made it more feasible to provide gardens for exercise. Edward Wakefield, visiting in 1815, noted that most of the male patients were outside, with some working in the garden.[152] Overall, there were very limited attempts to provide indoor activities, and these were primarily directed at people deemed convalescent. At Newcastle in 1810, Paul saw convalescent patients assisting in the kitchen as well as helping to look after other patients.[153] There was also evidence at the York Asylum of selected patients assisting the keepers, though this probably had more to do with poor staffing levels than any conceptions of therapeutic occupation.[154]

There were attempts at St Luke's to provide some sort of occupation. John Howard in 1789 observed some 'calm and quiet' women doing needlework in the company of the matron, Mrs Dunston, and similar activities were observed in 1815.[155] Thomas Dunston would periodically engage male patients to assist the 'servants' in practical tasks. For example, in 1799, several helped to white-wash and clean the building, and there was a similar initiative in 1816. The chief motivation, however, appears to have been the 'considerable expense' saved from not employing outside contractors.[156] Dunston told the 1807 select committee that the convalescent patients 'assist in performing the household work'.[157] Some were also directly helping the keepers in caring for other patients, which Dunston admitted was partly because of low staffing levels, though insisting that there were clear therapeutic benefits for 'the best doctor they have is employment'.[158] Dr Sutherland also acknowledged the mixed motives for, whilst convalescents were 'exceedingly serviceable' to other patients, their assistance served to reduce the numbers of keepers required.[159]

The opportunities for occupational activities were evidently more developed at St Luke's than in some other voluntary institutions. Nevertheless, the overall impression is that work and other related pursuits were usually little more than diversions for patients, to help pass the time, engage their attention, or render them more tractable. Sometimes there was the significant additional motive of providing assistance to hard-pressed staff in their more routine tasks. However, the elevation of work to become a rationalized central element of therapy and rehabilitation in public lunatic asylums would not come until the early 1820s, with the Tuke-influenced efforts of William Ellis at the Wakefield Asylum.[160]

RESTRAINT AND COERCION

The use and abuse of mechanical restraint, and its eventual abolition, became one of the great issues in nineteenth-century psychiatry. However, serious questioning of practices did not begin before the exposures of the 1815 select committee, and it was not until the late 1830s that proponents of 'non-restraint' were able to mount an effective challenge.[161] Until then, restraint in its various guises remained a corner-stone of patient management in public and private institutions. It was accepted as a necessary adjunct to medical and 'moral' treatment, with objectives that overtly combined the therapeutic and the custodial. Restraint and other forms of coercion were intended to ensure the individual patient's compliance to his regimen of treatment, whilst protecting him and others from harm and ensuring the orderly operation of the institution. As John Haslam succinctly put it, experience had taught that 'restraint is not only necessary as a protection to the patient and to those about him, but that it also contributes to the cure of insanity.'[162] Retrospective condemnations of the widespread employment of mechanical restraint have tended to miss the point that the practical options for containing the more violent and destructive behavioural manifestations were extremely limited. It is significant, and sometimes overlooked, that restraint was accepted as a part of normal practice at the York Retreat; even Samuel Tuke himself referred to it as a 'necessary evil'.[163]

In the same way that the practitioner had to gain an ascendancy over the individual patient as a preliminary to implementing a treatment plan, so there was a perceived need for an overall milieu of physical control in the institution. Restraint instruments accompanied high walls, enclosed airing courts, unglazed windows with bars, and heavy wooden doors with iron bolts, in creating and maintaining an environment in which all would feel secure and controlled. This was partly about the minimization of actual harm and damage. There was also a strong message to be delivered as to where the power lay and who was in control. With those essentials established, the accoutrements of restriction and restraint could be construed as actively beneficial in the attempt to initiate curative treatment.

Thomas Arnold bluntly summarized the argument when suggesting that, without some form of bodily or mental restraint or both, 'we may attempt to very little purpose the cure of the insane'. Some required 'powerful opposition and coercion' because they were as 'violent and dangerous wild beasts', whilst others were like 'irrational and thoughtless children' and consequently needed 'steady guidance and judicious control'.[164] Fellow practitioners concurred with the need to impose control, by coercive measures if necessary, before active treatment could begin. In Currie's description of the 'furious' L.I., the initial response after admission had to be 'very powerful methods of coercion' before any medical remedies could be applied.[165] Ferriar, though a somewhat reluctant advocate, recognized that where a patient was in 'the furious state', his arms and maybe also his legs 'must be confined'. This was a part of the essential process of imposing discipline.[166] Therapeutic arguments were later advanced by John Davis, a former governor of the Liverpool Lunatic Asylum, who contested that the 'real value' of coercion was in promoting the patients' recovery by 'keeping them quiet, and preventing them sinking into a state of exhaustion'. However, he went on to acknowledge the wider punitive aspects, for it was also 'highly salutary' in correcting 'mischievous behaviour' and 'subduing a disposition to riot and outrage'.[167]

In all of the provincial lunatic hospitals the rules laid down guidance on the application of restraint and the use of other coercive measures. These could be quite revealing as to what was considered acceptable practice. Quite early in the life of the Manchester Lunatic Hospital it was enjoined that:

No Stripes or Beatings, no painful coercion whatsoever, more than what is necessary to restrain the Furious from hurting themselves or others, shall be inflicted or made use of by the Keeper or any of the Servants unless by a special Order in writing from the Physician.[168]

The responsibility for sanctioning coercive measures normally lay with the physician, though at St Luke's it was completely delegated to Thomas Dunston.[169] At the lunatic hospitals in Manchester, Hereford and Liverpool it was stipulated that if any patient was 'pertinaciously refractory' the physician was to be informed so that he could give directions on the measures to be taken.[170] At Exeter the requirements were more specific: no patients were to be chained or handcuffed without the knowledge and approval of the physician or apothecary.[171] Rules also included precautions to be taken where patients were confined, with a standard requirement that the feet of people lying in straw, chained, or subject to other coercion were to be regularly examined and rubbed, and covered with flannel during cold weather, in order to guard against mortification of the extremities.[172] The general inclusion of these injunctions in printed rules provides some indication of the ubiquity of mechanical restraint.

Lunatic hospitals were routinely equipped with all the paraphernalia of restraint, such as chains, leg-locks, hand-cuffs, strait waistcoats, and straps and belts made of leather, as well as specially adapted chairs and beds. The precedents had been well established at Bethlem, and also at the Norwich Bethel where an inventory of 1743 showed the presence of a range of instruments.[173] This became the accepted norm for public as well as privately managed institutions. In 1750, prior to the opening of St Luke's, the governors sanctioned the purchase of twelve pairs of handcuffs and twelve leg-locks.[174] Surviving inventories give some indication of the extensive reliance on restraint implements. At the Hereford Asylum in 1801, prior to its passage into private hands, there were at least four pairs of handcuffs, eight leg-locks and two strait waistcoats, as well as a number of straps.[175] At Exeter in 1803 there were ten strait waistcoats, ten sets of hand and leg irons, and a dozen straps, in addition to four crib beds equipped with fastenings.[176] In both cases the implements would have potentially provided for a significant proportion of the patients who were there at the time.

The preparations made for the opening of the Leicester Lunatic Asylum in 1792, under Arnold's guidance, were particularly interesting and significant. He provided the infirmary governors with a fully costed list of what he considered necessary to equip the house to receive twenty patients. All forty-eight windows, 'for the safety of the patients', had to be well secured with 'strong, iron bars placed pretty close to each other'. There were to be twenty strait waistcoats, or one for each patient. In addition, Arnold wanted 'a great number of appropriate Straps, Locks, and other fastenings and securities', as well as 'Chairs of a peculiar construction for particular purposes', and a special room to house the instruments when not in use. The governors felt they could not afford it all and agreed to equip the asylum initially for only ten patients. They did, however, accept the principle of ample restraint implements to provide for each patient.[177] Arnold had argued for the creation of a veritable fortress with prison features. The enforcement of close control and security evidently far outweighed the sorts of therapeutic considerations that he elucidated in 1809.

The system established at Leicester was far from unique. Samuel Tuke in 1815 complained that security was the only object in 'most of the older erections of this kind', manifested in cells with massive bolts on the doors and high shuttered windows.[178] St Luke's certainly conformed to this description, despite attempts to distance it from practices at Bethlem. The 1815 investigations were kinder to St Luke's than to its illustrious predecessor but none-the-less revealed a regime that made extensive use of strait waistcoats, chains, handcuffs, and so on. In some cases, patients were both put in a strait waistcoat and manacled because, according to Thomas Dunston, 'they will burst the waistcoat out and tear it to pieces'. For this reason he favoured chains as the safer and more effective option, but he was also mindful of other incidental advantages: 'the idea of the chain is half the confinement to them, and it gives them more liberty, and does not stop the circulation of the blood'. He was forced to admit that 'outrageous maniacs' were sometimes chained in their beds for several days at a time.[179] Dunston's views on the preferability of chains and manacles were shared by Dr Alexander Sutherland. In the warmer months, in particular, he thought a strait waistcoat could have an irritating effect by making the patient too hot. Handcuffs were 'decidedly better' in keeping him 'uniformly cool and comfortable', whilst manacles had the advantage of not interfering with the circulation. Sutherland, however, was careful to point out that he would not use irons in one of his private establishments, for 'it creates alarm perhaps of the friends, and would not be submitted to', considerations that clearly did not apply in St Luke's.[180]

The picture drawn by Edward Wakefield was rather more stark than Dunston's somewhat defensive evidence. On the several occasions he had visited St Luke's he had seen 'persons chained to a bed nearly naked', covered with only a rug, in many of the cells. Apart from those chained in their cells, there were others 'violent without being noisy' chained in the day rooms. He conceded, however, that these measures were often necessary, citing one particularly graphic case in illustration:

> There is a very remarkable man in Saint Luke's, a sailor, who is leg-locked and handcuffed, but I do not make this remark at all by way of complaint, as I consider him one of the most dangerous animals whom I have ever seen; fastened as he is, he flies at you, and would seize anybody within his reach with his teeth. Such a man as that must be chained.[181]

Although fairly critical, by and large Wakefield considered the regime at St Luke's to be relatively mild and benevolent in comparison to that at Bethlem.

The actual extent to which mechanical restraint was employed at St Luke's is difficult to gauge accurately, as figures given were very probably under-stated. In 1807 Dunston said he could not be definite but thought that three patients out of twenty required a 'continuance of coercion', due to a disposition to 'injure themselves or others'.[182] With about 300 patients in St Luke's at the time, this would mean at least forty-five under regular restraint. In 1816, when asked how many were chained or in strait waistcoats, he was again unable to be exact but suggested that 'there may be sixteen or eighteen, or there may be two or three more'. He denied that any were confined without clothes, contrary to what Wakefield had observed.[183] Little had changed by 1827, to judge from evidence given by the hospital's resident apothecary John Thomas. If anything the amount of restraint had increased for, although Thomas claimed that 'we restrain them as little as possible', he conceded that there would be perhaps four or five patients under restraint in each gallery containing about thirty-five patients, which meant about forty in total. When asked what modes were employed, Thomas confirmed that 'We have almost all that are in use', including handcuffs, muffs, strait waistcoats, and belts. Patients were also frequently chained in their beds.[184] In this respect, St Luke's was evidently still far from being considered a model establishment, though viewed as considerably superior to the much criticized Bethnal Green madhouses.

The situation in the provincial lunatic hospitals was almost certainly comparable to that at St Luke's, with the use of mechanical restraint part of normal practice as their printed rules indicated. At the Newcastle Lunatic Hospital, for example, restraint had been employed extensively from the outset. Before the reforms of the mid-1820s, the house was characterized by 'chains, iron-bars, and dungeon-like cells', with coercion said to be the basis of the 'medical treatment'. When the new physician took over in 1824, there were found to be 'six miserable wretches' chained down in their 'melancholy cells'.[185] Edward Wakefield's positive impression of the regime at the Exeter Asylum in 1814 was not diminished by his observation of the use of chains. Although he saw a young man who was constantly handcuffed and lying naked upon straw, he accepted that this was appropriate as he demonstrated 'extreme maniacal violence' towards others and had 'extraordinary athletic powers'.[186]

Wakefield's tacit acceptance that the use of chains was justifiable in certain types of case reflected the perspective of even the most reform-minded commentators. In their exposures of abuses and ill-treatment in public and private asylums, the select committees of 1815 and 1816 highlighted what appeared to be the excessive use of mechanical restraint, though they did not condemn the practices in themselves. As Andrew Scull has argued, any debate was around what were the most humane methods of restraint rather than whether it ought to be used at all.[187] Moves towards actual abolition were still twenty years away. However, attempts were being initiated to reduce some of the associated harshness and discomfort. At St Luke's, for example, there was a recognition that chaining to the bed should be time limited, and that those confined should be able to change positions or move around as freely as possible.[188]

Thomas Arnold had also been considering the most satisfactory methods of restraint, arguing that coercion should always be 'as gentle and easy, as the nature and degree of the violence of the insane person will admit.' Unlike Dunston, he favoured the strait waistcoat or otherwise strong straps that were 'purposely made soft and easy'.[189] However, Arnold's reservations against the use of chains were highly conditional, for he suggested bluntly that they that they 'should never be used but in the case of poor patients, whose pecuniary circumstances will not admit of such attendance as is necessary to procure safety without them.'[190] Elsewhere, tentative steps were being taken toward making the means of restraint more palatable. At the York Asylum, despite Dr Charles Best's clear failings in other areas, he had actually reduced the use of chains toward the point of abolition by 1814.[191] At the Liverpool Asylum, by the early 1820s, the governor John Davis claimed to have achieved success 'in abolishing the cruel system of using chains, iron leg-locks, and hand-cuffs'. These were replaced by leather items, considered to be 'less irritating' to the feelings of the patients and 'milder and more humane' in their application, as well as 'greatly superior' in assisting recovery.[192]

It was at the infant Lincoln Lunatic Asylum, however, that the most studied moves were made to abate the more problematic aspects of mechanical restraint. In the first few years after opening in 1820, it operated on a basis at least as custodial as any of its predecessors. All manner of restraint was routinely employed, including strait waistcoats, muffs, belts, chains, handcuffs, leg-irons and restraint chairs. One of the three physicians, Dr Edward Charlesworth, started protesting about the system as early as 1821, arguing that greater classification would reduce the need for some male patients to be 'kept almost constantly in manacles'.[193] Important reforms began in 1828, driven by Charlesworth. The restraint instruments were removed from the keepers and collected together, their use to be closely monitored. Some of the heaviest iron implements and several strait waistcoats were destroyed.[194] A singular event in February 1829 proved particularly influential. A pauper patient, William Scrivenger, died from strangulation while strapped to his bed in a strait waistcoat. After the resulting outcry, the use of the waistcoat was discontinued unless on the specific instruction of the physician.[195] A serious process of introspective examination followed among the governors and physicians. One casualty was the asylum's 'director', Thomas Fisher, whose dismissal in 1830 was partly brought about by his stubborn resistance to Charlesworth's drive to reduce the amount of mechanical restraint.[196] With a new director in post, Charlesworth and his supporters speeded up the process. Considerable progress had been made several years before the dramatic announcement in 1838 that its total abolition had been achieved, for the first time, at the Lincoln Lunatic Asylum.[197]

CONCLUSIONS

By the end of the eighteenth century a new system of therapeutics was being forged in the treatment of mental disorder, in response to what Andrew Scull has referred to as the changing 'cultural meaning of madness'.[198] That system brought together the use of physical treatments which aimed to address symptomatology and the application of psychological techniques that were intended to influence behaviour. These developments were taking place in a context where considerations of curative treatment had still to be balanced against a requirement to ensure the safety and security of the sufferer, of those looking after him, and of the wider public. As yet, the more custodial aspects of institutional care were not being seriously questioned. Treatment and management continued to comprise overt elements of control, manifested most clearly in the continuing utilization of the paraphernalia of mechanical restraint. However, there was a perceptible shift emerging in the balance between custodial and curative considerations. As Anne Digby has acknowledged, the ostensibly new approach of the York Retreat reflected developments elsewhere, not least in the lunatic hospitals, under the influence of physicians like Battie, Currie and Ferriar.[199]

From the physicians' perspective, insanity constituted another 'disease' to be diagnosed and treated by medical means. The treatments that mad-doctors were employing did not constitute a break with the practices of their predecessors. The drugs they prescribed, and most of the physical methods they applied, were drawn from the established armoury of physic and surgery. Practitioners were exhibiting, however, a greater preparedness to experiment and to take risks in dealing with the manifestations of mental disorder. This showed itself in a pragmatic approach where different remedies were tried in sequence. If one seemed to work, it was continued; if it failed, it was discarded and replaced by another. Although emetics and purgatives continued to be the drugs of first recourse, others were gaining currency, notably opium-based sedatives and digitalis. Physical treatments also combined the use of established techniques, like bleeding and blistering, with the employment of newer therapies, notably those utilizing warm or cold water. At the same time, mad-doctors were demonstrating a growing awareness of the subsidiary psychological effects of some of their medical treatments, as they found that actual behaviour patterns could be influenced or even altered in response to the experience of the treatment.

The conscious use of reinforcement techniques in association with physical treatments was steadily bringing together the approaches identified respectively as those of 'medicine' and 'management'. By and large, the reinforcement offered was negative, concentrating on the inducement of fear and apprehension. It was, however, in the area of what became known as moral management that paradoxical influences were most evident. Concepts of authority, ascendancy, discipline and obedience retained a central place in patient management. Concurrently, other notions were gaining ground — that patients should be treated with 'tenderness' and 'indulgence'; that their self-esteem or sense of honour should be promoted; and, that they should be encouraged to develop self-control and to display rational behaviour. Intrinsic to this aspect of management was the relationship established between practitioner and patient, whereby direct influence could be exercised toward the goal of recovery.

In retrospect, the continuing prevalence of mechanical restraint appears to rest uneasily with the new therapeutics. However, until the second decade of the nineteenth century, the use of restraint and coercion was barely questioned and remained intrinsic to the management both of the institution and of the individual disturbed patient. Any debate was only over the most effective, humane methods that ought to be applied. Advocates of restraint were seeking to accord it a therapeutic rationale, whereby it provided the necessary controls to prevent self-injurious behaviour or the expenditure of excessive energy, in order to enable restorative treatment to be applied. As practitioners saw it, there had to be order and control for the institution to function effectively, and for them to implement their medical treatment and their management techniques. The individual patient was perceived to require a sense of security, an understanding of boundaries, and a clear recognition of the authority of keepers and medical men, if the conditions were to be right for effective treatment. This did not mean necessarily that management and treatment systems had to be overtly repressive, but the circumstances were undoubtedly present which meant that they might be.

7 Aspiration to actuality

By the end of the eighteenth century, voluntary hospitals funded by public subscription had become a recognized and important part of the national fabric. Lunatic hospitals, although only one part of the network, were of growing significance as existing ones expanded, new ones continued to open, and others were in the stages of planning and projection. The model that had emerged was perceived as worthy of imitation. Sir George Onisephorus Paul had adopted it for the proposed lunatic asylum for the western counties, and then more significantly in 1807 for his influential blueprint for a national system of public asylums.[1] Nevertheless, by 1800, despite the optimistic indications, significant problems were beginning to be revealed. These culminated in the exposures of practices at the York Lunatic Asylum, which formed one of the main elements of the investigations of the Select Committees on Madhouses of 1815 and 1816. The situation at York had developed into a national scandal, and the Asylum was probably singular in the extent of its defects, but it was no isolated phenomenon. Difficulties of a not dissimilar nature had emerged at several of the other lunatic hospitals.

The lunatic hospitals had been established with proclamations of ideals of humanity and of the rescue, relief and restoration of troubled souls. There is nothing to suggest that these intentions were anything other than honestly conceived and genuine, tempered as they may have been by 'mercantilist' goals of enabling men to return to productive work or women to their proper place in a functioning domestic economy.[2] Humanitarian and curative objectives were regularly re-stated and reiterated. In 1782, speaking about the York Asylum, Rev. R.B. Dealtry commented that 'all is Gentleness, Attention and Comfort; each Struggle of Reason is watched, is encouraged' and that for those 'sad objects' who could not be cured 'a place of retreat is given, free from trouble'.[3] Even as late as 1813, with the storm about to break, the asylum's annual report assured the public that:

> The objects it has in view are, To secure to the patients admitted, the moral and medical treatment, best suited to their several cases.
> — To afford them the accommodations, the comforts, and the humane

attentions, which so materially assist in effecting the restoration of reason. — To prevent them from committing any acts of violence either on themselves and others. — To seclude them from public observation and the intrusion of idle curiosity...[4]

It would only be a short time before these principles, probably still sincerely held by the asylum's governors, were shown to have been seriously compromised.

There were several reasons why good intentions, at York and elsewhere, did not completely translate into practice. These included both material factors and those related more directly to human failings. The fabric of buildings naturally deteriorated, at the same time as higher standards were being expected regarding their appearance, facilities and equipment. Apart from the unique case of St Luke's, finance was a significant problem at all the lunatic hospitals, and the pursuit of economy in operation would have been a necessity even if not viewed as intrinsically worthwhile. The management and containment of disturbed and, at times, violent patients brought its own difficulties for medical men with limited treatment options and for staff who were poorly remunerated, lacking in status, and subject to the normal range of human failings. Less tangible, though not without influence, were the manifestations of inefficient, complacent, neglectful, oppressive, or downright corrupt practices that seemed to become inevitable as Georgian institutions progressed from infancy to maturity and beyond, which Roy Porter comprised under the banner of 'Old Corruption'.[5]

To summarize the whole development of the voluntary movement in lunacy provision as characterized by abuses, corruption and deterioration would, however, be a serious misrepresentation. The therapeutic efforts of men like Ferriar at Manchester and Currie at Liverpool, and the genuine endeavours of many well-intentioned lay people, paid and unpaid, challenged negative generalizations. The foundation of the new voluntary lunatic asylums at Exeter and later at Lincoln and Oxford, as well as the joint asylums at Nottingham, Stafford, Gloucester and Bodmin, showed the continuing dynamism of the voluntary model.[6] Published and unpublished statements of the numbers of people 'cured' or 'relieved', with all their shortcomings, confirmed that the lunatic hospitals were achieving at least some demonstrable success. Even the fact of the exposures and scandals showed that they were not completely closed institutions, impervious to scrutiny and change. There were even positive benefits to emerge from the evidence of decline, dilapidation and deterioration, for in most cases revelations would precipitate fundamental reform.

Lunacy 'reform' is an issue that has aroused considerable interest, and some controversy, among historians. Kathleen Jones made it the central reference point in her pioneering study of the development of psychiatric institutions and the laws that governed compulsory detention and treatment. Her approach was to view the reform movement, composed mainly of evangelical Christians and Benthamite radicals, as providing a logical and robust humanitarian response to abuses that had been clearly exposed.[7] Jones' later critics, led by Andrew Scull, have tended to characterize her work as a 'whiggish' and over-simplified account of steady progress from a harsh and repressive system toward one that was ostensibly humane and enlightened. Scull's more critical position, whilst acknowledging the real advances that were made, viewed lunacy reform as one aspect of the imposition of a more subtle and sophisticated set of controls on socially deviant individuals.[8] More recent scholarship has related lunacy reform to wider currents within English society. Akihito Suzuki has interpreted it in the context of changing attitudes to insanity and the means employed to manage it in both private and public spaces.[9] Michael Brown has placed asylum reform within a wider politico-cultural context, as a representation of factional conflict.[10] Whatever the perspective adopted, there has been a recognition that the investigations and reports of the various parliamentary select committees, and particularly those of 1815–16, were of great significance both in providing evidence of the state of provision for the insane and also in shaping public attitudes toward the problems and issues.[11]

GROWTH AND DEVELOPMENT

In the half-century or so after the founding of St Luke's, as shown in chapter five, there was a steady expansion in the numbers of patients resident in the voluntary lunatic hospitals. In order to provide for the growing demand, new accommodation had to be made available. Normally this would mean the construction of extensions or additional buildings. However, the central urban location of most of the lunatic hospitals placed inevitable limits on the amount of expansion feasible. Most of any additional accommodation provided in the provincial institutions was, consequently, by means of piecemeal alterations and additions. Ultimately, any significant growth would require re-location to a less congested area, solutions that were eventually adopted in Liverpool, Leicester, and Manchester, as well as in London.

The governors of St Luke's, with the benefit of their ample financial resources, were able in the 1780s to undertake a wholesale replacement of the original hospital by means of the construction of a much larger edifice. By 1800, St Luke's contained slightly in excess of its capacity of 300 patients, a level not subsequently exceeded.[12] Although the building itself had been subjected to criticism from the outset because of its formidable prison-like aspect, there was no doubting its imposing presence on the edge of the City of London, with *St Luke's Hospital for Lunaticks* strikingly emblazoned in large letters in the stone-work across the entrance in Old Street.[13] To most observers it was a 'noble hospital', with its exterior possessing a 'simple grandeur'. Its interior, consisting of four stories if the

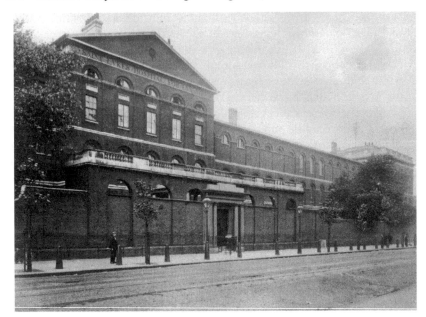

Figure 7.1 St Luke's Hospital, late 19th century.
Source: Camden and Islington Mental Health and Social Care Trust. My thanks
　　to Sylvia Mannering, Medical Records Manager.

basement was included, was seen to 'serve as a model for every similar charity'.[14]

In the provinces, growth had taken place on a much more *ad hoc* basis. At the Manchester Lunatic Hospital a series of enlargements began in 1772, to be followed by others in 1781, 1788, and early in the nineteenth century.[15] Separate accommodation of a higher standard, with gardens attached, was created for private patients and the division was made into lunatic hospital and lunatic asylum.[16] Further expansion, however, was restricted by its location, and by 1801 the physicians were recommending that the lunatic hospital be moved. However, the infirmary trustees resisted and opted instead to carry out some improvements on the buildings.[17] The move out to Cheadle had to wait almost fifty years; in the mean time, any prospect of significant expansion was checked.[18]

The York Lunatic Asylum, though located quite near the city centre, was not constrained by any lack of space for expansion.[19] The original building, designed for fifty-four people, remained adequate to meet the needs for several years. Its critics, though, continued to maintain that it was over-ostentatious: to Rev. William Burgh it was a 'sumptuous edifice', and Rev. William Mason compared it to 'the villa of a nabob'.[20] The first extension, for twenty-four patients, was constructed in 1788.[21] A further large detached block was added in 1800, with a view both to providing additional accommodation and to 'keeping the different classes of patients distinct from each other'.[22] It was this annex that was destroyed in the disastrous fire of 1813, by which time the asylum contained almost 200 patients. The period of enforced overcrowding that ensued contributed materially to the institution's acute difficulties. In the context of the subsequent radical reform programme, a replacement two-storey building for female patients was provided in 1817, leaving the main building for men only. Further accommodation was added over the next few years, first for private patients and then in 1828 for fourteeen people deemed particularly violent or refractory.[23]

Some expansion clearly took place at the Newcastle Lunatic Hospital, in order to cater for the doubling in patient numbers between 1767 and 1810, though its exact nature is unclear.[24] The Exeter Lunatic Asylum saw significant growth within a few years of its opening. In 1804 a new wing was added, branching off from Bowhill House at a ninety degree angle, thus creating a 'T' shaped building which could accommodate at least fifty patients. With its 'salubrious' semi-rural location, its three gardens and three airing grounds, in all comprising several acres, Exeter may well have served as an example for later public asylums of the advantages of a site away from the town. The building itself and its facilities gained the admiration of the lunacy reformer Edward Wakefield in 1814.[25] The further addition in 1823 of a new block parallel to the original transformed it into an 'H' shape and raised the asylum's capacity to 70 patients.[26]

Elsewhere in the provinces growth was rather less marked. At the Leicester Lunatic Asylum, with its unusually long gestation period and financial constraints that prevented complete opening in 1794, the building never actually provided for its original planned capacity of twenty patients; a maximum of eighteen was reached in 1830.[27] The alternatives offered by Arnold's private asylum, and then the opening of the Nottingham Asylum in 1811, presumably siphoned off much of the potential demand. The Liverpool Lunatic Asylum had also been subject to initial financial difficulties, and it took a few years for the numbers of patients to build up. It had, though, been constructed large enough to contain up to seventy people, and no further expansion was required.[28] If more capacity had been needed, the constricted site in the city centre would not have been conducive to further building. However, expansionary pressure was not the primary reason for the move a mile or so up the road in 1831, for the new asylum was built with space for only sixty-four patients.[29] By this time, it would seem, most of Lancashire's pauper lunatics were going directly to the county asylum at Lancaster.

In addition to the growth in the existing provincial lunatic hospitals, there was also further capacity becoming available in the new voluntary and joint asylums that opened after 1810. The Lincoln Lunatic Asylum was able to provide places for at least fifty patients when it opened in 1820.[30] Additions and alterations in 1827-8 allowed for a further twenty patients, as part of a general reorganization of the building which promoted greater classification and separation of different types of patients.[31] The original plans for the Oxford Lunatic Asylum envisaged a building large enough to accommodate between sixty and one hundred, though the actual capacity on opening in 1828 was nearer forty.[32] At the Nottingham Asylum, the first based on the joint endeavours of subscribers and county justices, the voluntary element accounted for about half of its initial capacity of eighty people.[33] At Gloucester, the original intention was also that half of the 120 patients would come under the charity, though it took several years for anything like this to materialize.[34] The proportions allocated at Stafford and Bodmin were rather smaller.[35] Between them, however, the various new public asylums contributed a significant addition to charitable provision.

THE DETERIORATING INSTITUTION

According to the physician Sir Andrew Halliday in 1828, St Luke's Hospital was 'much worse than useless as an hospital for curable lunatics'. It possessed 'none of the advantages' by then considered necessary for promoting recovery, and was 'only fit to become a prison for confirmed idiots'.[36] By that time the building was more than forty years old. It had been constructed to designs and standards deemed modern and relevant in the 1780s, when conceptions about the nature of insanity and the proper means to manage and treat the lunatic were very much in a state of transition. Although the second St Luke's had itself been extremely influential on the design and construction of the new group of county asylums that had followed the Act of 1808[37], the development of the newer institutions was rendering St Luke's and the other lunatic hospitals increasingly obsolete. Changing norms and expectations combined with the natural processes of institutional deterioration to contribute to the sorts of difficulties highlighted in the 1815 select committee's deliberations. At most of the provincial lunatic hospitals matters descended toward some sort of crisis point which would lead eventually to a major upheaval.

The original St Luke's structure had been noted for its plainness and functionality. The quality of its construction was probably also rather basic. Within a few years the building was showing clear signs of deterioration. By the early 1770s, money was regularly being spent on 'curing the House of Bugges'.[38] In 1778, after less than thirty years of operation, the building was observed to be 'so much decayed' as to require replacement.[39] When the second St Luke's opened in 1787, it was a model institution. Inherent shortcomings, nevertheless, became increasingly apparent. Not least, its city location on Old Street placed a severe constraint on alterations or expansion, and restricted any possible intention to develop outside recreational or occupational facilities for the patients. The only significant structural development was a considerable increase in the number of iron bars on the windows in December 1813.[40] Edward Wakefield visited several times in 1814 and commented on 'radical defects', including many cells with unglazed windows and 'increasingly offensive' internal privies, as well as the absence of facilities for classification. Furthermore, adjoining the hospital was a parish burial ground: from the galleries the patients could hardly avoid 'almost daily instances of interment occurring under their very eyes'.[41] The equally critical asylum architect James Bevans remarked on the inadequate size of the day rooms, poor sanitation, and the lack of protection against fire, as well as the complete absence of heating or ventilation in the 'the sleeping apartments'.[42] The inexorable process of decline was evident well before Halliday's strictures in 1828.

The problems associated with the ageing of buildings would be compounded by the damage caused by some patients. Difficulties of one sort or another became manifest in virtually all the provincial institutions. It took only two years from opening in 1799 for John Nash's Hereford Lunatic Asylum to become 'delapidated', attributed partly to mismanagement as well as to 'the defects of the original building'. The Hereford Infirmary governors took the opportunity offered to support their inclination to offload the awkward appendage.[43] The Leicester Lunatic Asylum had been in trouble almost from the outset, its situation hardly helped by ten years of disuse. Even when it did open in 1794, the infirmary governors could only afford to accommodate ten patients, rather than the twenty originally intended. The fact that it never achieved its anticipated capacity was more to do with the poor condition of the building than any lack of demand. By 1815 the deterioration was considerable. One of the men's airing courts had been closed due to being unusable. The privies were in a bad state, with one being used as a rabbit house. Some cell doors had no locks, and four men's cells were considered 'scarcely habitable'. The ventilation of the men's ward 'appeared to be very imperfect', and conditions on the women's ward were similar. The accommodation allowed for no separation of different types of patient, with the maniacal and 'those of a milder cast' intermingled. The resignation of the ageing Dr Arnold as the asylum's physician, and the offer to him of the role of 'Physician Extraordinary', suggested that he was the focus of much of the blame for the general picture of neglect and decline.[44]

The difficulties that arose at the Manchester Lunatic Hospital were rather less pronounced. Its administrative integration with the main infirmary, and its high profile central location, provided some insurance against scandal and malpractice. In fact the location was the main source of its problems, preventing expansion and severely restricting facilities for patients' outdoor exercise. By 1800, in the wake of a series of fatal fever epidemics in the Manchester district, the infirmary physicians were becoming increasingly concerned about the lunatic hospital's siting, arguing that 'its situation is become highly objectionable, in consequence of the great increase of building, and population in the Neighbourhood.' They claimed also that its 'plan' was 'very defective'. Their proposed remedy, to convert the building into fever wards and to erect a replacement 'at a convenient distance from the Town', provoked intense argument.[45] No action followed, however, and the lunatic hospital was left to struggle along on its congested site, its patient numbers in steady decline.

The decline into squalid dereliction that occurred at the Newcastle Lunatic Hospital was a long and gradual process. The 1767 house retained the essence of its original character for more than half a century. Externally it may not have appeared to Sir George Paul in 1810 like a 'place of confinement', but inside there were all the common custodial features. Although fairly enthusiastic about aspects of the hospital's operation, there were defects apparent even to Paul. Due to its age it was not, he conceded, 'an object of architectural imitation'. He was not impressed with the day rooms, the airing-yards, and the adjoining cells for violent patients. Paul was also unsure about the emphasis of the physician Dr Wood on a strict system of discipline and his consequent rejection on principle of 'chearful galleries'.[46] There was significant degeneration over the next few years, much of it blamed posthumously on the unfortunate physician Dr Glenton who died in early 1824, having himself only succeeded Wood after his death in 1822. A scathing report to the Newcastle Common Council in June 1824 concluded that the lunatic hospital was 'entirely unfit for the accommodation of lunatics of any description or rank of life'.[47] The deficiencies were later detailed graphically:

> it then consisted of one airing Court for females, with a damp and most unwholesome day Room and 21 Sleeping Rooms without fire places and in the most wretched state. In another Court were placed, detached from the principal Building, nine sleeping Cells for males with a Day Room, and nine Cells for females without a Day Room. The whole were without Fire places and the Court yard was common to both sexes. There was no other access to these miserable apartments than from the open Court. These Cells were damp, unventilated, cold, filthy, and in short unfit habitations for any human being.[48]

According to another contemporary, the building had been 'ill calculated' for its purpose. It was frequently 'crowded to excess', with little attention given either to cleanliness or proper ventilation. The combination of 'chains, iron-bars, and dungeon-like cells' gave it all the worst characteristics of a prison, whilst being 'highly injurious to their health and lives'. Many of the patients' cells were 'close, dark, cold holes (less comfortable than cow-houses)'.[49] These were descriptions matching the worst exposures of madhouses or asylums by the select committees of 1815 or 1827.

The notorious case of the York Asylum and the abuses that occurred there has, along-side the exposures of Bethlem Hospital, become almost emblematic of the perceived evils of the *ancien regime* in institutions for the insane.[50] The censures of York emphasized the failings of individuals rather than a general institutional decline. It was evident, though, that phenomena apparent elsewhere were also manifesting themselves in the York Asylum. The architect James Bevans in 1815 described it as being 'on a very bad construction throughout'.[51] Having been built in the 1770s, it was predictable that defects would become increasingly apparent. Critical comment before 1813, however, appears surprisingly lacking. Indeed, Sir George Paul was generally complimentary after his 1810 visit, observing that the asylum 'is constructed with more regard to comfort, and has less the appearance of a place of restraint, than any other house, for the like purpose, which I have visited.' He had wanted to emphasize the advantages of the voluntary model, but he did have to concede that the airing yards were 'inconveniently situated', being detached from the day rooms, and that they contained no seats or covered walkways.[52] Paul's generally positive perspective was at considerable variance to what Samuel Tuke described only three or four years later. He portrayed a crowded and turbulent scene of listless patients herded unsupervised into grim and gloomy day rooms, deprived of light from the high shuttered windows, and with any considerations of cheerful surroundings sacrificed to the needs of security.[53]

The deficiencies of the York Asylum were greatly magnified by the effects of the destructive fire of 1813. The resulting concentration of patients into the original building precipitated a rapid deterioration of its physical fabric. Many patients were required to sleep two in a bed. Larger numbers had to be crowded into already defective airing courts in which there was little shelter, or into inadequate and airless day rooms. Throughout much of the building an 'utter neglect of ventilation and cleanliness' was apparent, rendering many parts 'disgusting and unwholesome'. One particular area, known as the 'low grates', was especially 'damp and offensive'; the supply of light to several of its rooms was blocked by the presence outside of pig-styes 'and other disagreeable offices'.[54] It would have been erroneous, however, to attribute all these problems to the fire and its consequences.

By the same token, the fire alone could not have accounted for what Godfrey Higgins and his associates dramatically 'discovered' in the basement. The appalling state of the allegedly hidden group of cells to which they gained access, and of the patients they saw in the day room, provided perhaps the most evocative scenario of the whole York Asylum scandal. A picture of darkness, stench, filth, and nudity, with piles of urine-soaked straw and air holes blocked up with excrement, gave zealous reformers the ammunition to convince both local and national opinion that dreadful things had been happening.[55] The apparently plausible protestations of Dr Best that these were the cells used specifically for dirty or violent patients, and therefore could hardly be expected to be in a clean and healthy state despite daily cleaning, failed to convince the critics and the sceptics.[56]

The dirt, squalor and neglect that had overtaken the York Asylum were part of a wider malaise, the other symptoms including a range of corrupt and abusive practices. In essence, there had been a steadily escalating failure of effective governance over a number of years. The seeds for the crisis of 1813–15 were probably laid as early as the 1780s, with Dr Alexander Hunter's achievement of dominance over the management and philosophical ethos of the asylum. His upholding of the interests of the non-pauper poor against those of parish paupers appears to have been largely driven by sincere conviction. The same could conceivably be argued for his promotion of the admission of lucrative private patients, with the profits used to subsidize the admission of the poor. Hunter's critics may have overstated their case in accusing him of promoting his own selfish interests and of trying to operate the asylum like a private establishment, but he did clearly consider himself entitled to some personal gain, even if this compromised some of the founders' original principles. Later claims by Godfrey Higgins, based on access to financial records, indicate that Hunter became greedy in his old age, for he was earning very large sums from the asylum, amounting to several thousand pounds per year. Much of this money came from the comfortably accommodated 'physician's patients', for whom he paid a fixed price to the asylum whilst receiving substantially more from their individual fees. Hunter's successor Dr Charles Best continued on a similar basis, sometimes making even larger amounts of money.[57]

The arrangements that had emerged at York were certainly unique among the voluntary lunatic hospitals. Although the charges against Hunter of seeking private emolument or even of establishing a 'lunatic hotel' had been stridently refuted by him and his supporters, by the early years of the nineteenth century he had really done just that within an enclave of the asylum.[58] Many of the dangers anticipated by his critics of unregulated private practice within a public institution had come to pass. The governors had effectively turned a blind eye to the insidious development. Any semblance of visitation and inspection by the governors had been abandoned in the 1790s, leaving Hunter in complete control. By the time that Dr Best inherited the mantle, there was a virtual management vacuum. Although Best accepted some limited responsibility for the overall direction of affairs, the day to day running of the asylum was in the hands of the apothecary Charles Atkinson and the elderly steward William Surr.[59] Without effective monitoring by the governors or the physician, they were unable to prevent the permeation of a whole range of corrupt, neglectful and abusive practices among the junior staff, which sullied the proper operation of the institution.

The public exposures demonstrated malpractice at every level within the York Asylum. This was clearly not a situation of sudden onset. One of the leading activists among the reforming contingent, Samuel Nicoll, astutely assessed matters in the context of a natural process of institutional development and decline:

I do not charge this conduct to harshness or apathy on the part of the Governors —they did nothing, because they believed there was nothing to be done — the institution had attained the last stages through which human institutions are commonly found to pass — in the commencement there is energy — to energy confidence succeeds — to confidence abuse — the opinions and feelings of the Governors were in the second stage, the institution itself on the very close of the last — for sooner or later, from abuse reform will spring. A more compact or extended concatenation of confidence has rarely been known — the Governors had confidence in the Physician — the Physician had confidence in the inferior officers — the officers in the keepers — the keepers in the patients themselves; who were hence rarely troubled with either attention or restraint.[60]

As Nicoll demonstrated, the governors had become complacent. After the defeat of Hunter's critics in 1795 there was no serious questioning of the asylum's management. The governors had thenceforth found it convenient to accept outward appearances and to 'think all was right', not noticing any indications to the contrary.[61] Based on his analysis, the whole saga had unfolded with a degree of inevitability.

The erosion of effective governance identifiable at York was a phenomenon also becoming manifest at other lunatic hospitals. The situation at Newcastle had long been unusual, and its status as a public lunatic hospital had become questionable. Apart from in its early years, subscriptions never provided a significant element of its finances. Solvency had been maintained by the fees paid by parishes and patients' relatives, augmented by a small annual contribution from Newcastle Corporation. There was no formal body of subscribers or governors. The corporation maintained some supervisory interest, but direction and management was essentially by the respective physicians, Hall, Wood and then Glenton. As at York, charges were made that the physician was using his role as a means of private profit. Public concerns were raised in 1817, to be followed eventually by an investigation in 1824. The corporation concluded that the lunatic hospital was operating like a private asylum, though without any of the statutory licensing protections available if that had been its formal status.[62] The absence of clarity on responsibility for the hospital's management was undoubtedly a significant factor in the process of steady decline into squalor and neglect that occurred.

At St Luke's there was no exposure of flagrant abuse comparable to York and Bethlem. However, the extreme longevity in post of Thomas Dunston, and his over-riding control of most aspects of the hospital's operation, brought a risk of complacency. Whilst Dunston continued to receive much credit for his work, there were inferences that the regime at St Luke's was becoming stale and that established practices were stagnant. There were also insinuations of Dunston's involvement in activities bordering on the corrupt, in the form of a business relationship with a private madhouse and, more particularly, close links with Thomas Warburton of the

Bethnal Green madhouses, whence many uncured St Luke's patients were transferred at the end of their year's stay.[63] Sir Andrew Halliday's strong criticisms in 1828 of the hospital's fitness for purpose came at the end of Dunston's half-century of dominance over the affairs of St Luke's.

Both at York and at St Luke's there was an over-concentration of power into the hands of a single individual. This also proved to be the case at the Leicester Asylum, where problems in its management became apparent. The infirmary governors were content to leave direction of the asylum's operation to Dr Thomas Arnold, whose high reputation as a mad-doctor was unassailed. He managed to prevent any arrangements for regular visitation and inspection by the governors. Serious questions do not appear to have been asked about the asylum's management until early 1814, some twenty years after it opened. The governors had to check the constitution of the infirmary in order to discover that their responsibilities related equally to the asylum. They proceeded to arrange a visit by a deputation, then to be followed up on a quarterly basis.[64] The poor state of affairs uncovered led on to a wider investigation by a special committee. It concluded that the asylum had hitherto been 'for the most part closed against public inspection; and the authority of some of its officers has been left undefined.'[65] The governors were clearly embarrassed by the evidence of general neglect. They had to acknowledge a degree of responsibility and felt impelled toward taking steps to re-exert control.

Oversight by the governors of a lunatic hospital attached to an infirmary was always problematic, when most of them had limited interest in the insane or in the treatment of mental disorder. The tendency would be for them to concentrate on the concerns of the main hospital. It could take a scandal, such as that befalling the Liverpool Asylum in 1825, to propel the lunatic institution into the consciousness of the board of governors. The exposures, which even reached the national press, involved the excessive and capricious use of mechanical restraint and unchecked acts of violence, cruelty and harassment toward patients by the keepers. It was apparent that the former matron, Mrs Davis, was at least complicit in some of the malpractices whilst her husband, the nominal 'governor', was evidently unable to exercise adequate control of the situation. Despite John Davis' rebuttals of the worst allegations, there was still plenty of ammunition for particular individuals with grievances against the infirmary governors and physicians. The affair clearly illustrated avoidance by the governors and negligence by the physicians, entailing risks to patients, to staff, and to their own reputations. The crisis did at least, however, lead directly to a review of the asylum's governance.[66]

In virtually all of the lunatic hospitals, deficiencies in the structures and practices of management had been exposed, with undesirable consequences that threatened to compromise and undermine the original ideals of the founders. Samuel Nicoll's characterization of an inevitable cycle of institutional decline proved a close approximation to what actually occurred in several places, as well as in York itself. The dictum later propounded by Nicoll that 'the keeper must himself be kept' addressed the fundamental part of the problem.[67] Physicians and salaried officers were in positions of power, with opportunities to make benevolent use of that power, or to abuse it if there were not proper mechanisms for regulation and oversight. These considerations applied equally to the more junior staff who exercised much of the direct personal contact with the patients.

THE SERVANT PROBLEM

The role of the servants or keepers, the onerous and demanding nature of their duties, and the material rewards they received, were considered in chapter three. With pay and conditions as they were, institutions for the insane were unlikely to attract staff of the highest calibre. The attributes of those employed tended to consist of physical strength and an imposing presence, as well as the sort of personality that accepted authority and was prepared to impose order and discipline.[68] Their role was, nevertheless, crucial in the implementation of both the custodial and the curative aspects of the lunatic hospital's regime. For most inmates the keepers were the real face of the institution, with the power to determine the nature of their experience as patients. Many, doubtless, did the job to the best of their ability, with diligence, humanity and compassion. Others, however, evidently took the opportunity to be callous, oppressive and exploitative. Staff imperfection was far from being a new problem. As Andrews has shown in regard to eighteenth-century Bethlem, up to one fifth of its basketmen and maidservants were dismissed for misconduct.[69]

It was often the case that the lowly keeper would be 'entrusted with the sole management of the unhappy sufferer'. However, critics considered that few were 'worthy of such a charge'.[70] A body of evidence accumulated which focused a good deal of the blame on junior staff for the shortcomings of both private and public asylums. According to 'Medicus' in 1806, most keepers, even those in the 'best regulated institutions', were 'sullen, unfeeling and cruel' and treated patients worse than animals. The keeper's conduct was 'only guided by caprice' and he was liable to make indiscriminate use of 'the lash'.[71] Samuel Tuke drew similar conclusions, though in more measured language, recognizing that the circumstances in which the keeper was placed might leave him with few alternatives. Where there were large numbers of patients, with little differentiation as to their individual condition, a lack of occupation, and few staff to supervise them, 'it becomes necessary for the attendant to rule...with an iron hand' to keep them in order.[72] Having 'uncontrolled authority', Tuke suggested that the 'inferior servant' would be inclined to make his own working life easier and keep 'personal exertion' to a minimum. The temptation toward 'neglect, oppression, and cruelty' was continual.[73]

There were certainly examples to support those sorts of contention, and not only from the York Asylum. Problems arose in the early years of the Manchester Lunatic Hospital. In October 1773, only six months after being appointed, John Hilton was dismissed and then prosecuted for 'sundry Misdemeanours', along with the governor Richard Wilding. Not long afterwards, strict new rules were imposed regarding, among other things, the use of 'Stripes or Beatings' and forcible baths without an order from the physician.[74] A few months later, allegations of 'shocking barbarities' at Manchester appeared in the London newspapers, following a parliamentary speech by Thomas Townsend in the debate on the bill for regulating madhouses. According to Townsend, the fatal stabbing of a keeper by a patient was followed by the recruitment of a new keeper from London, 'who prescribed a severe beating to any of them that should appear disorderly', resulting in one patient being beaten to death and another sustaining a broken arm in trying to defend him. The infirmary trustees declared the allegations to have 'no foundation in truth', though they conceded that a keeper was 'unfortunately Stabbed by one of the patients', that a new patient had committed suicide, and that another patient did have his arm broken by a blow from a 'servant'. The physicians signed a somewhat unconvincing declaration that the keepers in the lunatic hospital 'have never to our knowledge, treated the Patients with any undue Severity, without being justly reprehended and punish'd by the Board of Trustees'.[75]

In 1809, the death of another Manchester patient, Richard Browne, led to a murder charge against a keeper, William Bell, who spent several months in prison on remand. Browne had suffered fractured ribs and a broken breast-bone which, before his death, he reportedly alleged had been inflicted by Bell. The evidence, however, was inconclusive. Bell had worked in the lunatic hospital for five years and was given 'a good character for his humanity' by Dr Winstanley, one of the physicians, as well as by John Sanderson, the governor. He was acquitted after the judge had directed that the hearsay evidence of a dying man could not be accepted.[76] Nevertheless, some unanswered questions remained.

The records of St Luke's Hospital reveal only occasional instances of misconduct by staff. In 1761, Richard Hay was dismissed for having 'used some of the Patients ill by beating them'.[77] In 1810, Edward Dowding was sacked for seducing a female patient whilst delivering beer to her gallery.[78] Serious accusations were made in 1817 by George D'Aranda, the house apothecary, that the patients were 'knocked about like Beasts in Smithfield'. On investigation, the allegations were deemed to have been malicious and without foundation and he was forced to resign.[79] A claim the following year, after the death of an incontinent, apoplectic female patient, that her posterior had been 'beat rotten' and that there were marks of 'very severe Stripes', was also proved to be unfounded.[80] The lack of other recorded evidence, however, tends to suggest a low incidence of serious abuses at St Luke's.

The same could hardly be said for the York Asylum, to judge from the literature emerging from the scandals of 1813–15. The problems were not of sudden onset. In 1797, for example, the keeper James Backhouse had made a female pauper patient pregnant. He evidently acknowledged paternity and paid maintenance to her parish overseers, but was never dismissed.[81] The investigations of 1814 revealed a whole catalogue of abuses by the keepers.[82] These included various incidents of violence towards patients, in the form of beatings, kicking, and general manhandling, as well as widespread neglect. Reverend John Schorey, a curate admitted to York Asylum three times, was physically abused on several occasions, particularly by Benjamin Batty. In response to his wife's remonstrance that, as a clergyman, he should not be pushed and kicked, Batty retorted that 'he's now no more than a dog'.[83] It was evident from the extensive allegations made against staff that a culture of violence and intimidation had become embedded, and that there was something approaching a rule of fear by the keepers. Dr Charles Best's protestations to the select committee that he never permitted them to strike or flog the patients, and that he had introduced regulations stating that ill treatment would lead to dismissal, were not accorded much credence.[84]

Part of the problem at the York Asylum appears to have been a complete erosion of supervisory structures, partly due to the failing health of William Surr, the elderly steward. The consequence was 'the almost total want of subordination and vigilance'. The keepers had effectively seized much of the power within the institution. Little notice was taken of the housekeeper Mrs Atkinson (the apothecary's wife), who nominally controlled the keys. For several years she had been unable to prevent the keepers going and coming as they chose, and had long since stopped locking the back door at night. She had also lost control, to one of the male keepers, of the keys for the house's beer and bread, and could only exercise 'partial and contested authority', much of it usurped by the female head keeper.[85] The plight of the head male keeper, Thomas Blackadder, was at least as unfortunate. His authority had been completely undermined by the other keepers who, according to the enquiry report, 'refused to obey his orders'.[86] Rules restricting leave of absence were being ignored, with several keepers often simultaneously out late without permission. Corruption, verging on extortion, was endemic. The four male keepers divided payments of seventy-four guineas from male patients of the 'superior classes', and the female keepers shared £25 from private women patients. There were also profits from the sale of manure and 'cast clothes'.[87] The resulting situation demonstrated how far keepers could misuse their power and position. Doubtless they had taken some cues from their superiors and from a climate in which self-interest, contempt for authority, and abuse and exploitation flourished.

There was evidence that some of the transgressions at York were replicated elsewhere. At the small Leicester Asylum the keepers seem also to have begun to act with relative impunity. Their working conditions, it must be said, were far from favourable. From the outset, they were expected to sleep two to a bed.[88] By 1815, with the amount of habitable accommodation having reduced, the keepers had to sleep either in the kitchen or in the day room.[89] Even after building alterations and reforms in the asylum's management, they were evidently prone to various malpractices. In 1816, they were collectively admonished for neglecting the patients and one man, William Pack, was dismissed after proof of 'repeated acts of cruelty'.[90] A few months later, in June 1817, all four keepers were 'solemnly reproved' after a woman was found confined 'in a dark and damp cell', with a threat that immediate dismissal would follow any repetition of 'such cruelty'.[91] However, their general conduct continued to cause concern to the infirmary governors. In August, they had to be directed to stop their practice of keeping fowl and rabbits. In November the two male keepers, John Tompkin and Thomas Hurst, were again 'solemnly reproved', this time for endangering the security of patients by allowing them to go too far from the asylum on their walks.[92] An advertisement in 1822 for a new male and female keeper gave some indication of the shortcomings that the governors had to address. Those appointed would require 'Characters as to Sobriety, Integrity, and command of temper'.[93]

An apparently entrenched system of abusive and oppressive practices by the Liverpool Lunatic Asylum's keepers was exposed in 1825, following the investigation of claims made by some articulate middle class patients, several of whom were military officers. Evidence was also taken from two former female keepers, Jane Carlow and Mary Jones. The alleged misbehaviours included unprovoked violence, intimidation and taunting. The patients claimed they had been beaten, kicked, pushed around, and forcibly and painfully restrained for having expressed dissent. The allegations concerned particularly the two male keepers, Alfred Doward and James Ashurst. The testimonies of Carlow and Jones also directly implicated the matron, Mrs Davis, who had recently resigned. Doward, who was eventually dismissed, came in for particular criticism in the enquiry. Even his apologist Dr Renwick conceded that his qualities lay mainly in strength and fortitude, whilst suggesting revealingly that Doward's 'roughness of manners and expressions' rendered him suitable to work only with the 'poorer sort' of patients.[94]

Even at the newly established Lincoln Lunatic Asylum, the inadequacies of staff soon became apparent. In its early years, most of the male keepers found themselves in trouble. In September 1820, the director Thomas Fisher complained to the governors that John Kelp had refused to obey instructions, and two months later he was reprimanded and threatened with dismissal for 'improper conduct'.[95] In September 1821, a female nurse received a 'severe reprimand' for 'culpable neglect' and misrepresentation after the death of a patient.[96] In October 1822, Thomas Ashlin, previously warned for intoxication, was reprimanded for allowing a patient to escape. However, he proved a habitual offender, for in April 1823 he let another patient escape whilst inebriated. The board of governors still only gave him a final warning, but his inevitable dismissal came in October after repeated complaints of drunkenness and 'other misconduct'.[97] In September 1826, a male and a female keeper were both dismissed for unspecified misconduct.[98] In May 1827, following complaints from Dr Cookson, William Hurd was dismissed and another keeper, Edward Hill, was reprimanded, apparently for lack of vigilance in preventing a patient's self injury.[99] In March 1828, John Green was sacked for 'improper drinking'.[100] Evidently, the standards and personal qualities of many of those appointed at Lincoln were poor. Regular reprimands and dismissals persisted over the next few years, continuing through into the era of non-restraint.[101]

There is, of course, a danger of imputing a disproportionate amount of blame onto the subordinate staff for the lunatic hospitals' increasingly evident deficiencies. It was inevitably the case that bad practices by servants or keepers were much more likely to be recorded for posterity than any more praiseworthy contributions. The lack of direct evidence for better practices does not mean that they did not routinely occur. There were doubtless men and women who diligently upheld the letter and the spirit of the institution's rules, having entered the work with genuine humanitarian considerations. Even one of the much-maligned keepers at the York Asylum in 1813, Henry Dawson, was acknowledged to have shown considerable heroism by risking his life to rescue patients from the great fire.[102] Some years earlier Margaret Hughes, a keeper at St Luke's, had sustained serious injuries and put her own life in danger to save a patient who had set herself on fire.[103] The keeper Abraham, at the Manchester Lunatic Hospital in 1801, showed genuine Christian understanding and fellowship to the patient Hugh Williams, offering him 'sweet council' as they 'meditated on the word', despite the risk of losing his position.[104] It was, however, the dishonest, corrupt, neglectful or abusive activities that were more likely to be reported and to influence perceptions of the quality and demeanour of those who staffed the lunatic hospitals.

REFORM AND IMPROVEMENT

The exposures of conditions and practices at the York Asylum and elsewhere had a profound effect on public opinion. They occurred within the context of a rising movement that questioned existing methods of dealing with madness and advocated major reform.[105] The campaign for asylum reform was, in turn, only one small part of a far wider movement for the correction of abuses and for the reform both of the political system and of penal, educational, and philanthropic organizations. The inspiration came from evangelical Christians, as well as from Benthamite radicals.[106] Among the lunacy reformers' early achievements had been the deliberations and conclusions of the 1807 select committee. Significantly, that committee had promoted the practices of St Luke's and the funding arrangements of the York Asylum as being worthy of emulation.[107] The ensuing Wynn's Act of 1808, arguably the first major practical accomplishment of the lunacy reform lobby, provided for the incorporation of the voluntary model into a county institution, by giving authorities the option to establish a lunatic asylum on their own, or in conjunction with other counties or voluntary subscribers.[108] Crucially, however, the Act signified that government, both central and local, now had to acknowledge and accept a key role in ensuring appropriate provision for the insane. Over the next few years, several counties embarked on the establishment of an asylum, the first to complete being Nottinghamshire, Bedfordshire, Norfolk, and Lancashire.[109]

It was in this climate of reforming zeal that Samuel Tuke's seminal *Description of the Retreat* appeared in 1813.[110] In a straightforward account of both the physical fabric of the small voluntary Quaker institution, and of its treatment and patient management techniques, Tuke provided practitioners with a model that was both transparently humane and attractively simple. This provided a gift for the reformers, who now had a template against which to appraise practices in other asylums, public and private. The book also had the incidental, and maybe unanticipated, consequence of precipitating the crisis of York's other voluntary institution for the insane. Dr Charles Best's interpretation of the *Description* as being a thinly disguised attack by insinuation on his asylum, and his ill-judged decision to go into print in protest, only served to suggest to the city's intellectual and reforming elite that there might be something to hide behind the York Asylum's grand facade.[111] The inquisition and the rush to judgment soon followed.

Nationally, the lunacy reformers' next major milestone was the collection and presentation of a large body of detailed evidence in the reports of the select committees of 1815 and 1816.[112] The deficiencies of Bethlem Hospital and the York Asylum received most of the critical coverage. They were contrasted with practices at St Luke's and the new county asylum at Nottingham, and at some of the better managed private madhouses. Although the select committees may not have produced tangible legislative results, their influence on attitudes was considerable. The evidence received extensive publicity, and helped to set standards around what would be considered acceptable or unacceptable in institutions for the insane. It also led directly on to more localized examination of facilities for lunatics, and in some cases to the implementation of measures for reform.

In York, the righteous indignation excited by Godfrey Higgins, Samuel Tuke and others would bring about a thorough cleansing of what Higgins characterized as the 'Augean stable' and 'this *filthy temple* of MOLOCH' well before the select committee had even met.[113] Following the initial revelations in 1813 a large number of interested people paid their subscription of £20, which entitled them to become governors. These included, as well as Godfrey Higgins, Samuel and William Tuke, Jonathan Gray, and

Samuel Nicoll.[114] A committee of enquiry was set up, which produced a thorough report on the asylum's affairs.[115] It not only detailed and analyzed recent occurrences but also provided a comprehensive summary of events since the original plan for a lunatic hospital in 1772. The fund of background information was supplemented by the publication a few months later of Gray's *History*, which also laid considerable stress on the manner in which past incidents and developments had contributed directly to the debacle.[116]

In the wake of all the revelations, accusations and insinuations, it was inevitable that heads would roll. The intemperate Godfrey Higgins published a letter to the governors in August 1814, proclaiming 'I call for justice', and urging them to attend a general meeting and take retribution on behalf of those people who had allegedly died violent or unrecorded deaths in the asylum.[117] At the ensuing court of governors, the apothecary Charles Atkinson and his wife, the matron, were both dismissed, along with the steward William Surr and several of the keepers. Dr Best retained his post for a while, though he eventually resigned, ostensibly on grounds of ill health, in 1815.[118] At the end of 1814, Higgins was able to declare that 'the institution is now placed on the best footing, as to management'.[119] New appointments were made, a comprehensive revised set of rules, regulations and safeguards was adopted, and the replacement of the destroyed annex was set in train.[120] A new physician, Dr Baldwin Wake, was appointed and the reforming group, including the Tukes, Nicoll and Gray, continued to retain a close involvement with the asylum's affairs. Over the next few years the York Asylum was established on similar footing to the better managed county asylums, such as that at Wakefield which served the West Riding from 1818.[121]

The 1815/16 select committees' activities and findings proved very influential at several provincial lunatic hospitals, even though their affairs had not been directly investigated. At Leicester the infirmary governors acknowledged explicitly in 1815 that their internal 'Special Committee' had taken advice from various sources, including the 'directors of similar institutions' at York and Manchester, but 'above all from a Report of the Committee of the House of Commons'.[122] The Leicester committee dealt first with the more blatant material deficiencies — ensuring sufficient light and pure air, proper exercise facilities, and only one patient to each cell. The main part of its recommendations, however, covered managerial aspects. It called, in particular, for 'vigilance and activity' by the governors to guard against the recurrence of abuses that had become endemic:

> The Asylum has been hitherto for the most part closed against public inspection; and the authority of some of its officers has been left undefined. Your Committee propose that this mistake shall be rectified, being of opinion that Institutions of this nature should be conducted on the broad principle of challenging, entreating, and securing

the most careful, watchful, and vigorous inspection which is consistent with prudence.

Probably with Dr Thomas Arnold in mind, it was declared that 'no Officer should be invested with an unascertained & uncontrolled power.' The main remedy proposed was a reassertion of control by the infirmary governors, with a view to proper oversight and the elimination of any suspicion of 'fraud, oppression, and barbarity.' Medical supervision was henceforth to be by the infirmary's medical officers, rather than left to 'the kind offices of those who may have devoted themselves exclusively to this particular species of medical practice' (i.e. Arnold).[123] In recognition of the asylum's inadequacy to meet the needs of the city and county, however, it recommended that the only real solution would be for the governors to join with the magistrates to develop a county asylum under the 1808 Act.[124]

The conditions that had developed at the Newcastle Lunatic Hospital were conceivably still more deplorable than those at Leicester. Although the select committee did not have such immediate influence in bringing about actual change, the climate of opinion created brought an acknowledgement that there were problems to address. In October 1817 the city council sought advice on the 'peculiar situation' of the lunatic hospital and on how it might be placed on a 'proper footing'.[125] However, it was another seven years before any proper action was taken. Following Dr Glenton's death in 1824, the mayor established a committee to investigate and report. Its damning conclusions led to drastic changes. By the end of 1825, a total of £4400 had been spent on 'magnificent improvements', and it was proclaimed that the 'Establishment has been made one of the most perfect in the Kingdom'.[126] Those improvements included proper ventilation and heating arrangements, considerably expanded exercise and recreation facilities, enlarged galleries, new day rooms, boarded floors, water-closets and baths, and a new kitchen and wash-house. The sleeping accommodation was completely overhauled, so that 'even the paupers are accommodated with warm, clean, separate beds', though there were still two or four in a room. Staffing levels were increased and the worst forms of mechanical restraint, by chaining people down, were abandoned.[127]

The managerial changes implemented at Newcastle, however, bore more resemblance to Hereford in 1801 than to Leicester in 1815. Without a base of subscribers to the lunatic hospital, the Newcastle Common Council was forced to consider commercially viable options. Following advice taken from the York Asylum, they saw part of the solution in providing some accommodation for 'patients of a higher rank in life', their payments to be applied 'to relieve and lower the payments of the poor'. However, the council could not justify the expense of directly financing and managing the operation itself and opted to raise the necessary funds by taking a loan, the interest to be repaid by the physician Dr Smith. A fifty-year lease at a nominal rent was granted to Smith, with additional land allocated to provide recreation for the patients. The entire management of the hospital was devolved to him, subject to regular inspection by the council and the town's magistrates. The council retained the option to set minimum payment rates for poor patients, as well as some nomination rights. It continued to pay its annual subscription of ten guineas 'for the sake of better preserving their station as patrons of the hospital'.[128] In effect, the transition of the New-castle Lunatic Hospital to a private asylum, albeit closely regulated by the local authorities, had been formally confirmed.

Elsewhere, the processes of review and reform were less pronounced. The select committees had been relatively kind to St Luke's Hospital, which probably induced a further degree of complacency among its governors and officers. As a consequence, no significant changes would take place there for many years.[129] At Manchester, new rules were published with a view to improving practices.[130] However, the spatial restrictions on sig-nificant alteration to the building provided a continuing justification for minimal change. At Liverpool, the scandal of late 1825 probably spurred on developments already in the offing. The removal of the asylum to a new building in 1831 gave the opportunity to implement a practical pro-gramme of reform.[131] By this time, however, the voluntary lunatic hospi-tals were increasingly finding themselves in the shadow of the larger and more favourably regarded post-1808 county asylums. The newer lunatic hospitals, at Lincoln and Oxford, could only gain their reputations by the implementation of approaches that made them distinctive — at Oxford by the exclusion of paupers, and at Lincoln by the liberalization of patient management techniques, leading ultimately to the abolition of mechanical restraint.[132]

THE GOAL OF CURE

The achievement of cure, in the form of a 'restoration of reason', became the great *sine qua non* of the lunatic hospitals. To an extent the impetus toward cure emanated from the broader voluntary hospital movement. The successful treatment and recovery of hospital patients was publicized as an encouragement to the public to subscribe. As argued by scholars such as Mary Fissell and Kathleen Wilson, from a 'mercantilist' perspective of economic utility the cure of the sick was invested with a wider significance, by enabling people to return to productive labour and relieving their fami-lies from dependence on poor relief.[133] Although similar motives of a wider social interest may also have influenced the projectors of lunatic hospitals, they were rarely stated explicitly. That there was, however, a continuing preoccupation with 'cure' is the only conclusion that can be drawn from the regular presentation to subscribers and the wider public of returns and statistics that dwelt on the numbers who were discharged cured, in relation to the numbers admitted. The constitution of St Luke's, whereby people were discharged after a year if uncured, was the prime representation of the curative goal.

Statistics detailing admissions, discharges and cures were notoriously problematic. Discharges would normally be divided into those 'cured', or 'recovered', and those 'uncured'. The actual nature of cure was, however, rarely defined. The term was probably used to comprise both cases of complete recovery and those of elimination of the more distressing symptoms. A recognition of differences in degree was apparent with the emergence of a new category of discharged 'relieved' or 'improved' on some returns.[134] In publishing their statistics, governors were seeking to demonstrate the success of their institution, and the consequent justification for donations or subscriptions. Prestige was also at stake, as they sought to show that their own hospital or asylum was proving particularly successful at achieving cures in comparison to other places, both public and private.

The performance of St Luke's Hospital, along with Bethlem and the York Retreat, tended to be set up as the standard against which others were judged. The St Luke's figures of admissions and discharges, both in manuscript records and in published returns showed a gradually falling rate of cures. In the first ten years of the hospital's operation, the numbers of recorded cures were approximately fifty per cent, with 410 discharged cured out of 832 admitted onto the curable list.[135] Ten years later, in 1772, the percentage cured had fallen to under forty-seven per cent, or 846 out of 1816 admitted.[136] This trend was to continue both in the old and the new hospitals. The 'average' figures given by Thomas Dunston to the 1807 select committee showed annual admissions as 263, of which 108 were discharged cured and one hundred uncured, with the rest either having died or been discharged as being 'unfit' for various reasons.[137] This gave a percentage cure rate of forty-one percent a figure that was exactly replicated in returns for the years 1811–13 that Dunston submitted to the 1815 select committee, based on 358 cures set against admissions of 870.[138]

The cure rates claimed at the Manchester Lunatic Hospital initially matched those at St Luke's remarkably closely. Figures published in 1773 for the first six years of its operation showed ninety-seven cured out of 193 admitted, or virtually fifty per cent.[139] By 1781, the percentage had fallen to forty-eight percent, based on 458 admissions and 220 discharged as cured.[140] Returns for 1801 showed that there had been a continuing steady fall down to forty per cent. Out of a total of 1521 admissions since 1766, 615 had been discharged cured. However, a further 211 people (or fourteen per cent) were described as having been discharged 'relieved'.[141] That category had not been enumerated at St Luke's, thus rendering direct comparison somewhat problematic. Published returns for the York Lunatic Asylum in the late 1780s and 1790s also contain a 'relieved' category, and show similar trends. 466 patients had been admitted from the asylum's opening in 1777 until the beginning of 1788. Out of those 213 (forty-six per cent) had been discharged cured and 116 (twenty-five per cent) relieved.[142] By

1793 the claimed figures represented an increase in cures to forty-eight per cent (or 360 out of 745), with a fractional fall in the numbers deemed relieved.[143] It has to be questionable, however, whether the York Asylum was really producing a higher incidence of patient recovery, or whether Alexander Hunter was determining 'cured' and 'relieved' differently to his colleagues at the Manchester Infirmary.

The difficulty of drawing clear conclusions due to the vagaries of recorded figures is illustrated by the information to be gained from the Liverpool Infirmary's annual reports. In the year March 1794–95, twelve patients out of twenty admitted (sixty-six per cent) to the lunatic asylum were discharged as cured, as well as a further four (twenty per cent) relieved.[144] These exceptionally high figures were based on small numbers of patients and were hardly sustainable. In the year 1795–96 there had been a sharp fall in those cured to twenty-two out of sixty-three admitted (thirty-five per cent).[145] However, by the end of the 1790s, cure rates were reaching over fifty percent — from forty-nine per cent in 1797, to sixty per cent in 1798, and sixty-one per cent in 1799.[146] In the early 1800s, the recorded numbers discharged as cured were unusually high, rising from sixty per cent in 1801 to eighty per cent in 1802, and then eighty-four per cent in 1808.[147] It is unclear, though, whether this was related to distinctive recording methods or to some dramatic therapeutic achievements. By 1813, the figures had settled at a more realistic fifty per cent (thirty-four admissions, seventeen discharged as cured).[148] Thereafter they fell below forty per cent, although they were distorted by the particular circumstances of large numbers of patients being transferred each year after 1818 to the county asylum at Lancaster.[149]

The outcomes of admissions to the Newcastle Lunatic Hospital from its opening until 1817 have been fortuitously preserved in a single surviving document, which was probably produced for a review of the hospital's affairs being undertaken by the city's Common Council.[150] The data has been summarized in Table 7.1. The figures show a cure rate of between thirty to thirty-five percent for the first three decades of the hospital's existence, which was low compared to the other lunatic hospitals. This may have been related to the governors' early acknowledgement of a responsibility to accept 'incurable' patients.[151] Between 1796 and 1806 the rate fell even further, to below one quarter. However, in that decade there was a significant increase in the numbers of those discharged as 'better', a category presumably corresponding to that of 'relieved' elsewhere, which would seem to suggest some changes in the way records were being kept. Over the following decade the numbers of those discharged 'better' fell back, while the percentage of cures had risen to a more respectable thirty-nine percent. The accompanying report sought to illustrate the recent relative success of the hospital in comparison to others such as Bethlem, St Luke's, and the York Retreat, despite its acceptance of incurable patients and even those close to death.[152] In the circumstances, and in the light of the prevalent conditions in the hospital, its figures appeared reasonably impressive.

Table 7.1 *Newcastle Lunatic Hospital — admissions, dischrages, and cures, 1764–1817*

	Admissions			Discharges		
Years	Numbers	Cured	% Cured	Better	By Desire	Dead
1764–74	172	60	35	10	74	28
1774–84	286	86	30	2	139	59
1784–94	258	85	32.5	19	107	44
1794–6	64	21	33	9	23	9
1796–1806	280	68	24	55	76	66
1806–17	402	158	39	49	69	67

Note: The category 'By Desire' refers to those discharged either by the wishes of their 'friends' or of their parish.
Source: Newcastle City Library, 'An Account of Patients Admitted, Discharged, and Remaining at the Lunatic Hospital, Newcastle Upon Tyne, From July 18th, 1764, to July 18th, 1817'.

Newcastle was not alone in seeking to place the most favourable interpretation on its discharge figures. The directors of the various lunatic hospitals set out to demonstrate their respective therapeutic achievements. Within a few years of opening, the governors of the Exeter Lunatic Asylum stated 'with the highest satisfaction' that they had 'good grounds' to believe that the number of people 'restored to the enjoyment of reason', in proportion to those admitted, had 'much surpassed that of any similar establishment'.[153] Although Dr Thomas Arnold did not make such a direct claim for Leicester, he did assert in 1809 that a cure rate of two thirds was being achieved both at his private asylum and at the Leicester Lunatic Asylum. An unspecified additional number were 'sent home *relieved*'.[154] If accurate, these contentions would have meant that the Leicester Asylum was the most successful of all the lunatic hospitals in the achievement of cures. The statistics published by the infirmary governors do actually appear to confirm Arnold's claims, an indication perhaps of the greater effectiveness of a small institution with an unusually high staff-patient ratio.[155] Allowance, however, has probably to be made for commercial hyperbole, with Arnold seeking both to demonstrate his own therapeutic credentials and to promote the advantages of Belle Grove Asylum.

It remains problematic to measure the success of the lunatic hospitals on the basis of their claimed achievement of cures, due to the limitations of the figures themselves and the difficulties of interpretation. Historians have tended to express skepticism about claims of high rates of cure, with suggestions that many of those people deemed cured or recovered were in fact examples of spontaneous remission.[156] This is clearly a factor to be taken into account in any assessment. However, the assumption by many later practitioners and commentators that few were successfully treated in Georgian institutions for the insane, and that those who recovered did so despite rather than because of the treatment they received, is too simplistic. At best, it is based on a misplaced retrospective judgment, emanating from altered concepts of the nature of therapeutics and standards of practice. The combination of the assorted statistical evidence, with all its limitations, and the published case material of several reputable practitioners provides sufficient evidence that some patients at least did make good recoveries and were enabled to return to family and community.

CONCLUSIONS

In virtually every case, the lunatic hospitals had been established amidst currents of idealism and optimism. The founders and subscribers had been actuated by the genuine aspiration to provide relief to distressed and damaged people. As time went on, however, good intentions became compromised, and even in some cases betrayed. Some of the problems that emerged were almost unavoidable. Buildings that had been up-to-date when constructed became outmoded and suffered the natural processes of decline toward obsolescence. They were subjected in most cases to particularly heavy wear and tear from the insane inmates, accelerating the onset of decay. Prominent locations in or near city centres compounded the difficulties by confining patients within restricted spaces and offering limited scope either for expansion or for provision of outdoor exercise and recreation facilities.

The gradual deterioration of material surroundings was accompanied by the consequences of failures of governance. As Paul Langford, Anne Borsay and others have shown, the voluntary hospital model was intended to replace the inefficient, oligarchic direction of institutions with a system that was more open, democratic and accountable, administered by men who conspicuously sought to exercise social responsibility.[157] Nevertheless, as time went on, management regimes within some of the lunatic hospitals descended into complacency and sterility. The shortcomings became clearly evident, and not only at York where the whole fiasco was laid before an incredulous public. Weak and supine governors, intent on maintaining their privileges but often with limited knowledge or interest in mental disorder, avoided sullying themselves with direct involvement in the ongoing management of their institutions. The checks and balances on medical men and officers that lay governors might provide were generally not imposed, and assertive individuals were apparently able to exercise unfettered power. At best, benign neglect was the likely consequence. Even at St Luke's, with its high public profile, Sir Andrew Halliday in 1828 had to condemn the 'close borough system' on which it was managed.[158] The analysis of the York lawyer Samuel Nicoll, concluding that there was an inexorable systemic process of deterioration and decline in a public institution, proved extremely apposite to lunatic hospitals.[159]

The maintenance of financial solvency was essential. However, without the sort of ample subscription base enjoyed by most voluntary general hospitals and by St Luke's, the provincial lunatic hospitals operated within a significant constraint. Treatment and care, as well as board and lodging, had to be paid for by weekly charges. The desire of subscribers and governors to provide subsidized care for the deserving non-pauper poor meant that further monies had to be raised. The solution of accepting private patients and charging them commercial rates introduced a clear business element into the operation of voluntary institutions. This posed serious risks of a fundamental alteration to their ostensibly charitable character. Where there was oversight by the governors of a parent voluntary hospital, as at Manchester and Liverpool, reasonable safeguards existed against any malpractice. Elsewhere, however, the door was opened to the temptations and corruptions of private practice. At the York Asylum profiteering and exploitation became endemic at all levels. Although it provided the most blatant examples, the undesirable consequences of the profit motive were evident elsewhere, as at Newcastle where the situation was finally regularized by a constitutional change. St Luke's itself was far from immune to dubious practices, for some of Thomas Dunston's extraneous activities were indicative of motives that were not entirely charitable.

The keepers and servants of the lunatic hospitals, untrained, ill-equipped and poorly paid as they were, could hardly be other than prone to human frailties. In a context of inadequate governance, as at York, where supervisory structures had become eroded, insubordination, malpractice and abuse could flourish. Its junior staff took their cue from what was happening in the higher echelons and indulged themselves at the expense of the institution. Once again York was the extreme example, but the shortcomings of some keepers were evident in other places. Nevertheless, attempts to attribute a high degree of responsibility to the people in the most subordinate roles for the developing ills of the lunatic hospitals were inappropriate, especially as many undoubtedly carried out their duties to the best of their ability.

According to Samuel Nicoll's construction of the organic life cycle of an institution, the descent into the depths of abuse and malpractice would be followed naturally by fundamental reform.[160] Historians have concurred that the exposures of scandalous conditions and practices at York and Bethlem were, indeed, the precipitants of a process of reform. There has been less agreement, however, on its meaning and significance. According to interpretation, asylum reform was either a humanitarian attempt to eliminate proved abuses or a pragmatic response which sought to render a failing system workable and to maintain the status quo.[161] The most recent analysis by Michael Brown, based on the circumstances at York, is particularly persuasive. His contention is that the socio-political context was paramount, with the public disputes about the asylum's affairs reflecting a more profound ideological struggle between competing class and interest groups.[162] It was almost certainly the case that similar dynamics prevailed at Leicester, where the arguments over reform in the asylum occurred in the context of a revival of the conflict between the Arnold and Vaughan camps.[163] Whichever version of events is adopted, 1815 has to mark a clear watershed in the development of public, as well as private, lunatic asylums. Rapid transformations subsequently occurred at York and elsewhere, based on renewed standards for the management of institutions and of their inmates.

The high aspirations of the lunatic hospitals' founders were always going to be difficult to fulfill, even if the institutions had consistently operated efficiently. With all the evident deficiencies that became increasingly apparent, however, there were severe hindrances to provision of an effective service. Cure and recovery, nevertheless, remained the primary objectives. The consistently replicated claims by governors and medical men that around half of the people who were admitted went on to enjoy a good recovery do not appear to have been greatly affected by the state of the institutions or their regimes at any given time. This can either confirm the elusiveness of the concept of cure or, alternatively, indicate that it was the actual processes of removal and incarceration that mattered, rather than what actually took place within the walls of the hospital or asylum.

Conclusion
The restoration of reason

The Liverpool physician and campaigner Dr James Currie contended that the ultimate objective of a lunatic hospital was 'restoring reason itself'.[1] This ambitious goal exemplified an apparently unbounded optimism that characterized the liberal intellectual elite in late eighteenth-century England. The remarkable transforming developments occurring in the commercial and industrial fields, as well as in the built environment, were being matched by the emergence of a sophisticated pattern of responses to all manner of social and cultural needs. Prominent among those responses was organized collective charitable endeavour, utilizing the mechanism of public subscription, which constituted one of the truly great legacies of the Georgian era. Arguably, its most effective representation was the impressive network of voluntary hospitals, which by 1800 covered the whole country.[2] The physical evidence, in bricks, mortar and the printed word, of the additions to the national fabric and of what had been accomplished over five or six decades made even grand aspirations like Currie's appear achievable.

As well as being among the most significant material representations of 'urban renaissance', the voluntary hospitals were also an important element of the emerging 'public sphere' in England. Their construction and development indicated an acknowledgement of public responsibility for dealing with the consequences of social and economic ills, and particularly their effects on the health and well-being of the poorer classes.[3] Within the developing voluntary hospital system, provision for lunatics became an increasingly important constituent. However, the 'public' nature of the lunatic hospitals was conceivably yet more pronounced than that of the general hospitals, for their establishment was essentially a direct counterpoise to the growing prevalence and influence of private provision for the insane. Private madhouses, with their connotations of exploitation, greed, and abuse of the defenceless, clearly created a degree of unease greater than was associated with private provision in other areas of medically related practice. Under-pinning the case for the lunatic hospitals was a conception that the care of the insane should be a public responsibility, and this received its formal expression in the 1807 Select Committee on Pauper and Criminal Lunatics and Wynn's Act of 1808.

Despite their proclaimed philanthropic ideals the lunatic hospitals could not exist in a vacuum, unsullied by commercial considerations and influences. With the notable exception of St Luke's Hospital, their funding bases were consistently too weak to enable them to function like other voluntary hospitals and provide free care for the poor. Arrangements for charging for board, lodging and treatment became accepted practice from the outset. The need to balance the books remained a key determinant both of admission policies and of institutional organization. Whilst the lunatic hospitals had been ostensibly established to provide for those who were 'poor and mad', financial considerations necessitated the extension of the facilities to people in what were euphemistically described at York as 'easy circumstances'.[4] The rationale was, of course, put forward that those of moderate means were also entitled to charitable attention, as well as protection from the depredations of greedy and unscrupulous madhouse keepers.[5] At York, and to a lesser extent at Exeter, the doctrine was extended to make a positive charitable virtue out of the attraction of wealthy patients, in order to earn profits that could be applied to subsidize the care of the less well off. Whatever the justification advanced, the consequence was that commercial influences spread throughout, typified by the widespread implementation of arrangements for the payment of physicians that were quite out of keeping with what happened in the voluntary general hospitals. In its extreme the result was the actual privatization of a public facility, as occurred at Hereford and later at Newcastle.

The lunatic hospitals, particularly those in the provinces, came to be in an increasingly paradoxical position. They were, on the one hand, intimately connected with the wider voluntary hospital movement of which they formed a distinct part. At the same time they had an uneasy, though unavoidable, relationship with the private sector. The drive to attract paying patients brought the lunatic hospitals into direct rivalry with the madhouses. Governors and physicians employed discourses of moral principle and of medical integrity to assert the superiority of their institutions over those directed by profit-seeking private proprietors. Nevertheless, the charitable lunatic hospitals had little alternative but to operate alongside the madhouses, as part of an emerging 'mixed economy of care'.[6] Those who directed their affairs found themselves in a complex situation as participants in two alternative systems of provision, with quite different orientations and motivations.[7]

Whilst the lunatic hospitals were part of a wider medico-economic network, their status as public medical institutions was endorsed by their direct associations with voluntary general hospitals, in origins and in management arrangements. Two distinct models of lunatic hospital became established — the integrated, and the independent. At Manchester and Liverpool, and to a lesser extent at Leicester, the connections with the parent infirmary remained intimate. Their lunatic hospitals continued to be managed and operated as an integral part of the main institution, with a sharing of administration, financial direction, catering, pharmacy services and, most importantly, medical oversight. Where the lunatic hospital had been constituted as an independent entity, the influences of predecessor general hospitals were, none-the-less, apparent in the formation of rules and of management structures. Whichever the model, the control and direction of affairs were based on a process of ongoing negotiation, particularly between lay governors and medical men. Historians such as Mary Fissell and Anne Borsay have demonstrated the complexity of changing power relationships within the voluntary general hospitals.[8] In the lunatic hospitals the position was normally more straightforward, for the lack of knowledge of insanity and treatment exhibited by most governors meant an easier concession of responsibility to the physicians or, in the case of St Luke's Hospital, the salaried manager. This relinquishment carried the inherent risk that the checks and balances enshrined in constitutions would not be effective, thus contributing materially to the scandals at York and the problems that emerged at Leicester and Newcastle.

The lunatic hospitals were the product of a singularly remarkable period in the history of British psychiatry. As Porter, Scull and others have shown, the latter part of the eighteenth century saw fundamental changes in the understanding of mental disorder and in ideas as to how it should be treated and managed.[9] Perceptions of the madman as approaching bestiality, and requiring severe corrective treatment and containment, were gradually superseded by notions of his essential humanity and the concomitant hope that he could be restored to some semblance of rational thought and behaviour. Insanity was, however, still being clearly viewed as a disease, comparable to other diagnosable physical conditions. Treatment methods, whether medical or 'moral', were perceived to require implementation under medical supervision. At the same time there was an increasing adherence to the doctrine that removal from family and community was an essential pre-requisite for restorative treatment. The rationales for committal to a specialist medically orientated institution, whether private madhouse or public lunatic hospital, became established as fundamental therapeutic requirements.

Changing attitudes and ideas regarding insanity and the insane were reflected in the development of more sophisticated treatment and patient management practices within institutions. Psychological techniques were increasingly taking their place alongside the more established pharmacological remedies and other physical treatments. Rooted in the rational, creative currents of thought characteristic of the era of Enlightenment, the new emphasis on methods of 'moral treatment' and 'management' represented a distinct alteration of direction. Liberally educated physicians, like John Ferriar and even Thomas Arnold, enthusiastically adopted and propounded the new therapeutics. Ferriar's idea of the promotion of 'hope' in the patient paralleled the cultivation of 'esteem' at the York Retreat. However, the associated interpersonal techniques did not provide adequate solutions to the problem of containment of violent, destructive, or chaotic behaviour in the lunatic hospitals. Physical coercion and the paraphernalia of mechanical restraint remained integral elements in the treatment regime, and continued to receive therapeutic justification for their contribution to calming the patient as a precursor to the recovery process. Even some of the increasingly popular newer treatments, like warm and cold baths and showers, were recognized to exercise much of their 'moral' benefit by means of punishment, deterrence, and the inducement of fear.

The apparently contradictory strands in the developing treatment regimes highlighted the continuing dilemma as to the real nature and purpose of treatment in a lunatic hospital. At its heart was the issue of whether the primary purpose of a public institution for the insane was to treat and cure people suffering distressing maladies, or to protect them, their relatives and the wider community from the consequences of dangerous or anti-social behaviours.[10] The public and professional discourse recognized both the custodial and the curative elements and sought to resolve the dilemma by an uneasy accommodation between therapeutics and containment. Arguably, the emphasis was moving slowly toward the former. The issues, however, were profound and the debates became more intense after the revelations of 1815. The public lunatic hospitals were at the forefront of the sites for attempting to reconcile the practical dilemmas inherent in the paradox of promoting curative treatment in a context of close control. Any resolution came with the achievement of a delicate balance between medical treatment, moral management, and the manifestations of restraint and coercion.

Physicians, individually and collectively, were accorded a leadership role in the lunatic hospitals, by virtue of the acknowledged acceptance that insanity had to be treated by medical means. The dominant position they achieved was more pronounced even than had been the case in the voluntary general hospitals.[11] Their authority stemmed not only from the professional expertise in diagnosis and treatment that was attributed to them, but also from their direct participation in policy formation and in practical management of the institution and its staff. Although some of the newer 'moral' treatment and management approaches were not intrinsically 'medical' in orientation, several of the key physicians were astute enough to adopt and even to advocate them. Indeed, their adherence to progressive ideas accorded well with the image of the intellectual and culturally aware gentleman-physician that an Edinburgh medical education promoted, and that their prominence in the urban community enabled them to cultivate.

The physicians' situation in lunatic hospitals, however, became increasingly unusual. The creation of charging structures on the basis of patients' and families' ability to pay, and the deliberate attraction of a lucrative private clientele, brought in a range of commercial considerations. Physicians, who initially gave their services *gratis*, found themselves faced with some of the inducements and temptations associated with participation in a medical market-place. Alexander Hunter's argument that his potential for outside work with private patients would be reduced if they were being admitted to the York Asylum on favourable terms, and that he was entitled to some recompense, contained a degree of justification.[12] At St Luke's, the voluntary principle was abandoned for different reasons. As the hospital's population grew, the demands on the physician for attendance became increasingly onerous, and it was not unreasonable that he should be rewarded with a regular 'gratuity', especially in light of the charity's considerable wealth. Nevertheless, in these circumstances a physician's public service principles were liable to become compromised by temptations to seek the maximum earnings from work within the lunatic hospital. The whole ideal of the gentleman-physician, with his liberal accomplishments and his disinterested service of the public interest, became that much harder to uphold.

The commercialization of the provincial lunatic hospitals, and competition with the private sector, was both effect and cause of a changing patient profile. Nevertheless, despite the moves to accommodate more people from the middling ranks, the majority of those admitted continued to emanate from the poorer classes. The most significant influence in determining patterns of admission appears to have been geographical. From the outset the provincial lunatic hospitals operated as regional facilities, attracting patients mainly from their surrounding hinterlands. Although St Luke's Hospital continued to function as a national institution, the great majority of its patients came from London and the south-east of England. The specified criteria for admission became gradually more refined, as governors gained more experience and physicians developed their specialist expertise. Whilst perceived curability was not a precondition, other than at St Luke's, the sorts of questions asked of referrers of prospective patients were designed to ascertain possible areas for restorative treatment interventions. Nevertheless, the conditions of many of those admitted were clearly chronic, with little prospect of anything other than containment and the meeting of their basic needs. Published cure rates of around fifty per cent indicated that the prospects for a significant number of lunatic hospital inmates were distinctly unpromising, similar to what proved to be the case in later generations of public asylums.[13]

At a time when the numbers of places in private madhouses and public institutions were still relatively limited, the people admitted were generally those too risky and anti-social to be supported in family or community. Despite the influences of the new therapeutic approaches, the options for managing the disturbed and destructive behaviours exhibited by many lunatic hospital patients remained limited. The common responses included the widespread use of the implements of restraint and coercion, within buildings constructed largely on custodial principles. Spartan conditions became the prevailing norm. Constricted urban sites rendered expansion, or improvement in facilities, problematic. Wear and tear caused by the inmates, combined with the ravages of time and obsolescence, contributed to a steady process of deterioration and decay in the material fabric of the buildings. At several of the lunatic hospitals, but at York, Leicester, and Newcastle in particular, matters became critical.

There was a clear linkage between the physical degeneration of the lunatic hospital buildings and the squalor, neglect and abuse that became evident at York and elsewhere. Much of the responsibility lay with deficient organizational structures. Shortcomings became evident at all levels within the institutional hierarchy. Governors and trustees overlooked their responsibilities, at best relinquishing them to the physician or a salaried director. They in turn delegated to more junior officers and staff, who were ill-equipped and insufficiently rewarded to carry out effectively their often onerous duties. In the extreme case of the York Asylum, managerial failings resulted in corrupt and abusive practices permeating downwards from the physicians via the senior officers to the keepers. The fire that had occurred in 1813 may have greatly worsened the internal situation in the asylum, but it provided the precipitant for the exposures that followed, which led in turn to the ensuing public outcry and the response to it.

Graphic revelations of squalid conditions and maltreatment excited moral outrage and the call for root-and-branch reform. The lunacy reform movement had received its inspiration from two main sources. Sir George Onisephorus Paul, who contributed significantly to the 1807 select committee and hence to the Act of 1808, had been one of the most prominent figures in practical prison reform.[14] The key reforming measure of the 'Ministry of All the Talents' in 1807, however, had been the abolition of the slave trade.[15] Some of the language of shock and indignation associated with revelations of unacceptable conditions in some madhouses and asylums bore similarities to that employed in the anti-slavery campaign. The Evangelicals and radicals who combined to advance lunacy reform received a propaganda gift with the disclosures of women herded together in filth and squalor in a hidden, subterranean room at the York Asylum, causing respectable magistrates to retch at the stench. Even more resonant was the spectre of James Norris, encased in an iron cage at Bethlem, and apparently receiving treatment comparable to the worst meted out to recalcitrant black slaves.[16]

The evidence produced by the 1815 select committee was not, however, wholly condemnatory of public provision for the insane. There was a brief but relatively favourable report on the Exeter Lunatic Asylum.[17] More particularly, the Nottingham Asylum, established jointly by the county and voluntary subscribers, appeared to be admirably conducted by current standards and had a management regime much influenced by that at the York Retreat.[18] At the same time, the private sector was even more discredited by revelations of appalling conditions in several madhouses, despite evidence that some others were well conducted. The conclusion to be drawn was that proper regulation was required rather than any particular model of provision.

Although legislation did not follow from the findings of the select committees, their influence was clear. At York, where local political influences and tensions had been much in evidence, significant changes in the management and operation of the asylum were being embedded well before its scandals reached national attention in 1815, and this process continued over the next few years. Improvements at Leicester, Newcastle and elsewhere followed. By the 1820s, the lunatic hospitals were increasingly being aligned with the newer post-1808 county and joint asylums, as exemplars of well-managed public provision. They now formed part of the wider mixed economy of care, which also incorporated the increasing numbers of private lunatic asylums.[19] Nevertheless, governors sought to retain the distinctiveness of the lunatic hospitals' status as voluntary institutions, illustrated by a continuing resistance to attempts to include them within regulatory legislation.[20] The risk, in adopting that approach, was the perpetuation of the sort of 'close borough system' of management that Sir Andrew Halliday condemned at St Luke's.[21]

Despite any evident shortcomings, the model of enlightened charity organized into voluntary activity continued to retain considerable attraction. This had accounted for its incorporation into the legislation of 1808, with the encouragement to county magistrates to combine with voluntary subscribers in order to provide a public lunatic asylum based on the principles established by the lunatic hospitals. Far from being eclipsed by the rate-funded county pauper asylums, the voluntary movement was given a significant boost. The new asylums at Nottingham, Stafford, Bodmin and Gloucester all contained an important charitable element, whilst those opened at Lincoln and Oxford in the 1820s, and Northampton in the 1830s, were purely voluntary establishments.[22] The lunatic hospital would retain a significant presence within the tapestry of institutional provision for the insane for many decades to come. Indeed, several of the eighteenth and early nineteenth-century foundations have survived to the present day. St Luke's Hospital and the Warneford Hospital (originally the Oxford, or Radcliffe, Lunatic Asylum) continue within the National Health Service. Cheadle Royal Hospital (formerly the Manchester Lunatic Hospital) and St Andrews Hospital (formerly the Northampton General Lunatic Asylum) still operate as private psychiatric hospitals.[23]

By any measure, the voluntary lunatic hospital movement had made a key contribution to the emergence and establishment of a national system of institutional care for mentally disordered people in England. The question has been posed as to whether the network of lunatic hospitals that was established itself constituted a cohesive 'system', in the same way as did the succeeding generations of public asylums. Chris Philo, in his recent work, has certainly argued convincingly that it merited this description.[24] Although relatively few in number, the commonalities in their establishment and their constitutions, their distinctive modes of operation, and the great influence they wielded on subsequent institutions for the insane, confirm that the lunatic hospitals were of sufficient significance to constitute an important entity in their own right. Their prominent place in the historical development of British mental health services deserves due acknowledgement.

Notes

Introduction

1. A. Scull, *Museums of Madness; the Social Organization of Insanity in Nineteenth-Century England*, London: Allen Lane, 1979.
2. 8 and 9 Vict. Cap 126; 9 Vict. Cap 100; K. Jones, *A History of the Mental Health Services*, London: Routledge & Kegan Paul, 1972, pp. 132–49.
3. 48 Geo.III, cap 96. For a study of the asylums developed under the provisions of the 1808 Act, see L. D. Smith, *'Cure, Comfort and Safe Custody'; Public Lunatic Asylums in Early Nineteenth Century England*, London: Leicester University Press, 1999.
4. R. Porter, *Mind Forg'd Manacles; A History of Madness in England From the Restoration to the Regency*, Cambridge, University Press, 1987 — in this seminal work on the eighteenth century, Porter devotes only a small section to the lunatic hospitals; A. Scull, *The Most Solitary of Afflictions; Madness and Society in Britain, 1700–1900*, London and New Haven: Yale University Press, 1993. The exception is Chris Philo, whose recent book has devoted a full chapter to the lunatic hospitals — *A Geographical History of Institutional Provision for the Insane from Medieval Times to the 1860s in England and Wales: the Space Reserved for Insanity*, Lampeter: Edwin Mellen, 2004.
5. Scull, *The Most Solitary of Afflictions*, pp. 56–64.
6. R. Porter, 'Being Mad in Georgian England', *History Today* 31, 1981, 42–8; Porter, 'Shaping Psychiatric Knowledge: the Role of the Asylum', in R. Porter (ed.), *Medicine in the Enlightenment*, Amsterdam: Rodopi, 1995, pp. 255–73; A. Ingram, *The Madhouse of Language: Writing and Reading Madness in the Eighteenth Century*, London: Routledge, 1991.
7. W. Battie, *A Treatise on Madness*, London: J. Whiston and B. White, 1758; J. Monro, *Remarks on Dr Battie's Treatise on Madness*, London: John Clarke, 1758; T. Arnold, *Observations on the Nature, Kinds, Causes, and Prevention of Insanity, Lunacy, or Madness*, Leicester: G. Ireland, 1782–6; W. Pargeter, *Observations on Maniacal Disorders*, Reading: for the Author, 1792.
8. St Luke's Hospital (SLH) Archives, General Court Book 1750–1779, 'Considerations Upon the Usefulness and Necessity of Establishing an Hospital, by Subscription, as a Farther Provision for Poor Lunaticks'; Manchester Royal Infirmary (MRI) Archives, 'An Account of the Proceedings of the Trustees of the Public Infirmary, in Manchester, in Regard to the Admission of Lunaticks into that Hospital' (c. 1763).
9. Porter, *Mind Forg'd Manacles*, Ch. 2.

10. C. Stevenson, 'The Architecture of Bethlem at Moorfields', in J. Andrews, A. Briggs, R. Porter, P. Tucker, K. Waddington, *The History of Bethlem*, London: Routledge, 2000, pp. 230–59.

11. M. Winston, ' The Bethel at Norwich: an Eighteenth Century Hospital for Lunatics', *Medical History* 38, 1994, 27–51.

12. W. L. Parry-Jones, *The Trade in Lunacy; a Study of Private Madhouses in England in the Eighteenth and Nineteenth Centuries*, London: Routledge Kegan Paul, 1972, pp. 6–9, 131; Porter, *Mind Forg'd Manacles*, pp. 136–40.

13. Porter, *Mind Forg'd Manacles*, pp. 117–8; Jones, *History of Mental Health Services*, pp. 25–8.

14. P. Bartlett and D. Wright (eds.), *Outside the Walls of the Asylum: the History of Care in the Community 1750–2000*, London: Athlone Press, 2000; A. Suzuki, 'Lunacy in Seventeenth- and Eighteenth-Century England: Analysis of Quarter Sessions Records', Part I, *History of Psychiatry* 2, 1991, 437–56, Part II, *History of Psychiatry* 3, 1993, 29–44; Suzuki, 'The Household and the Care of Lunatics in Eighteenth-Century London', in P. Horden and R. Smith (eds.), *The Locus of Care: Families, Communities, Institutions and the Provision of Welfare Since Antiquity*, London: Routledge, 1998, pp. 153–75. Following contemporary parlance, the term 'lunatics' will here refer to people with a mental illness, and 'idiots' to people with a learning disability.

15. Porter, *Manacles*, pp. 155, 221; Battie, *A Treatise on Madness*, pp. 68–9; Monro, *Remarks on Dr Battie's Treatise*, pp. 37–8.

16. N. McKendrick, J. Brewer, and J.H. Plumb, *The Birth of a Consumer Society: the Commercialization of Eighteenth-Century England*, London: Europa, 1982; Porter, *Manacles*, pp. 138–68.

17. *York Courant*, 15 September 1772; *An Earnest Application to the Humane Public, Concerning the Present State of the Asylum Erected Near York for the Reception of Lunatics*, York: 1777, pp. 4–5.

18. D. Owen, *English Philanthropy 1660–1960*, London: Oxford University Press, 1965, pp. 11–16, 36–68.

19. P. Borsay, *The English Urban Renaissance; Culture and Society in the Provincial Town, 1660–1770*, Oxford: Oxford University Press, 1989.

20. K. Wilson, 'Urban Culture and Political Activism in Hanoverian England: the Example of Voluntary Hospitals', in E. Hellmuth (ed.), *The Transformation of Political Culture; England and Germany in the Late Eighteenth Century*, Oxford: Oxford University Press, 1990, pp. 165–84; P. Langford, *Public Life and the Propertied Englishman, 1689–1798*, Oxford: Clarendon, 1991, pp. 490–500.

21. A. Digby, *Madness, Morality and Medicine: a Study of the York Retreat, 1796–1914*, Cambridge: Cambridge University Press, 1985.

22. *Gentleman's Magazine* XLIII, 1773, p. 185.

23. A. Digby, *Making a Medical Living; Doctors and Patients in the English Market for Medicine, 1720–1911*, Cambridge University Press, 1994.

24. For discussion of the 'custody versus cure' question, see A. Digby, 'Changes in the Asylum: the Case of York, 1777–1815', *Economic History Review*, 2nd Series 36, 1983, 218–39, and also Smith, 'Cure, Comfort and Safe Custody', pp. 5, 179–80, 218, 247, 284–7.

25. Jones, *A History of the Mental Health Services*, Chs 3–6; Scull, *The Most Solitary of Afflictions*, Chs 2-3; M. Donnelly, *Managing the Mind: A Study of Medical Psychology in Early Nineteenth Century Britain*, London: Tavistock, 1983; P. McCandless, 'Insanity and Society: a Study of the English Lunacy Reform Movement, 1815–1870', PhD thesis, University of Wisconsin, 1974; A. Digby, *From York Lunatic Asylum to Bootham Park Hospital*,

York: University of York, Borthwick Papers 69, 1986, pp. 15–27; M. Brown, 'Rethinking Early Nineteenth-Century Asylum Reform', *The Historical Journal* 49,2006, 425–52.

26. BPP 1807, Vol. II, *Report of the Select Committee into the State of Criminal and Pauper Lunatics.*
27. BPP 1814–15, Vol. IV, *Select Committee on the State of Madhouses;* BPP 1816, Vol.VI, *Select Committee on Madhouses.*
28. B. Abel-Smith, *The Hospitals 1800-1948,* London: Heinemann, 1964; J. Woodward; *To Do the Sick No Harm; A Study of the Voluntary Hospital System to 1875,* London: Routledge Kegan Paul, 1974.

Chapter 1

1. C. Stevenson, *Medicine and Magnificence; British Hospital and Asylum Architecture, 1660–1815,* New Haven and London: Yale University Press, 2000, pp. 33–41, 63–65; C. Stevenson, 'The Architecture of Bethlem at Moorfields', in J. Andrews, A. Briggs, R. Porter, P. Tucker, and K. Waddington, *The History of Bethlem,* London: Routledge, 1997, pp. 230–59.
2. *York Courant,* 5 September 1772, cited in A. Digby, *From York Lunatic Asylum to Bootham Park Hospital,* York: University of York, Borthwick Papers No.69, 1986, p. 1.
3. C. Wilson, *England's Apprenticeship,* London: Longman, 1965; N. McKendrick, J. Brewer, and J.H. Plumb, *The Birth of a Consumer Society: the Commercialization of Eighteenth-Century England,* London: Europa, 1982; D. Owen, *English Philanthropy 1660–1960,* London: Oxford University Press, 1965, Chs. 1–4; D. T. Andrew, *Philanthropy and Police; London Charity in the Eighteenth Century,* Princeton and Oxford: Princeton University Press, 1989; R. Porter, 'The Gift Relation: Philanthropy and Provincial Hospitals in Eighteenth Century England', in L. Granshaw and R. Porter (eds), *The Hospital in History,* London: Routledge, 1989, 149–78.
4. P. Langford, *Public Life and the Propertied Englishman, 1689–1798,* Oxford: Clarendon, 1991, pp. 490–98; K. Wilson, *The Sense of the People; Politics, Culture and Imperialism in England, 1715–1785,* Cambridge: Cambridge University Press, 1995, pp. 73–82. .
5. J. Woodward, *To Do the Sick No Harm; A Study of the Voluntary Hospital System to 1875,* London: Routledge Kegan Paul, 1974; J. Pickstone, *Medicine and Industrial Society; A History of Hospital Development in Manchester and its Region, 1752–1946,* Manchester: Manchester University Press, 1985.
6. Andrews et al, *The History of Bethlem,* Chs. 2–3.
7. Ibid., Ch. 7.
8. Ibid., Chs. 5, 7, pp. 111, 124.
9. Ibid., Ch.10.
10. Ibid., p. 149.
11. J. Andrews, 'Bedlam Revisited: A History of Bethlem Hospital c1634–1770', University of London, unpublished PhD, 1991; Stevenson, *Medicine and Magnificence,* pp. 33–41.
12. Andrews et al, *History of Bethlem,* Chs.11–16; Andrews, 'Bedlam Revisited', Chs.2–4; R. Porter, *Mind Forg'd Manacles; A History of Madness in England From the Restoration to the Regency,* Cambridge: Cambridge University Press, 1987, pp. 121–29.
13. Another public facility, the lunatic ward of the French Protestant Hospital in London (known as 'La Providence'), opened in 1718, has been identified

by Chris Philo, *A Geographical History of Institutional Provision for the Insane from Medieval Times to the 1860s in England and Wales: the Space Reserved for Insanity*, Lampeter: Edwin Mellen, 2004, pp. 451–52.

14. Porter, *Mind Forg'd Manacles*, pp. 129–30; M. Winston, 'The Bethel at Norwich: an Eighteenth Century Hospital for Lunatics', *Medical History* 38, 1994, 27–51.

15. Winston, 'The Bethel at Norwch', pp. 28–32, 36.

16. Porter, *Manacles*, p. 130; R. Hunter and I. Macalpine, *Three Hundred Years of Psychiatry, 1535–1860*, London: Oxford University Press, 1963, p. 331; Philo, *A Geographical History*, pp. 452, 475; BPP 1814–15, Vol. IV, *Select Committee on the State of Madhouses*, p. 17, evidence of Edward Wakefield.

17. Porter, *Manacles*, pp. 136–47; W. L. Parry-Jones, *The Trade in Lunacy; a Study of Private Madhouses in England in the Eighteenth and Nineteenth Centuries*, London: Routledge Kegan Paul, 1972; Philo, *A Geographical History*, pp. 320–34.

18. B. Abel–Smith, *The Hospitals 1800–1948*, London: Heinemann, 1964, pp. 4–6; Woodward, *To Do the Sick No Harm*, Chs.2-3, pp. 147–48; J. Lane, *A Social History of Medicine; Health, Healing and Disease in England, 1750–1950*, London: Routledge, 2001, Ch.5; M. Fissell, *Patients, Power and the Poor in Eighteenth-Century Bristol*, Cambridge: Cambridge University Press, 1991, Ch.4.

19. J. Aikin, *Thoughts on Hospitals*, London: Joseph Johnson, 1771, p. 6.

20. Woodward, *To Do the Sick No Harm*, pp. 12, 17–22; Porter, 'The Gift Relation: Philanthropy and Provincial Hospitals in Eighteenth Century England', pp. 158–61; Abel–Smith, *The Hospitals*, p. 5; Lane, *A Social History of Medicine*, pp. 83–5, 88; Langford, *Public Life and the Propertied Englishman*, pp. 494–97; M. Fissell, 'The "Sick and Drooping Poor" in Eighteenth Century Bristol and its Region', *Social History of Medicine* 2, 1989, 35–58; A. Borsay, 'Cash and Conscience; Financing the General Hospital at Bath c1738–1850', *Social History of Medicine* 4, 1991, 207–29; A. Berry, 'Community Sponsorship and the Hospital Patient in Late Eighteenth Century England', in P. Horden and R. Smith, *The Locus of Care; Families, Communities, Institutions and the Provision of Welfare Since Antiquity*, London: Routledge, 1998, pp. 126–50.

21. Porter, 'The Gift Relation', pp. 152–55, 161, 172; A. Borsay, *Medicine and Charity in Georgian Bath; a Social History of the General Infirmary, c.1739–1830*, Aldershot: Ashgate, 1999, Ch.6.

22. Cited in Borsay, 'Cash and Conscience', p. 216.

23. Borsay, 'Cash and Conscience', p. 215; Fissell, 'The "Sick and Drooping Poor" ', p. 36; Fissell, *Patients, Power, and the Poor*, p. 78; Porter, 'The Gift Relation', p. 163; K. Wilson, 'Urban Culture and Political Activism in Hanoverian England: the Example of Voluntary Hospitals', in E. Hellmuth (ed.), *The Transformation of Political Culture; England and Germany in the Late Eighteenth Century*, Oxford: Oxford University Press, 1990, pp. 169–71.

24. Andrew, *Philanthropy and Police*, Ch. 1; Borsay, *Medicine and Charity in Georgian Bath*, Ch.7; Fissell, *Patients, Power, and the Poor in Eighteenth-Century Bristol*, p. 78.

25. Woodward, *To Do the Sick No Harm*, pp. 17–21; Porter, 'The Gift Relation', pp. 151–62; Borsay, 'Cash and Conscience', pp. 217–20; Wilson, *The Sense of the People*, pp. 73–80.

26. Abel-Smith, *The Hospitals*, p. 6; Woodward, *To Do the Sick No Harm*, pp. 38–9; Fissell, ' "The Sick and Drooping Poor" ' pp. 36–7; Fissell, *Patients,*

Power, and the Poor, pp. 74, 113–16; Pickstone, *Medicine and Industrial Society*, p. 16; Lane, *A Social History of Medicine*, p. 82.

27. Woodward, *To Do the Sick No Harm*, pp. 37–45; Abel-Smith, *The Hospitals*, pp. 12–13; Pickstone, *Medicine and Industrial Society*, p. 16; Lane, *A Social History*, pp. 82–83.

28. Borsay, *Medicine and Charity in Georgian Bath*, pp. 24–26; Porter, 'The Gift Relation', pp. 156–57; Woodward, *To Do the Sick No Harm*, p. 18.

29. Porter, 'The Gift Relation', p. 167; Borsay, *Medicine and Charity*, pp. 345–51; Fissell, *Patients, Power, and the Poor*, pp. 82–83; Lane, *A Social History*, p. 86.

30. Woodward, *To Do the Sick No Harm*, p. 23; Abel-Smith, *The Hospitals*, p. 6; Borsay, *Medicine and Charity*, Ch.4; Porter, 'The Gift Relation', pp. 161–62.

31. Abel-Smith, *The Hospitals*, p. 7; Woodward, *To Do the Sick No Harm*, p. 28; I. Loudon, *Medical Care and the General Practitioner, 1750–1850*, Oxford: Clarendon, 1986, pp. 20–27.

32. C.N. French, *The Story of St Luke's Hospital*, London: Heinemann, 1951, pp. 4–5; SLH, *General Court Book*, 'Considerations on the Usefulness and Necessity of Establishing an Hospital', 13 June 1750. At the time of writing the extensive St Luke's archive was held at the hospital in Muswell Hill; it has subsequently been re-located to the London Metropolitan Archives.

33. SLH, untitled volume, 'Reasons for the establishment and further Encouragement of St Lukes Hospital for Lunaticks together with the Rules and Orders for the Government thereof', pp. 5–6.

34. SLH, 'Considerations upon the Usefulness...'. The criticisms of Bethlem's limitations did not go unchallenged, and precipitated counter-claims regarding St Luke's and the motivations of its protagonists — see J. Andrews and A. Scull, *Undertaker of the Mind; John Monro and Mad-Doctoring in Eighteenth-Century England*, London: University of California Press, 2001, pp. 45–47.

35. *Gentleman's Magazine* 18, 1748, p. 199.

36. SLH, 'Considerations Upon the Usefulness'; French, *The Story of St Luke's*, pp. 5–6. For the principle of separation of the insane patient from family and placement with 'strangers', see Porter, *Mind Forg'd Manacles*, Ch. 3.

37. SLH, *General Court Book*, 13, 29 June, 12 September, 10, 26 October, 8 November 1750; *Gentleman's Magazine*, 23 October 1750; J. Noorthouck, *A New History of London, Including Westminster and Southwark, to Which is Added, A General Survey of the Whole; Describing the Public Buildings, Late Improvements, &c*, London: R. Baldwin, 1773, pp. 755–56; W. Harrison, *A New and Universal History, Description and Survey of London and Westminster*, London: 1778, pp. 543–44; French, *The Story of St Luke's*, pp. 6-10. French concluded, probably from a too-literal interpretation of the hospital minutes that the hospital building was adapted from an old foundry, but this is probably not correct. Dorothy Stroud, the biographer of the architect George Dance, son of the building's designer, ascertained that it was built on the site of houses adjoining the old foundry building, see D. Stroud, *George Dance, Architect 1741–1825*, London: Faber and Faber, 1971, pp. 49–50.

38. SLH, *General Court Book*, 12 September, 10 October 1750; French, *The Story of St Luke's*, pp. 7–9.

39. SLH, *General Court Book*, 13 June 1750; French, pp. 7–9.

40. Hunter and Macalpine, *Three Hundred Years of Psychiatry*, pp. 402–04; Andrews and Scull, *Undertaker of the Mind*, pp. 45–48.

41. 'Reasons for the Establishment and Further Encouragement of St Lukes Hospital for Lunatics'; *Reasons for the Establishment and Further Encouragement*

of St Lukes Hospital for Lunatics Together with the Rules and Orders for the Government Thereof, London: J. March and Son, 1790, pp. 3–6; A. Highmore, *Pietas Londinensis: the History, Design and Present State of the Various Public Charities in and Near London*, London: Richard Phillips, 1810, pp. 172–73; Andrews and Scull, *Undertaker of the Mind*, pp. 52–53, 283, note 26.

42. SLH, *General Court Book*, 31 October 1750. For Battie, see — Hunter and Macalpine, op. cit., pp. 402–10; R.A. Hunter, 'William Battie, M.D., F.R.S., Pioneer Psychiatrist', *The Practitioner* 174, 1955, 208–15; Andrews and Scull, pp. 11, 45–52. See also below, Ch. 4.
43. SLH, *General Court Book,* 8 November 1750.
44. SLH, *General Court Book*, 22 March, 22 June 1751.
45. SLH, *House Committee Minutes*, 26, 30 July, 2 August 1751; *General Court Book*, 26 June, 14 August 1751.
46. Stroud, *George Dance*, p. 50; Stevenson, *Medicine and Magnificence*, pp. 93, 99–100.
47. R. Dodsley, *London and its Environs Described*, London: 1761, cited in Stevenson, *Medicine and Magnificence*, p. 93; Noorthouck, *A New History of London*, p. 755.
48. Andrews and Scull, *Undertaker of the Mind*, pp. 45–46.
49. Andrews et al., *The History of Behlem*, pp. 317–20.
50. SLH, *General Court Book*, 8 November 1750; *House Committee Minute Book*, 30 July 1751.
51. By 1767 the hospital's funds stood at £24,000, when they were augmented by a huge bequest of £30,000 from Sir Thomas Clarke, the Master of the Rolls — French, *The Story of St Luke's*, p. 22. By the summer of 1775, the hospital's funds had reached over £75,000 — *General Court Book*, 2 August 1775. This was an almost astronomic figure in comparison to the funds raised by the provincial lunatic hospitals — see chapter two. Some of St Luke's Hospital's wealth emanated from somewhat unsavoury sources; for example, in February 1800 the Treasurer was required to arrange for the sale of some slaves in Dominica, who had formed part of a bequest — *General Court Book*, 12 February 1800.
52. SLH, *General Court Book*, 12 February, 12 August 1752.
53. *General Court Book*, 6 August 1753, 13 February 1754.
54. *General Court Book*, 13 February 1754; *House Committee Minute*, 14 June 1754; *Gentleman's Magazine*, February 1754. For the change in policy toward incurables, see J. Andrews, 'The Lot of the "Incurably" Insane in Enlightenment England', *Eighteenth Century Life* 12, New Series, 1, 1988, 1–18.
55. *General Court Book*, 11 February, 13 August 1755, 5 February 1756; *Incurable Patient Book*, commencing 28 June 1754.
56. *General Court Book*, 9 February 1763, 6 February 1765; *Incurable Patient Book*, 1765.
57. *General Court Book*, 14 February 1770.
58. *General Court Book*, 6 August 1770.
59. Parry-Jones, *The Trade in Lunacy*, pp. 43, 60, 244, 252; E. Murphy, 'Mad Farming in the Metropolis, Part 1: A Significant Service Industry in East London', *History of Psychiatry* 12, 2001, 245–82.
60. Harrison, *A New and Universal History, Description and Survey of London*, p. 544; J.Howard, *An Account of the Principal Lazarretos in Europe, and Additional Remarks on the Present State of Those in Great Britain and Ireland*, Warrington: William Ayres, 1789, p. 139.

61. SLH, *General Court Book*, 2 August 1775.
62. *General Court Book*, 14 August 1776; French, *The Story of St Luke's*, pp. 22, 26–27.
63. French, pp. 27–28.
64. SLH, *General Committee Book*, 8 January 1787.
65. *The Picture of London for 1818*, London: Longman, 1818, p. 201; French, p. 29 — he put the cost as being nearer £46,000.
66. Stevenson, *Medicine and Magnificence*, pp. 86, 101–02.
67. W.H. Yeandle, *A Corner of Finsbury*, London: W. Knott & Son, 1934, p. 55, citing Elmes, *Topographical Dictionary of the British Metropolis* (1831).
68. Stevenson, *Medicine and Magnificence*, pp. 97–104; Stroud, *George Dance*, pp. 141–42; H. Richardson (ed.), *English Hospitals 1660–1948*, Swindon: Royal Commission on Historical Monuments in England, 1998, p. 155; Andrews and Scull, *Undertaker of the Mind*, p. 45.
69. Cited in Stroud, *George Dance*, p. 142. See also — C. Stevenson, 'Carsten Anker Dines With the Younger George Dance, and Visits St Luke's Hospital for the Insane', *Architectural History* 44, 2001, 153–61; idem, 'Robert Hooke's Bethlem', *Journal of the Society of Architectural Historians* 55, 1996, 254–275.
70. *The Daily Universal Register*, 2 October 1786.
71. Ibid., 3 October 1786.
72. Howard, *An Account of the Principal Lazarettos in Europe*, pp. 139–40.
73. Stevenson, *Medicine and Magnificence*, pp. 100–02.
74. T. Markus, *Buildings and Power; Freedom and Control in the Origin of the Modern Building Types*, London: Routledge, 1993, pp. 130–31.
75. *The Times*, 1, 3 December 1788. This stated the funds to be £95,000; the higher figure comes from SLH, *General Court Book*, 7 February 1787.
76. *General Court Book*, 7 February 1787, 6 February 1788.
77. *The Times*, 15 February 1788; *General Court Book*, 4 February 1789.
78. *General Court Book*, 16 June 1794, 9 January 1800.
79. Ibid., 7 February 1787.
80. SLH, *Incurable Patient* Book, 1788-1800; *General Court Book*, 2 February 1791, 9 January 1800.
81. *General Committee Book*, 14 August 1800.
82. E.g. *Reasons for the Establishment and Further Encouragement of St Lukes Hospital for Lunatics*, 1790.
83. Andrews et al, *History of Bethlem*, pp. 277-78.
84. Porter, *Mind Forg'd Manacles*, pp. 130–32, 140. See below, Ch. 2.
85. A. Digby, *Madness, Morality and Medicine: a Study of the York Retreat, 1796–1914*, Cambridge: Cambridge University Press, 1985.
86. BPP 1807, Vol. II, *Report of the Select Committee into the State of Criminal and Pauper Lunatics*, pp. 21–24; BPP 1814–1815, Vol. IV, *Report from the Select Committee on Madhouses in England*, pp. 126–28, 131–37; BPP 1816, Vol. VI, *Select Committee on Madhouses*, pp. 28–34.
87. Stevenson, *Medicine and Magnificence*, pp. 97, 103; L. D. Smith, 'Cure, Comfort and Safe Custody'; *Public Lunatic Asylums in Early Nineteenth Century England*, London: Leicester University Press, 1999, pp 32–36.

Chapter 2

1. The inter-connection between lunatic hospitals and voluntary general hospitals is explored in some depth in C. Philo, *A Geographical History of Institutional Provision for the Insane from Medieval Times to the 1860s in England*

and Wales: the Space Reserved for Insanity, Lampeter: Edwin Mellen, 2004, pp. 466–71.

2. The term 'lunatic asylum' appears to have been first applied at York, where the institution was planned as a 'lunatic hospital', but had become known as the York Lunatic Asylum by the time it opened in 1777.

3. As I have shown elsewhere, several of the first group of county asylums that opened following Wynn's Act of 1808 were joint ventures between the county and voluntary subscribers. The Act had effectively made possible the completion of delayed projects at Nottingham (1811), Stafford (1818), and Gloucester (1823). See L. D. Smith, *'Cure, Comfort and Safe Custody'; Public Lunatic Asylums in Early Nineteenth Century England*, London: Leicester University Press, 1999, Ch.1.

4. SCRO, Q/A1c, 'Statutes and Constitutions of the Lunatic Asylum, in the Parish of St Thomas, Near Exeter', pp. 25-27. This includes an almost verbatim reproduction of the 'Reasons for the Establishment of St Luke's'.

5. J. Lane, *A Social History of Medicine; Health, Healing and Disease in England, 1750–1950*, London: Routledge, 2001, p. 86.

6. MRI Archives, 'An Account of the Proceedings of the Trustees of the Public Infirmary in Manchester, in Regard to the Admission of Lunaticks into that Hospital' (1763); Cheadle Royal Hospital Archives, 'Lunatick Hospital in Manchester, December 10, 1766'; *An Account of the Rise, and Present Establishment of the Lunatick Hospital in Manchester*, Manchester: J. Harrop, 1771, pp. 3–4; Lane, *A Social History of Medicine*, p. 83; J. Pickstone, *Medicine and Industrial Society; A History of Hospital Development in Manchester and its Region, 1752–1946*, Manchester: Manchester University Press, 1985, pp. 13–16.

7. J. Gray, *A History of the York Lunatic Asylum*, York: Hargrove and Co., 1815, p. 21; G. McLoughlin, *A Short History of the First Liverpool Infirmary*, London: Phillimore, 1978, pp. 31, 74 —the exclusion was published in 1748, in Rule 53. Philo also highlights the exclusion of the insane from voluntary hospitals, citing the Leeds Infirmary and the Norfolk and Norwich Infirmary — Philo, *A Geographical History*, p. 445.

8. *Newcastle Courant*, 21 May 1763.

9. 'An Account of the Proceedings of the Trustees of the Public Infirmary in Manchester'; N. Roberts, *Cheadle Royal Hospital: A Bicentenary History*, Altrincham: John Sherratt and Son, 1967, p. 6.

10. *An Account of the Rise, and Present Establishment of the Lunatick Hospital*, p. 4.

11. *York Courant*, 15 September 1772; A. Digby, *From York Lunatic Asylum to Bootham Park Hospital*, York: University of York, Borthwick Papers No.69, 1986, p. 1.

12. LCRO, *Leicester Infirmary — Annual Reports*, Year Ending 24 June 1794; *Leicester Journal*, 26 September, 3 October 1794; E.R. Frizelle, *The Life and Times of the Royal Infirmary at Leicester*, Leicester: Leicester Medical Society, 1988, p. 67. At Exeter in 1795, the proponents of an asylum may have looked at the Leicester appeal, for they too referred to 'the most helpless and pitiable Class of Mortals' — DCRO, 3992/F/H26, 'Outline of a Plan for a Lunatic Asylum', 16 March 1795.

13. McLoughlin, *A Short History of the First Liverpool Infirmary*, pp. 48–49; J. A. Shepherd, *A History of the Liverpool Medical Institution*, Liverpool: Liverpool Medical Institution, 1979, pp. 18, 37–9, 64–67. Currie authored political publications, as well as medical. He also was the first authorized biographer of Robert Burns. For Currie, see below, Ch. 4.

14. *Gore's Liverpool General Advertiser*, 20 August 1789; *Williamson's Liverpool Advertiser*, 24 August 1789.
15. *Newcastle Courant*, 21 May 1763.
16. 'An Account of the Proceedings of the Trustees of the Public Infirmary in Manchester'; 'Lunatick Hospital in Manchester', 1766; J. Aikin, *Thoughts on Hospitals*, London: Joseph Johnson, 1771, pp. 66–68; *An Account of the Rise, and Present Establishment of the Lunatick Hospital*, p. 3.
17. *York Courant*, 15 September 1772; *An Earnest Application to the Humane Public, Concerning the Present State of the Lunatic Asylum Erected Near York for the Reception of Lunatics*, York, 1777, p. 4.
18. *Leicester Journal*, 26 September, 3 October 1794; LCRO, Leicester Infirmary, Annual Report, Year Ending 24 June 1794.
19. W. Battie, *A Treatise on Madness*, London: J. Whiston and B. White, 1758, pp. 68–69; R. Porter, *Mind Forg'd Manacles; A History of Madness in England From the Restoration to the Regency*, Cambridge University Press, 1987, p. 155. The term 'mad-doctor' was in general currency as a description of specialist physicians engaged in the treatment of the insane.
20. Battie, *A Treatise*, p. 68.
21. J. Monro, *Remarks on Dr Battie's Treatise on Madness*, London: John Clarke, 1758, p. 37.
22. T. Arnold, *Observations on the Nature, Kinds, Causes, and Prevention of Insanity, Lunacy, or Madness*, Leicester: G. Ireland, 1782–6, Vol. I, pp. 9–10.
23. *Newcastle Courant*, 21 May 1763.
24. 'An Account of the Proceedings of the Trustees of the Public Infirmary'; *Manchester Mercury*, 22 January 1765.
25. *An Account of the Rise, and Present Establishment of the Lunatick Hospital*, p. 3.
26. Philo has referred to them as 'medical spaces'—*A Geographical History*, pp. 443.
27. 'An Account of the Proceedings of the Trustees of the Public Infirmary'; *An Account of the Rise, and Present Establishment of the Lunatick Hospital*, p. 5; Aikin, *Thoughts on Hospitals*, p. 69.
28. Included in J. Marsden, DD, *A Sermon Preached at York, on Thursday the 27th of March 1783, for the Benefit of the Lunatic Asylum*, York: A. Ward, 1783.
29. W. Mason, *Animadversions on the Present Government of the York Lunatic Asylum in Which the Case of Parish Paupers is Distinctly Considered in a Series of Propositions*, York: Blanchard, 1788, pp. 2–3 —Mason acknowledges that the York resolutions were directly copied from Manchester; *Gentleman's Magazine* 43, 1773, p. 185; Aikin, *Thoughts on Hospitals*, pp. 69–70; *An Account of the Rise, and Present Establishment*, p. 5; 'Lunatick Hospital, in Manchester'; *Report of the Committee of Inquiry in to the Rules and Management of the York Lunatic Asylum*, York: Thomas Wilson and Sons, 1814, p. 21; Digby, *From York Lunatic Asylum*, p. 2.
30. *Gore's Liverpool General Advertiser*, 20 August 1789; *Williamson's Liverpool Advertiser*, 24 August 1789.
31. Mason, *Animadversions*. For fuller discussion of this issue, see below, Chs. 4, 6.
32. *Newcastle Courant*, 21 May 1763, 17 May 1766; J. Hall, *A Narrative of the Proceedings Relative to the Establishment &c of St Luke's House*, Newcastle: J. White and T. Saint, 1767, pp. 8–17.

33. P. Carpenter, 'Thomas Arnold: A Provincial Psychiatrist in Georgian England', *Medical History* 33, 1989, 199–216. Arnold subsequently transferred his business to the Belle Grove Asylum. For Arnold, see below, Ch. 4.
34. Lane, *A Social History of Medicine*, pp. 82–6.
35. *Newcastle Courant*, 21 May 1763.
36. *Gore's Liverpool General Advertiser*, 20 August 1789; *Williamson's Liverpool Advertiser*, 24 August 1789.
37. *Manchester Mercury*, 22 January 1765; 'Lunatick Hospital, in Manchester', 1766.
38. For admission arrangements and processes see below, Ch.5.
39. *York Courant*, 5 September 1772; *An Earnest Application to the Humane Public*, p. 4; Digby, *From York Lunatic Asylum to Bootham Park Hospital*, p. 2. These assertions had much similarity to those of the St Luke's governors in 1750.
40. The Bethel Hospital at Norwich had been established some fifty years previously. However, it was originally financed by an individual charitable bequest rather than by public subscription. See M. Winston, 'The Bethel at Norwich: an Eighteenth Century Hospital for Lunatics', *Medical History* 38, 1994, pp. 28–33.
41. J. Woodward, *To Do the Sick No Harm; A Study of the Voluntary Hospital System to 1875*, London: Routledge Kegan Paul, 1974, p. 148; J. Le Gassicke, 'History of Psychiatry on Tyneside', in *Medicine in Northumbria; Essays in the History of Medicine in the North East of England*, Newcastle: Pybus Society for the History and Bibliography of Medicine, 1993, p. 277 — this gives the date of the opening of the Infirmary as 1753.
42. *Newcastle Courant*, 21 May 1763.
43. *Newcastle Courant*, 25 June, 2 July 1763; Tyne and Wear Archives, *Newcastle Common Council Minutes 1743–66*, fo.380, 16 June 1763; Newcastle City Library, hand-bill, 'An Account of Patients Admitted, Discharged, and Remaining at the Lunatic Hospital from July 18th, 1764, to July 18th, 1817'; Hall, *A Narrative of the Proceedings*', p. 17.
44. *Newcastle Courant*, 25 June 1763. It appears that the Norwich Bethel Hospital had been charging weekly fees, for paupers and others, by 1730 — Winston, 'The Bethel at Norwich', pp. 35–36.
45. Le Gassicke, 'History of Psychiatry on Tyneside', pp. 277–79; P. M. Horsley, *Eighteenth Century Newcastle*, Newcastle: Oriel Press, 1971, p. 124.
46. Hall, *A Narrative*, pp. 7, 17; *Newcastle Common Council Minutes*, fos.421-22, 7 October 1765; J. Brand, *History of Newcastle Upon Tyne*, London: B. White and Son, 1789, Vol. I, pp. 421–22. The site, on Bath Lane, was very close to where St James's Park (Newcastle United) football ground now stands.
47. Hall, pp. 7–11, 14–15, 17, 37; *Newcastle Courant*, 17 May, 28 June 1766, 19, 26 September, 3–31 October, 7–28 November, 5–24 December 1767, 2–30 January, 2 July, 29 October, 31 December 1768. As Philo has suggested, there has hitherto been some confusion regarding the relative status of St Luke's House and the lunatic hospital – Philo, *A Geographical History*, pp. 505-06 (note 142). There has also been a mistaken belief, unfortunately perpetuated by Roy Porter, that the Newcastle Lunatic Hospital was subject to privatization within a few years of its opening — *Mind Forg'd Manacles*, p. 132.
48. Hall, p. 17.
49. Newcastle City Library, Local Tracts, 111A, 'Rules of the Hospital for Lunaticks, for the Counties of Northumberland, Newcastle Upon Tyne, and Durham'.

50. J. Harvey, *A Sentimental Tour Through Newcastle; By a Young Lady*, New-castle: D. Akenhead, 1794, p. 6.
51. Northumberland CRO, ZBL 269/69, 'A Sketch of a Ground Plan of an Hospital for Lunaticks'; E. Mackenzie, *A Descriptive and Historical Account of the Town and County of Newcastle Upon Tyne*, Newcastle: Mackenzie and Dent, 1827, Vol. II, p. 525; Lane, *A Social History*, p. 103.
52. Pickstone, *Medicine and Industrial Society*, pp. 13–14; W. Brockbank, *Portrait of a Hospital, 1752–1948; to Commemorate the Bi-centenary of the Royal Infirmary Manchester*, London: Heinemann, 1952, pp. 6–16.
53. *An Account of the Rise and Present Establishment of the Lunatick Hospital in Manchester*, p. 3.
54. 'An Account of the Proceedings of the Trustees'; MRI Archives, Manchester Infirmary, Weekly Board, 1 August, 22 September 1763, Annual Report, XIII, 24 June 1764 to 24 June 1765; *An Account of the Rise and Present Establishment*, p. 4; Brockbank, *Portrait of a Hospital*, p. 21.
55. 'An Account of the Proceedings of the Trustees'; *Manchester Mercury and Harrop's General Advertiser*, 22 January 1765.
56. *Manchester Mercury and Harrop's General Advertiser*, 8, 22, 29 October, 3, 24 December 1765, 22 April 1766; 'Lunatick Hospital, in Manchester, December 10, 1766'.
57. 'Lunatick Hospital, in Manchester'; *Manchester Mercury*, 13, 20 January 1767; MRI Archives, Manchester Infirmary, Annual Reports, XIV, 24 June 1765 to 24 June 1766, XV, 24 June 1766 to 24 June 1767; Roberts, *Cheadle Royal Hospital*, pp. 11–12.
58. 'Lunatick Hospital, in Manchester'; Manchester Infirmary, Annual Reports, XIII, XV, Weekly Board, 26 September 1765; Brockbank, *Portrait of a Hospital*, p. 21.
59. *An Account of the Rise and Present Establishment*, p. 10.
60. Manchester Infirmary, Weekly Board, 26 September 1765; Brockbank, p. 21.
61. *An Account of the Rise and Present Establishment*, p. 9; Roberts, *Cheadle Royal Hospital*, p. 12.
62. Annual Report, XIV, 1765-66.
63. Annual Report, XV, 1766-67.
64. Annual Report, XVI, July 21, 1768 — the first to be entitled 'The Report of the Infirmary and Lunatic Hospital in Manchester'.
65. Annual Report, XIII, 1764-65; *An Account of the Rise and Present Establishment*, p. 6.
66. *Manchester Mercury*, 29 April, 6, 13, 20, 27 May, 10, 17, 24 June, 1, 15 July 1766; *An Account of the Rise and Present Establishment*, p. 7.
67. *York Courant*, 11, 25 August 1772.
68. *York Courant*, 1, 8 September 1772; York Reference Library, Bowen MSS, letter W. Burgh to William Wilberforce MP, 10 November 1791—I am grateful to Anne Digby for this reference.
69. *York Courant*, 15 September 1772 — REASONS for the Establishing a Lunatic HOSPITAL'; Mason, *Animadversions*, p. 2.
70. *York Courant*, 29 September, 13 October 1772.
71. See below, Chs. 3, 4, 7.
72. Woodward, *To Do the Sick No Harm*, p. 148.
73. Alexander Hunter, *Silva; or, a Discourse of Forest-Trees, and the Propagation of Timber in His Majesty's Dominions*, York: Wilson and Sons, Fourth Edition, 1812, xi–xii, 'A Memoir of the Life of Alexander Hunter, M.D.'
74. *York Courant*, 6 December 1773; Digby, *From York Lunatic Asylum*, pp. 2–3.

75. Digby, p. 3; University of York, Borthwick Institute, BOO 3/10/2/1, Subscription List, 1772 — among the larger subscribers were the Marquis of Rockingham, Lord Bingley, the Earl of Carlisle, the Company of Merchant Adventurers of York, and the Mayor and Corporation of Doncaster; *York Courant*, 15 September, 13, 20 October 1772, 27 July 1773.
76. *Report of the Committee of Inquiry into the Rules and Management of the York Lunatic Asylum*, Appendix, p. 22.
77. Bowen MSS, Burgh to Wilberforce, 10 November 1791; Digby, p. 3.
78. Harriet Richardson (ed.), *English Hospitals 1660–1948*, Swindon: Royal Commission on Historical Monuments of England, 1998, p. 156; Digby, p. 4.
79. Bowen MSS, Burgh to Wilberforce; Digby, pp. 3–4.
80. Richardson, *English Hospitals*, p. 156; *York Courant*, 21 March 1774; Bowen MSS, Burgh to Wilberforce.
81. Digby, p. 4; *York Courant*, 26 August, 23 September 1777; Burgh to Wilberforce.
82. Digby, p. 6; Jonathan Gray, *A History of the York Lunatic Asylum*, York: W. Hargrove and Co., 1815, p. 24.
83. Digby, p. 4; *Report of the Committee of Inquiry*, pp. 27–28.
84. *York Courant*, 21 March 1774.
85. *York Courant*, 26 August 1777; Bowen MSS, Burgh to Wilberforce.
86. McLoughlin, *A Short History of the First Liverpool Infirmary*, p. 22.
87. Surprise at Manchester's example not having been followed earlier was expressed by a correspondent to the Liverpool newspapers — *Williamson's Liverpool Advertiser*, 28 September 1789; *Gore's Liverpool General Advertiser*, 1 October 1789.
88. MRI Archives, Manchester Lunatic Hospital Register, 1773–77.
89. LRO, 614 INF 1/1, Minutes of Board of Trustees of Liverpool Infirmary, 19 August 1789; *Williamson's Liverpool Advertiser*, 3, 24 August 1789; *Gore's Liverpool General Advertiser* 20 August 1789.
90. LRO, 614 INF 1/1, 7 September 1789.
91. W.W. Currie, *Memoir of the Life, Writings, and Correspondence of James Currie, M.D., F.R.S., of Liverpool*, London: Longman, Rees, Orme, Brown, and Green, 1831. For Currie see below, Ch. 4.
92. *Gore's Liverpool General Advertiser*, 20 August, 15 October 1789; *Williamson's Liverpool Advertiser*, 24 August, 19 October 1789. The significance of these letters was reinforced by their being later re-published in full — J. Currie, *Medical Reports on the Effects of Water, Cold and Warm, as a Remedy in Fever and Febrile Diseases*, Vol. II, London: Cadell and Davies, 1805, Appendix II, pp. 19–39; W.W. Currie, *Memoir of the Life, Writings, and Correspondence of James Currie*, Vol. I, Appendix.
93. *Gore's Liverpool General Advertiser*, 15 October 1789; *Williamson's Liverpool Advertiser*, 19 October 1789.
94. Philo, *A Geographical History*, pp. 467–69. Philo also highlights the influence of the medical model on the urban location of the lunatic hospitals at Liverpool and elsewhere.
95. LRO, 614 INF 1/1, 7 December 1789; 614 INF 5/2, Liverpool Infirmary, Annual Report, 2 March 1789 to 1 March 1790.
96. *Williamson's Liverpool Advertiser*, 21 December 1789.
97. *Williamson's Liverpool Advertiser*, 2 November 1789.
98. LRO, 614 INF 1/1, 1 March 1790; 614 INF 5/2, Annual Report, 2 March 1789 to 1 March 1790.
99. 614 INF 5/2, Annual Report, 1 March 1790 to 2 March 1791.

100. 614 INF 5/2, 1 March 1792 to 2 March 1793, 1 March 1793 to 2 March 1794; SCRO, Q/A1c, Box 1, Letter 11 March 1812, J. Squires to C. Aylesbury.
101. 614 INF 5/2, 1 March 1793 to 2 March 1794.
102. 614 INF 5/2, 3 March 1794 to 2 March 1795.
103. 614 INF 5/2, 3 March 1795 to 5 March 1796.
104. 614 INF 5/2, Annual Reports, 1798–1801.
105. See also L. Smith, 'Doctors and Lunatics; the Enigma of the Leicester Asylum, 1781–1837', in *Midland History*, forthcoming.
106. Frizelle, *Life and Times of the Royal Infirmary at Leicester*; Woodward, *To Do the Sick No Harm*, p. 148.
107. LCRO, 1L3 D54/1, Leicester Infirmary Minutes, 21 June 1781; J. Throsby, *The History and Antiquities of the Ancient Town of Leicester*, Leicester: J. Brown, 1791, p. 314; *Leicester and Nottingham Journal*, 23 June 1781.
108. *Leicester and Nottingham Journal*, 7, 14, 21 July 1781.
109. LCRO, 13 D54/1, 10, 28 September, 5 October, 11 December 1781; *Leicester and Nottingham Journal*, 22, 29 September, 6, 13 October 1781.
110. Vaughan came from a medical family. His grandfather had been a royal physician. His second son, Sir Henry Halford (after marrying an heiress and inheriting a baronetcy), went on to become President of the Royal College of Physicians — see Carpenter, 'Thomas Arnold', p. 202.
111. Throsby, *History and Antiquities of Leicester*, p. 314. The bequest came from a Mrs Topp.
112. LCRO, 13 D 54/1, 20 June 1782, 19 June 1783; Frizelle, *Life and Times*, p. 63.
113. *Leicester and Nottingham Journal*, 26 October, 8 November 1783.
114. LCRO, 13 D 54/1, 16 September 1783.
115. LCRO, 13 D54/1, 17 June 1784; *Leicester and Nottingham Journal*, 19 June 1784.
116. LCRO, 13 D54/1, 23 June 1785; Frizelle, *Life and Times*, p. 64.
117. Carpenter, 'Thomas Arnold', pp. 202-6. For the quarrels between Arnold and Vaughan, see Ch. 4.
118. For more on Arnold's background, see Ch. 4.
119. Carpenter, 'Thomas Arnold', p. 203.
120. Ibid., pp. 203–04.
121. *Leicester and Nottingham Journal*, 13 March 1782.
122. LCRO, 13 D54/1, 17 June 1784; Carpenter, p. 205.
123. Throsby, *History and Antiquities*, p. 314.
124. J. Throsby, *Select Views in Leicestershire*, Leicester, 1789, Vol. II, p. 35.
125. *Leicester and Nottingham Journal*, 7 May, 18 June 1785
126. *Leicester and Nottingham Journal*, 25 June, 2 July 1785; LCRO, 13 D54/1, 23 June 1785.
127. *Leicester and Nottingham Journal*, 14 March 1794 — this advertisement was dated June 3, 1790, when it evidently first appeared.
128. LCRO, 13 D54/2, Infirmary Minutes 1787–1808, 22 January 1788, 28 September 1792.
129. LCRO, 13 D54/2, 18 September 1792.
130. 13 D54/2, 28 September 1792.
131. 13 D54/2, 28 September 1792, 11 January, 20 June 1793.
132. 13 D54/2, 11 September, 19 December 1793, 21 January 1794; *Leicester and Nottingham Journal*, 3 January 1794.
133. 13 D54/2, 29 April 1794; *Leicester and Nottingham Journal*, 9, 16 May 1794.
134. 13 D54/2, 15 August 1794; *Leicester and Nottingham Journal*, 11 July, 1, 8 August 1794.

135. 13 D54/2, 16 September 1794; *Leicester and Nottingham Journal*, 26 September, 3 October 1794.
136. 13 D54/2, 19 June, 15 August 1794.
137. *Leicester and Nottingham Journal*, 14 March, 6 June 1794.
138. SCRO, Q/A1c, Box 1, letter from Secretary to Leicester Asylum, dated 13 March 1812.
139. LCRO, Leicester Infirmary, Annual Reports, 1795–1808.
140. LCRO, 13 D54/2, 17 September 1795, 20 June 1799; Annual Report, Year Ending June 24, 1800.
141. Woodward, *To Do the Sick No Harm*, p. 148.
142. J. Adams, 'The Mixed Economy for Medical Services in Herefordshire c.1770–c.1850', unpublished PhD thesis, University of Warwick, 2004, pp. 210, 215.
143. *Gloucester Journal*, 3 March 1777, cited in T. Arnold, *Observations on the Nature, Kinds, Causes, and Prevention of Insanity*, Vol. II, Leicester: G. Ireland, 1786, pp. 249–50.
144. Herefords CRO, 560/25, Hereford Infirmary, Governors' Meetings, 11 October 1792; *The British Chronicle, or Pugh's Hereford Journal*, 17 October 1792; Adams, 'The Mixed Economy for Medical Services', p. 216.
145. Herefords CRO, 560/25, 11 April, 6 June 1793; *Hereford Journal*, 25 December 1793; Adams, 'The Mixed Economy', p. 217.
146. 560/25, 24 April 1798.
147. 560/25, 22, 26 March 1799.
148. *Rules for the Government of the Lunatic Asylum in Hereford*, Hereford, 1799 (copy in Hereford Public Library).
149. Herefords CRO, 560/26, Minutes of Governors of Hereford Infirmary, 30 October 1823, 'Report of Committee Appointed to Investigate the State of the Lunatic Asylum'; W. L. Parry-Jones, *The Trade in Lunacy; a Study of Private Madhouses in England in the Eighteenth and Nineteenth Centuries*, London: Routldge Kegan Paul, 1972, pp. 63–64
150. Herefords CRO, 560/26, 28 May, 6, 29 June 1846.
151. Herefords CRO, 560/25, 17 August 1815, 560/26, 28 August 1845, 28 May 1846; Pateshall Mss, A95/V/Ju/11, 17, 19, 33.
152. BPP 1839, Vol. IX, *Report from SC on the Hereford Lunatic Asylum*; Herefords CRO, Q/AL/137–44, Visiting Magistrates Reports 1823–36; Parry-Jones, *The Trade in Lunacy*, pp. 263, 274–75. For the later history of the Hereford Asylum see J. Adams, 'The Campaign for a Public Asylum in Hereford, 1836-1839', forthcoming in *Midland History*.
153. Woodward, *To Do the Sick No Harm.*, p. 148.
154. DCRO, 3992/F/H1/1, Committee of Governors, Minutes, 16 March 1795; SCRO, Q/A1c, Box 1, letter 10 March 1812, Rev. Manning to Secretary of Stafford Infirmary; *Ninth Report of the Commissioners in Lunacy to the Lord Chancellor*, 1855, Appendix B, pp. 48–49; N. Hervey, *Bowhill House; St Thomas's Hospital for Lunatics, Asylum for the Four Western Counties, 1800–69*, Exeter: University of Exeter, 1980, p. 12.
155. DCRO, 3992/F/H26, 'Outline of a Plan for a Lunatic Asylum, 16 March 1795'; *The Exeter Flying Post*, 2 April 1795.
156. SCRO, Q/A1c, letter 10 March 1812.
157. DCRO, 3992/F/H1/1, 29 July 1795; Hervey, *Bowhill House*, p. 13.
158. DCRO, 3992/F/H26, 29 July 1795; *Exeter Flying Post*, 6 August 1795.
159. *Exeter Flying Post*, 7 January 1796.
160. DCRO, 3992/F/H1/1, 16 September, 29 December 1796, 31 January, 21 March, 20 April 1798.

161. SCRO, Q/A1c, 10 March 1812; DCRO, 3992/F/H1/1, 11 July 1798, 3 April, 24 July, 23 September, 6 November 1799, 3992/F/H13, Sixth Annual Report, 1807.

162. 3992/F/H26, 'Statutes and Constitutions of the Lunatic Asylum, at Bow-hill-House, near Exeter, with the Rules and Orders for the Government and Conduct of the House', Exeter, 1801, 'Statutes and Constitution of the Lunatic Asylum, in the Parish of St Thomas, Near Exeter, with the Rules and Orders for the Government and Conduct of the House', Third Edition, Exeter, 1804.

163. DCRO, 3992/F/H26, 16 July 1800; 3992/F/H13, Sixth Report, 1807.

164. 3992/F/H26, 'The Plan of the Intended Lunatic Asylum'.

165. DCRO, 3992/F/H1/1, 10 August 1802.

166. Statutes and Constitution of the Lunatic Asylum, in the Parish of St Thomas', 1804 edition, pp. 27–29.

167. BPP 1814–15, *SC on the State of Madhouses*, evidence of Edward Wakefield, p. 20.

168. DCRO, 3992/F/H13, Sixth Report, 1807.

169. SCRO, Q/A1c, Box 1, letter 10 March 1812.

170. Woodward, *To Do the Sick No Harm*, p. 148.

171. Throsby, *Select Views in Leicestershire*, Vol. I, p. 265; Notts CRO, SO/HO/1/1/1, 5 October 1808.

172. Notts CRO, SO/HO/1/1/1, 1 November, 14 December 1803, 28 January 1804; *Nottingham Journal*, 8 October 1803, 31 March 1804. Atkinson had presumably been responsible for one of the wings added to York Asylum, as he was not the original architect.

173. Notts CRO, SO/HO/1/1/1, 12 July 1808.

174. Smith, *'Cure, Comfort and Safe Custody'*, pp. 25–26.

175. Notts CRO, SO/HO/1/1/1, 14 September 1808, 15, 29 November 1809, 4 October 1810; *Nottingham Journal*, 15 October, 19 November 1808, 26 August, 14 October, 25 November 1809, 3 January, 29 September 1810, 11, 18, 25 January, 8, 15 February 1812.

176. BPP 1807, Vol. II, *SC on the State of Criminal and Pauper Lunatics*.

177. For Paul and his work, see Smith, *'Cure,Comfort and Safe Custody'*, pp. 16, 20–25; Kathleen Jones, *A History of the Mental Health Services*, London: Routledge & Kegan Paul, 1972, pp. 55–59; E.A.L. Moir, 'Sir George Onisephorus Paul', in H. p. R. Finberg (ed.), *Gloucestershire Studies*, Leicester University Press, 1957, pp. 195–224; M. Ignatieff, *A Just Measure of Pain; the Penitentiary in the Industrial Revolution 1750–1850*, London: Penguin, 1978, pp. 98–101.

178. *An Abstract of Proceedings Relative to the Institution of a General Lunatic Asylum in or Near the City of Gloucester*, Gloucester: R. Raikes, 1794; G.O. Paul, *A Scheme of an Institution and a Description of a Plan for a General Lunatic Asylum for the Western Counties to be Built in or Near the City of Gloucester*, Gloucester, 1796.

179. Woodward, *To Do the Sick no Harm*, p. 148.

180. *An Abstract of the Proceedings Relative to the Institution of a General Lunatic Asylum*, pp. 3–4; *Gloucester Journal*, 22 July, 16 September, 9 December 1793.

181. Paul, *A Scheme of an Institution and a Description of a Plan*; *Gloucester Journal*, 17 March 1794.

182. Paul, *A Scheme of an Institution*, p. 1.

183. *Gloucester Journal*, 23 August, 13 September 1802, 24 March, 7 July 1806.

184. G.O. Paul, *Observations on the Subject of Lunatic Asylums, Addressed to a General Meeting of Subscribers to a Fund for Building and Establishing a General Lunatic Asylum, Near Gloucester*, Gloucester: D. Walker, 1812; G.O. Paul, *Doubts Concerning the Expediency and Propriety of Immediately Proceeding to Provide a Lunatic Asylum at Gloucester*, Gloucester: D. Walker, 1813.

185. Gloucs CRO, HO22/3/1, Gloucestershire County Lunatic Asylum, Minute Book of Justices and Subscribers, 19 February 1813–17 July 1823; *Gloucester Journal*, 30 June, 18 August 1823; A. Bailey, 'The Founding of the Gloucestershire County Asylum, now Horton Road Hospital Gloucester, 1792–1823', *Transactions of the Bristol and Gloucestershire Archaeological Society* 90, 1971, 178–91.

186. Woodward, *To Do the Sick No Harm*, p. 148.

187. Lincolnshire Archives, LAWN 1/1/1, Lincoln Lunatic Asylum, Committee Minutes, Vol. 1, 17 June 1807.

188. LAWN 1/1/1, 8 July, 12 August, 30 September 1807; DCRO, 3992 F/H13, Exeter Lunatic Asylum, Sixth Annual Report, 1807.

189. LAWN 1/1/1, 24 February 1808.

190. LAWN 1/1/1, 16 March, 4, 30 May, 11 June, 2 July, 3 August, 23 September 1808, 26 January, 2, 16 March, 6, 27 April, 25 May, 20 July, 25 August, 7, 21 September 1809. Ingleman was also the architect of the Nottingham Asylum and later the Oxford (Radcliffe) Asylum — see Smith, *'Cure, Comfort and Safe Custody'*, pp. 31–33, 35.

191. LAWN 1/1/1, 15 March, 31 May, 21 September, 1 November, 13 December 1810, 2 September   1811, 20 April, 5 August 1813.

192. 13, 24 September, 13 October 1813, 22 November 1814.

193. 12, 24 March 1817.

194. 11 August, 8 October 1817, 1 February, 3 May, 4, 15 November 1819.

195. 15 November 1819, 7 January, 18 February, 3, 5, 10 April 1820.

196. Lincoln Reference Library, U. P. 876, 'Third Report of the Lincoln Lunatic Asylum'.

197. For the later history of the Lincoln Asylum, see Smith, *'Cure, Comfort, and Safe Custody'*, particularly Ch. 8, and L.D. Smith, 'The "Great Experiment": the Place of Lincoln in the History of Psychiatry', *Lincolnshire History and Archaeology* 30, 1995, 55–62.

198. Woodward, p. 148.

199. *Minutes of Proceedings Relative to a Proposal for Establishing a Lunatick Asylum in the Vicinity of Oxford, by Voluntary Contributions Under the Sanction and Direction of the Governors of the Radcliffe Infirmary*, p. 5. — cited in D. Bowes, 'Who Cares for the Insane? A Study of Asylum Care in Nineteenth Century Oxfordshire', unpublished M.A. thesis, Oxford Brookes University, 2000, p. 10; B. Parry-Jones, *The Warneford Hospital, 1826–1976*, Oxford: Holywell Press, 1976, p. 7.

200. *An Account of the Origin, Nature and Objects of the Asylum on Headington Hill, Near Oxford*, Oxford: J. Munday and Son, 1827, pp. 1–2.

201. Becher was one of the prime movers of the Nottingham Asylum and a key witness to the 1815 Select Committee on Madhouses.

202. *An Account of the Origin, Nature and Objects of the Asylum*, p. 2; Warneford Hospital Archives, W. P. 5, x, xi, xiii, xv, xvii, xxii.

203. Bowes, 'Who Cares for the Insane ?', p. 11; Parry-Jones, *The Warneford Hospital*, p. 11.

204. Warneford Hospital Archives, W. P. 26, i, x; Bowes, 'Who Cares for the Insane?', pp. 10–11; Parry-Jones, *The Warneford Hospital*, pp. 8, 11.

205. Parry-Jones, p. 8.
206. *An Account of the Origin, Nature and Objects of the Asylum*, p. 6.
207. *An Account*, pp. 8–20; *Useful Information Concerning the Origin, Nature, and Purpose of the Radcliffe Lunatic Asylum*, Oxford: W. Baxter, 1840; Bowes, p. 11. It was later re-named the Radcliffe Asylum, and subsequently the Warneford Asylum, after its main benefactor.
208. Parry-Jones, *The Warneford Hospital*, pp. 13, 17. The Warneford Hospital still operates as a psychiatric hospital, within the NHS.
209. Woodward, *To Do the Sick No Harm*, p. 148.
210. A. Foss and K. Trick, *St Andrew's Hospital, Northampton; the First One Hundred and Fifty Years (1838–1988)*, Cambridge: Granta, 1989, p. 7.
211. Ibid., pp. 7–11.
212. Ibid., pp. 12–26. St Andrew's Hospital still continues to function as an independent specialist psychiatric facility, outside the NHS.
213. New lunatic hospitals were later opened at Stafford, Nottingham and Gloucester, in the 1850s and 1860s. The original joint asylums built under the 1808 Act were split into their county pauper and voluntary constituents, with the paupers remaining in the original building and the charity and private patients moving into the new building — see Smith, 'Cure, Comfort and Safe Custody', p. 79.
214. SLH, General Court Book, 14 February 1787, 12 February, 16 June 1794. The same donor also gave £5000 to Bethlem Hospital.
215. *A Letter From a Subscriber to the York Lunatic Asylum, to the Governors of That Charity*, York: Wilson, Spence and Mawman, 1788, pp. 8–14; Gray, *A History of the York Lunatic Asylum*, pp. 13–15; *An Abstract of Proceedings Relative to the Institution of a General Lunatic Asylum in or Near the City of Gloucester*, pp. 3–5, 9, 11, 15; Paul, *A Scheme of an Institution*, pp. 2–4; SC on the State of Lunatics, 1807, p. 18; DCRO, 3992/ F/H14/8, 'Table of Rules for the Admission and Discharge of Patients'; 3992/ F/H13, 6th Annual Report, 1807, 19th Report, 1820, 22nd Report, 1823.
216. The model was eventually revived over a century and a half later in the 1970s, with the allegedly new and progressive idea of the psychiatric unit attached to a district general hospital, so that mental illnesses could be treated along-side physical illnesses. This approach has since been implemented in many towns and cities.
217. Significant exceptions were the major towns of Warwickshire, Worcestershire and Derbyshire.
218. SLH, Admission Books, 1751–1820. For an analysis of admissions to St Luke's see chapter 5.
219. Parry-Jones, *The Trade in Lunacy*.
220. The growth in numbers of patients, and the accompanying expansion of the lunatic hospitals, will be outlined in chapters 5 and 7.
221. 48 Geo.III, Cap. XCVI, *An Act for the Better Care and Maintenance of Lunatics, being Paupers or Criminals in England*.
222. Smith, 'Cure, Comfort and Safe Custody', pp. 22–32.

Chapter 3

1. R. Porter, 'The Gift Relation: Philanthropy and Provincial Hospitals in Eighteenth-Century England', in L. Granshaw and R. Porter (eds.), *The Hospital in History*, London: Routledge, 1989, 149–78.
2. The titles of 'superintendent' and 'director' were also used in the early nineteenth century.

3. By the early nineteenth century, male staff (and some female staff) were tending to be known as 'keepers'.
4. P. Langford, *Public Life and the Propertied Englishman, 1689–1798*, Oxford: Clarendon, 1991, pp. 495–97.
5. J. Lane, *A Social History of Medicine; Health, Healing and Disease in England, 1750–1950*, London: Routledge, 2001, pp. 82–88; J. Woodward, *To Do the Sick No Harm; A Study of the Voluntary Hospital System to 1875*, London: Routledge Kegan Paul, 1974, pp. 17–22, 38–39; Porter, 'The Gift Relation'; M. Fissell, *Patients, Power and the Poor in Eighteenth-Century Bristol*, Cambridge: Cambridge University Press, 1991, Ch. 4.; A. Borsay, 'Cash and Conscience; Financing the General Hospital at Bath c1738–1850', *Social History of Medicine* 4, 1991, 207–29; A. Berry, 'Community Sponsorship and the Hospital Patient in Late Eighteenth Century England', in P. Horden and R. Smith, *The Locus of Care; Families, Communities, Institutions and the Provision of Welfare Since Antiquity*, London: Routledge, 1998, pp. 126–50.
6. MRI Archives, 'Lunatick Hospital, in Manchester, December 1, 1766'; N. Roberts, *Cheadle Royal Hospital: A Bicentenary History*, Altrincham: John Sherratt and Son, 1967, p. 12.
7. *An Account of the Rise, and Present Establishment of the Lunatick Hospital in Manchester*, Manchester: J. Harrop, 1771, p. 8; *Gentleman's Magazine* 43, 1773, p. 185; SCRO, Q/A1c, Box 1, Manchester Infirmary Rules, 1791, p. 8.
8. MRI Archives, Manchester Infirmary, Weekly Board, 20 December 1773.
9. SCRO, Q/A1c, Box 1, 'Statutes, Laws, or Rules for the Government of the Leicester Lunatic Asylum', 15 August 1794, p. 3.
10. LCRO, 13 D54 / 3, 17 November 1815.
11. LRO, 614 INF 6/1, 'Liverpool Infirmary — Rules and Orders' (1813), p. 25.
12. *Rules for the Government of the Lunatic Asylum in Hereford*, Hereford, 1799, p. 3.
13. 'Lunatick Hospital, in Manchester'; *An Account of the Rise, and Present Establishment of the Lunatick Hospital*, p. 8.
14. Manchester Infirmary Rules, 1791, p. 8; Liverpool Infirmary Rules, p. 30.
15. *Rules for the Government of the Lunatic Asylum in Hereford*, p. 3.
16. Leicester Asylum Rules, p. 4.
17. SLH, 'Reasons for the Establishment and Further Encouragement of St Lukes Hospital for Lunaticks'.
18. SLH, General Court Book, 13 June, 10 October 1750; C.N. French, *The Story of St Luke's Hospital*, London: Heinemann, 1951, pp. 7–9; *Reasons for the Establishment and Further Encouragement of St Lukes Hospital for Lunatics Together with the Rules and Orders for the Government Thereof*, London: J. March and Son, 1790, p. 7.
19. According to *The Times*, 3 December 1788, St Luke's was one of the wealthiest hospitals in London. Much of this money was said to have come from bequests, which may only have provided governorships for the executors.
20. Newcastle City Library, Local Tracts 111A, 'Rules of the Hospital for Lunaticks, for the Counties of Northumberland, Newcastle Upon Tyne, and Durham' (c.1764).
21. *Report of the Committee of Inquiry in to the Rules and Management of the York Lunatic Asylum*, York: Thomas Wilson and Sons, 1814, p. 33; *A Letter From a Subscriber to the York Lunatic Asylum, to the Governors of That Charity*, York: Wilson, Spence and Mawman, 1788, p. 24.

22. DCRO, 3992/F/H26, 'Statutes and Constitutions of the Lunatic Asylum, at Bowhill-House, near Exeter, with the Rules and Orders for the Government and Conduct of that House', 1801, p. 3.

23. *Rules for the Lunatic Asylum at Lincoln, November 4th, 1819*, Lincoln: William Brooke, 1819, p. 3; *Rules of the Lincoln Lunatic Asylum*, Lincoln: W. Brooke, 1832, p. 5; Lincolnshire Archives, LAWN 1/1/1, 15 November 1819. The example that Lincoln most closely followed was from the joint county and voluntary asylum at neighbouring Nottingham, which opened in 1811 under the 1808 Act, where eligibility to be a governor was based on a benefaction of twenty guineas or annual subscription of two guineas —J.T. Becher, *Resolutions Concerning the Intended General Lunatic Asylum Near Nottingham*, Newark: S. and J. Ridge, 1810, p. 10.

24. Lane, *A Social History of Medicine*, p. 82; Fissell, *Patients, Power and the Poor*, pp. 75, 87, 113–16; Woodward, *To Do the Sick No Harm*, pp. 18–21.

25. SCRO, Q/A1c, Box 1, Leicester Asylum Rules, pp. 4–5.

26. *Report of the Committee of Inquiry*, p. 34.

27. At the Liverpool Infirmary, this sub-committee was called the 'Board of Economy'.

28. LRO, 614 INF 1/1–3, Liverpool Infirmary, Board of Governors' meetings, 614 INF 2/1–2, Board of Economy Minute Book; LCRO, 13 D 54/1–4, Leicester Infirmary Minutes; Herefords CRO, 560/25–26, Hereford Infirmary, Governors' Meetings. At Liverpool, the administration of the two institutions was clearly combined; the infirmary's annual reports comprised within them reports on the asylum. In 1812, the asylum's keeper John Squires, in giving advice to the secretary of Stafford Infirmary, whose governors were contemplating the establishment of an asylum, stressed the intimate connection between Liverpool's Infirmary and Asylum, as illustrated by their accounts not being kept separately — SCRO, Q/A1c, Box 1, 11 March 1812, J. Squires to C. Aylesbury.

29. 'Lunatick Hospital in Manchester', 1766; *An Account of the Rise, and Present Establishment of the Lunatick Hospital*, p. 8.

30. LRO, 614 INF 2/2, Board of Economy, 1 March 1820.

31. MRI Archives, Weekly Board, 1766-1830.

32. *Reasons for the Establishing, and Further Encouragement of St Luke's Hospital*, 1790, pp. 13–15. The 'domestick Servants' refers to all the subordinate staff, including those responsible for the direct care of the patients.

33. SLH, General Committee Book, 5 March 1783.

34. 'Rules of the Hospital for Lunaticks for the Counties of Northumberland, Newcastle Upon Tyne, and Durham', p. 1.

35. *Report of the Committee of Inquiry*, pp. 33–34.

36. Ibid., pp. 28-35; J. Gray, *A History of the York Lunatic Asylum*, York: W. Hargrove and Co., 1815, pp. 14–22; A. Digby, *From York Lunatic Asylum to Bootham Park Hospital*, York: University of York, Borthwick Papers No.69, 1986, pp. 6–13.

37. BPP 1814–15, Vol. IV, *Select Committee on the State of Madhouses*, p. 8.

38. Ibid., p. 144.

39. LCRO, 13D54/2/2, 1 February, 17 March 1814, 13D54/3, 29 August, 22 September, 15, 31 October, 17 November 1815. See below, Ch. 7.

40. DCRO, 3992/F/H26, 'Statutes and Constitution of the Lunatic Asylum, at Bowhill-House, near Exeter', p. 3.

41. *Rules for the Lunatic Asylum at Lincoln*, 1819, pp. 3–5.

42. L. D. Smith, *'Cure, Comfort and Safe Custody'; Public Lunatic Asylums in Early Nineteenth-Century England*, London: Leicester University Press,

1999, Ch. 8; L.D. Smith, 'The "Great Experiment": the Place of Lincoln in the History of Psychiatry', *Lincolnshire History and Archaeology* 30, 1995, 55–62.

43. See below, Ch.7.
44. *SC on the State of Madhouses*, 1814–15, p. 8, evidence of Godfrey Higgins, regarding the York Lunatic Asylum.
45. This will be discussed in more detail in Ch. 6.
46. For the Monro's, see — J. Andrews, A. Briggs, R. Porter, P. Tucker, and K. Waddington, *The History of Bethlem*, London: Routledge, particularly Ch. 16; J. Andrews and A. Scull, *Undertaker of the Mind; John Monro and Mad-Doctoring in Eighteenth-Century England*, London: University of California Press, 2001.
47. See Ch. 1.
48. See Ch. 2.
49. BPP 1807, Vol. II, *Report of SC on the State of Criminal and Pauper Lunatics*, p. 19.
50. G.O. Paul, *A Scheme of an Institution and a Description of a Plan for a General Lunatic Asylum for the Western Counties to be Built in or Near the City of Gloucester*, Gloucester, 1796, p. 12.
51. DCRO, 3992/F/H26, 'Statutes and Constitution of the Lunatic Asylum Near Exeter', p. 10.
52. Ibid., p. 19.
53. Ibid., pp. 21–22.
54. LCRO, 13D54/2, 28 September 1792.
55. LCRO, 13D54/2, 11 January 1793, 15 August 1794.
56. SCRO, Q/A1c, Box 1, Leicester Asylum Rules, p. 6.
57. Ibid., p. 8.
58. Ibid., pp. 10–1.
59. SLH, General Committee Book, 23 October 1751; *Reasons for the Establishing, and Further Encouragement*, 1790.
60. SLH, General Court Book, 8 November 1750.
61. SLH, House Committee Minutes, 2 August 1751
62. Ibid., 27 September, 25 October, 15, 29 November, 20,27 December 1751, 7, 20 March, 17 April, 8 May 1752.
63. Ibid., 23 August, 6 September, 8 November 1751, 10 January, 15, 29 May, 17 July, 14 August, 13 October, 3 November, 1 December 1752, 23 March 1753, 25 January 1754.
64. R. Hunter and I. Macalpine, *Three Hundred Years of Psychiatry, 1535–1860*, London: Oxford University Press, 1963, p. 404.
65. E. Raffald, *The Manchester Directory, for the Year 1772,Containing an Alphabetical List of the Merchants, Tradesmen, and Principal Inhabitants in the Town of Manchester*, London, Manchester, 1772, p. 52; Raffald, *The Manchester Directory, for the Year 1781*, Manchester: Raffald, 1781, p. 101; E. Holme, *A Directory of the Towns of Manchester and Salford for the Year 1788*, Manchester: J. Radford, 1788, p. 130; *Scholes's Manchester and Salford Directory*, 1794, Manchester: Sowler and Russell, 1794, xv–xvi — by this time there were five physicians; Hunter and Macalpine, *Three Hundred Years of Psychiatry*, pp. 543–46, 585–86.
66. SCRO, Q/A1c, Box 1, 'Rules for the Government of the Lunatic Hospital and Asylum in Manchester' (1791), pp. 12–13; Cambridge University Library, Hunter Collection, 'Rules for the Government of the Lunatic-Hospital and Asylum in Manchester', c.1816, pp. 34–38.

67. MRI Archives, Manchester Infirmary, Weekly Board, Minutes, 13, 27 July, 3, 17 August 1807. (The 'Keeper' was the senior member of staff, known elsewhere usually as the governor.)
68. Weekly Board, 7 September 1801.
69. LRO, 614 INF 6/1, 'Liverpool Royal Infirmary — Rules and Orders', pp. 25–28.
70. *Gore's General Advertiser*, 5 January 1826; *Liverpool Mercury*, 6, 13, 20 January 1826; *Morning Herald*, 12 January 1826. See Ch. 7.
71. See L. Smith, 'Doctors and Lunatics; The Enigma of the Leicester Asylum, 1782–1837', *Midland History* (2007); P. Carpenter, 'Thomas Arnold: A Provincial Psychiatrist in Georgian England', *Medical History* 33, 1989, 199–216.
72. Digby, *From York Lunatic Asylum to Bootham Park Hospital*, pp. 1–12. Digby aptly entitles one of her sections 'The Physician's Asylum'.
73. Digby, *From York Lunatic Asylum*, pp. 15-24; K. Jones, *A History of the Mental Health Services*, London: Routledge & Kegan Paul, 1972, pp. 45–46, 64–74; Gray, *A History of the York Lunatic Asylum*; *Report of the Committee of Inquiry*. The most recent scholarship is by M. Brown, 'Rethinking Early Nineteenth-Century Asylum Reform', *The Historical Journal* 49, 2006, 425–52. I am most grateful to Michael Brown for providing me with a copy of his important article prior to publication.
74. The controversy will be discussed further in Chs. 4 and 7. It is also dealt with by Brown, 'Rethinking Early Nineteenth Century Asylum Reform', in the context of local political struggles.
75. Rev. R.B. Dealtry, *A Sermon Preached at York on Wednesday the 10th of April, 1782, for the Benefit of the Lunatic Asylum*, York: A. Ward, 1782, p. 16. Dealtry was related to Hunter by marriage — W. Mason, *Animadversions on the Present Government of the York Lunatic Asylum in Which the Case of Parish Paupers is Distinctly Considered in a Series of Propositions*, York: Blanchard, 1788, p. 25.
76. Digby, *From York Lunatic Asylum*, pp. 1–2; *A Letter From a Subscriber*, pp. 17–18; Gray, *A History*, p. 12
77. *Report of the Committee of Inquiry*, p. 7.
78. *A Letter From A Subscriber*, p. 7.
79. Ibid., pp. 7–8, 23, Appendix II, letter dated 5 January 1788, p. 30.
80. *A Letter*, pp. 8–14, 23; Gray, *A History*, p. 14; *Report of the Committee of Inquiry*, p. 31.
81. *A Letter*, pp. 11–13, 23; Gray, pp. 14–17; *Report of the Committee*, pp. 29, 33; Digby, pp. 6–9. The receipt of fees by the physician from private patients was not, in itself, unprecedented. It was already the practice at the Manchester Lunatic Hospital — *An Account of the Rise, and Present Establishment of the Manchester Lunatic Hospital*, p. 9. Hunter was well aware of this, and reproduced the relevant part of the Manchester Rules in the appendix to the polemical history of the York Asylum that he published in 1792 — A. Hunter, *The History of the Rise and Progress of the York Lunatic Asylum*, York, 1792, p. 25. This *History* was reproduced in an appendix to W. White, M.D., *Observations on the Nature and Method of Cure of the Pthisis Pulomonalis....From Materials Left by the Late William White, and now Published by A. Hunter*, York: Wilson, Spence, and Mawman, 1792.
82. *York Courant*, 22 January 1788; Hunter, *The History of the Rise and Progress of the York Lunatic Asylum*; *A Letter From a Subscriber* (though ostensibly anonymous, it was well known that the author was Hunter), and Appendix I, letter dated 24 August 1787, Appendix II, letter dated 5 January 1788.

83. Mason, *Animadversions*; York Central Library, Bowen MSS, Letter 10 November 1791, Burgh to Wilberforce; Gray, *A History*, pp. 17–18.
84. Gray, pp. 18–22.
85. Hunter, *The History of the Rise and Progress*, p. 14.
86. Gray, pp. 21–22; *SC on the State of Madhouses*, 1814–15, pp. 8, 144.
87. Gray, p. 23.
88. Ibid., pp. 23–25.
89. See Ch.7.
90. Leicester Asylum Rules, p. 6; Manchester Lunatic Hospital Rules, 1791, p. 9.
91. 'Rules of the Hospital for Lunaticks for the Counties of Northumberland, Newcastle Upon Tyne, and Durham', p. 3; *Reasons for the Establishing, and Further Encouragement of St Luke's Hospital*, 1790, p. 19.
92. This changed in the group of lunatic asylums developed under the provisions of Wynn's Act of 1808; in several instances the house surgeon also acted as superintendent — Smith, '*Cure, Comfort and Safe Custody*', pp. 58–61.
93. Woodward, *To Do the Sick No Harm*, pp. 28–29; Fissell, *Patients, Power and the Poor*, pp. 126–27; A. Borsay, *Medicine and Charity in Georgian Bath; a Social History of the General Infirmary, c.1739–1830*, Aldershot: Ashgate, 1999, pp. 350–51; S.C. Lawrence, *Charitable Knowledge; Hospital Pupils and Practitioners in Eighteenth-Century London*, Cambridge: Cambridge University Press, 1996, p. 57.
94. SLH, General Committee Book, 23 October 1751; General Court Book, 13 February 1754.
95. Mason, *Animadversions*, p. 25.
96. *Report of the Committee of Inquiry*, p. 36.
97. *The Rules and Regulations of the York Lunatic Asylum, with a List of Governors, &c.&c.*, York: Thomas Wilson and Sons, 1820, pp. 19–20.
98. Paul, *A Scheme of an Institution*, p. 12.
99. DCRO, 3992/F/H26, 'The Plan of the Intended Lunatic Asylum', no.XIV.
100. DCRO, 3992/F/H26, 'Statutes and Constitutions of the Lunatic Asylum Near Exeter, with Rules and Orders for the Government and Conduct of the House', Third Edition, 1804, pp. 21–22.
101. See below.
102. Becher, *Resolutions Concerning the Intended Lunatic Asylum*, p. 11; *The Articles of Union, Entered Into and Agreed Upon, Between the Justices of the Peace for the County of Nottingham, the Justices of the Peace for the County of the Town of Nottingham, and the Subscribers to a Voluntary Institution for the Purpose of Providing a General Lunatic Asylum, Near Nottingham, Together With the By-Laws, Rules, Orders, Regulations, Established for the Management and Conduct of the Institution*, Nottingham: S. Bennett, 1825, pp. 19, 51–55.
103. P. Slade Knight, *A Letter to the Right Honourable Lord Stanley, and the Other Visiting Justices of the Lunatic Asylum for the County of Lancaster*, Lancaster, 1822, title page. It appears that Knight also held an M.D., though was evidently not practicing as a physician at the asylum.
104. SCRO, D550/1, Staffordshire General Lunatic Asylum, Minute Book of Visitors, 15 December 1817, 12 January, 13 April 1818.
105. *Rules for the Lunatic Asylum at Lincoln* (1819), pp. 12–14; *Rules of the Lincoln Lunatic Asylum* (1832), p. 16; Lincs Archives, LAWN 1/1/2, 14 October 1829–27 December 1830.
106. *Statutes and Constitutions of the Lunatic Asylum in the Parish of St Thomas, Near Exeter, with the Rules and Orders for the Government and Conduct of the House*, Exeter: S. Hedgeland, 1824, Fourth Edition, p. 12.

107. Smith, '*Cure, Comfort and Safe Custody*', pp. 261–69.
108. French, *The Story of St Luke's*, pp. 4, 24, 37–40, 45, 49–50, 118–120.
109. SLH, General Committee Book, 23 October 1751; General Court Book, 26 June 1751, 12 February 1752. It was evident that the keeper's responsibilities might be quite wide-ranging, including providing a pump for the beer cellar, arranging for 'curing the House of Bugges', getting the 'Necessaries' emptied, arranging repairs, and providing the material to be used to make strait-waist-coats — SLH, House Committee Minutes, 16 October, 6 November 1772, 12 November 1773, 21 June 1776, 28 June 1777.
110. The term 'keeper' was also sometimes used to describe the proprietor of a private madhouse. See L.D. Smith, 'Behind Closed Doors: Lunatic Asylum Keepers, 1800–60', *Social History of Medicine* 1, 1988, 301–27.
111. French, *The Story of St Luke's*, pp. 20, 23. Subsequently, and certainly by 1786, the post was being described as 'Head Keeper'— SLH, General Court Book, 24 November 1786.
112. French, p. 23.
113. SLH, General Committee Book, 6 February, 6 March 1782; French, pp. 23–24.
114. General Committee Book, 3 April 1782; French, p. 24.
115. General Court Book, 24 November 1786.
116. Ibid., 7, 14 February 1787.
117. Ibid., 7 October 1789. At this time, the apothecary was receiving the same salary as Dunston.
118. General Committee Book, 12 September 1805.
119. Ibid., 12 December 1811.
120. *SC on the State of Criminal and Pauper Lunatics*, 1807, pp. 21–24; *SC on the State of Madhouses*, 1814–15, pp. 126–28, 131–33; BPP1816, Vol. VI, *Third Report from SC on Madhouses in England*, pp. 28–34.
121. *SC on the State of Criminal and Pauper Lunatics*, 1807, pp. 21–24.
122. *SC on the State of Madhouses*, 1814–15, pp. 127–33.
123. Ibid., pp. 135–37.
124. *SC on the State of Madhouses*, 1816, pp. 28, 30, 32.
125. Ibid., pp. 28, 32.
126. Ibid., pp. 29–31. Although it was not raised directly by the Committee, Dunston's son John acted as surgeon to Warburton's houses. Thomas Warburton himself had told an earlier meeting of the Committee: 'My houses at Bethnal Green are medically attended by Mr Dunston, who has had great experience in cases of insanity, being the son of the Steward of St Luke's Hospital, and having been brought up in that establishment.' — *SC on the State of Madhouses*, 1814–15, p. 191. At the Select Committee in 1827, Warburton reported that he paid John Dunston £550 per annum. By this time, Dunston was also acting as surgeon to St Luke's — BPP 1826–27, Vol. VI, *Report of the Select Committee on the State of Pauper Lunatics in the County of Middlesex, and on Lunatic Asylums*, pp. 70, 72, 103–113.
127. SLH, General Committee Book, 10 February, 13 October 1814.
128. *A Picture of London for 1818*, London: Longman, 1818, pp. 202–03.
129. SLH, General Committee Book, 13 June, 11 July 1816. This would appear to be the first use of this title for the person in charge of a lunatic asylum.
130. Ibid., 11 September 1816, 6 February 1817, 30 January 1818.
131. *SC on Pauper Lunatics in the County of Middlesex, and on Lunatic Asylums*, 1827, pp. 167–68. Dunston himself acknowledged that 'my memory is not so good as it used to be.'
132. French, *The Story of St Luke's*, pp. 49–50, 120.
133. MRI Archives, 'Lunatick Hospital, in Manchester, December 1766'.

134. MRI Archives, 'The Report of the Infirmary and Lunatic Hospital in Manchester', XVIII, July 19 1770.
135. MRI Archives, Manchester Infirmary, Weekly Board, 25 October 1773.
136. Ibid., 20 December 1773.
137. Ibid., 7 March 1774; *General Evening Post*, 26 February, 15 March 1774; Roberts, *Cheadle Royal Hospital*, pp. 24–25. These events are considered further in Ch. 7.
138. Raffald, *The Manchester Directory, for the Year 1781*, p. 102. By 1788 Betty Craddock had been replaced by Mrs Jane Hopper Holme, *A Directory of the Towns of Manchester and Salford for the Year 1788*, p. 130.
139. Weekly Board, 16 November 1789.
140. Ibid., 22 March, 3 May 1790.
141. SCRO, Q/A1c, Box 1, Manchester Lunatic Hospital, Rules, p. 12.
142. *Scholes's Manchester and Salford Directory, 1794*, xvi.
143. Weekly Board, 1 December 1800.
144. Ibid., 18 January 1802.
145. Ibid., 26 January, 20 April, 13 July 1807; MRI archives, 'A Report of the State of the Infirmary, Dispensary, Lunatic Hospital, and Asylum, in Manchester', 1801–02, 1804–05, 1805–06, 1806–07.
146. Weekly Board, 27 July 1807. One of the physicians involved was Dr John Ferriar, author of *Medical Histories and Reflections*, London: Cadell and Davies, 1792–98, an acknowledged authority on the treatment of insanity — Hunter and Macalpine, *Three Hundred Years of Psychiatry*, pp. 543–46.
147. Weekly Board, 3, 17 August 1807. According to Roberts, Sanderson had previously been a weaver. He had been admitted to the infirmary as a patient after an accident in 1794; following his recovery he became an employee — *Cheadle Royal Hospital*, p. 23. A 'still man' worked as an assistant to the apothecary.
148. Roberts, *Cheadle Royal Hospital*, p. 23.
149. LRO, 614 INF 5/2, Liverpool Infirmary, Annual Reports, 3 March 1794 to 2 March 1795; G. McLoughlin, *A Short History of the First Liverpool Infirmary*, London: Phillimore, 1978, p. 53.
150. LRO, 614 INF 1/1, Board of Governors, 21 September 1812; 614 INF 5/2, Annual Reports, 1797, 1813; McLoughlin, p. 53 — he stated incorrectly that they left in 1818.
151. Board of Governors, 21 September 1812; Annual Report, 1813; McLoughlin, *A Short History*, p. 53.
152. *SC on the State of Madhouses*, 1814–15, pp. 102–04, cited in A. Ingram (ed.), *Patterns of Madness in the Eighteenth Century, A Reader*, Liverpool: Liverpool University Press, 1998, pp. 253–55. Haslam's avowal of King's innocence of the charges was not entirely convincing, especially as he went on to acknowledge that King tended to be frightened of the patients.
153. LRO, 614 INF 2/1, Board of Economy Minute Book, 22 April 1813.
154. Ibid., 25 January, 8 February 1816.
155. Ibid., 2 January 1817.
156. Ibid., 3 February 1820; Board of Governors, 3 January 1820.
157. LRO, 614 INF 6/1, 'Liverpool Royal Infirmary, Rules and Orders' (1813), pp. 25–33. The distinctions within the lunatic section are clearly explained on page 25 — 'The LUNATIC HOSPITAL being divided within, so as to accommodate different Classes of Patients, the better Apartments are denominated the ASYLUM.'
158. Board of Economy, 1 March 1820; Board of Governors, 3 July 1820.
159. *Gore's General Advertiser*, 5 January 1826; *Liverpool Mercury*, 6, 13 January 1826; *Morning Herald*, 12 January 1826.

160. *Liverpool Mercury*, 20 January 1826.
161. Herefords CRO, 560/25, 26 March 1799.
162. *Rules for the Government of the Lunatic Asylum in Hereford.*
163. Herefords CRO, 560/25, 17 August 1815; 560/26, 30 October 1823, 'Report of Committee Appointed to Investigate the State of the Lunatic Asylum'.
164. SCRO, Q/AIc, Box 1, letter 10 March 1812, Rev. James Manning to Charles Aylesbury; 'General Meeting of Governors of Exeter Lunatic Asylum, Held at Exeter Castle 11 April 1804'.
165. *SC On the State of Madhouses*, 1814–15, p. 22.
166. Ibid., p. 20; SCRO, Q/AIc, Manning to Aylesbury, 10 March 1812.
167. DCRO, 3992/F/H26, 'The Plan of the Intended Lunatic Asylum'; 'Statutes and Constitution of the Lunatic Asylum in the Parish of St Thomas Near Exeter', 1804 Edition., p. 23; Manning to Aylesbury, 10 March 1812.
168. DCRO, 3992 F/H1/2, 22 July 1806; 3992 F/H13, 37th Annual Report, 1838.
169. 'Lunatick Hospital, in Manchester, December 10, 1766'.
170. SLH, 'Considerations Upon the Usefulness and Necessity of Establishing an Hospital as a Further Provision for Poor Lunaticks'.
171. The terminology could be confusing. 'Servant' was the most commonly used term for the staff providing direct care, with 'maid' sometimes used for female staff. The term 'keeper' came into use increasingly by 1800. However, 'keeper' was still sometimes used as an alternative to 'governor' or 'master', describing the lay manager of the institution.
172. J. Andrews, 'Bedlam Revisited: A History of Bethlem Hospital c.1634–1770', University of London, unpublished PhD, 1991, pp. 344–56; Andrews et al, *The History of Bethlem*, pp. 292–94.
173. A background in domestic service appears to have been quite common, as was the case for Mary Jones who worked for several months at the Liverpool Asylum in 1825; after she left she resumed a career in service — *Morning Herald*, 12 January 1826.
174. Smith, 'Behind Closed Doors: Lunatic Asylum Keepers, 1800–1860', pp. 305–09; Smith, *'Cure,Comfort and Safe Custody'*, pp. 132–38.
175. Gray, *A History of the York Lunatic Asylum*, p. 11; *Report of the Committee of Inquiry*, pp. 12, 17; A New Governor, *A Vindication of Mr Higgins from the Charges of Corrector: Including a Sketch of the Recent Transactions at the York Lunatic Asylum*, York: Hargrove and Co., 1814, p. 37. ('A New Governor' was almost certainly a pseudonym for Samuel Tuke).
176. Manchester Infirmary, Weekly Board, 19 May 1766, 5 April, 20 December 1773.
177. Warneford Hospital Archives, W. P. 5 / xv, letter 7 April 1818.
178. SCRO, Q/AIc, Box 1, letter 11 March 1812, from John Squires; LRO, 614 INF 2/2, 18 November 1813.
179. G.O. Paul, *Observations on the Subject of Lunatic Asylums, Addressed to a General Meeting of Subscribers to a Fund for Building and Establishing a General Lunatic Asylum, Near Gloucester*, Gloucester: D. Walker, 1812, p. 28.
180. E. Mackenzie, *A Descriptive and Historical Account of the Town and County of Newcastle Upon Tyne*, Newcastle: Mackenzie and Dent, 1827, Vol. II, p. 526.
181. *SC on the State of Madhouses*, 1816, p. 53.
182. *SC on the State of Madhouses*, 1814–15, p. 127; *SC on the State of Madhouses*, 1816, p. 33.
183. *SC on Criminal and Pauper Lunatics*, 1807, p. 21; SLH, General Committee Book, 13 July 1809. The female numbers included a cook and two laundry

maids. The numbers of female patients admitted to St Luke's consistently exceeded males, particularly in the early years — see below, Ch. 5.

184. *SC on the State of Madhouses*, 1814–15, pp. 127–28. The general committee minutes indicate that there were six male keepers at this time - General Committee Book, 14 July 1814, 13 July 1815.
185. *SC on the State of Madhouses*, 1814–15, pp. 136–37.
186. General Committee Book, 8 July 1819.
187. SCRO, Q/AIc, Box 1, letter 10 March 1812, Manning to Aylesbury.
188. Smith, *'Cure, Comfort and Safe Custody'*, pp. 132–33.
189. Lincolnshire Archives, LAWN 1/1/1, 18 February 1820, 2 April 1821, 6 October 1823, LAWN 1/1/2, 26 July 1824, 27 March, 1 May 1826, 7 April, 1 September 1828; E. P. Charlesworth, *Remarks on the Treatment of the Insane and the Management of Lunatic Asylums. Being the Substance of a Return from the Lincoln Lunatic Asylum to the Circular of His Majesty's Secretary of State: With a Plan*, London: C. & J. Rivington, 1828, p. 23.
190. Andrews, 'Bedlam Revisited', p. 353; Andrews et al, *History of Bethlem*, pp. 293–94.
191. SLH, General Court Book, 7 October 1789; *The Times*, 19 October 1789.
192. SLH, General Committee Book, 14 January 1808, 13 July 1809, 8 July 1819; Smith, *'Cure, Comfort and Safe Custody'*, pp. 143–45.
193. Smith, 'Behind Closed Doors', pp. 310–11.
194. Manchester Infirmary, Weekly Board, 5 April, 20 December 1773. Amey White had the additional privilege 'that she eats from the Matron's Table at the Infirmary'.
195. DCRO, 3992 F/H1/1, 20 September, 8 November 1803, 25 December 1804.
196. SCRO, Q/AIC, Box 1, letter 13 March 1812, John Flint to Charles Aylesbury; LCRO, 13 D 54/4, 13 July 1819, 21 January 1823 — by this time wages were being paid on a weekly basis, at 7s and 4s.
197. LRO, 614 INF 2/1, Board of Economy Minutes, 18 November 1813.
198. Paul, *Observations on the Subject of Lunatic Asylums*, p. 33; Gray, *A History*, p. 29; *Report of the Committee of Inquiry*, pp. 12, 45, 48. Staff at York also received significant sums from 'perquisites' before the reforms from 1814 onwards.
199. Lincolnshire Archives, LAWN 1/1/1, 18 February 1820, 2 April 1821, 1, 6 October 1823, LAWN 1/1/2, 28 December 1829.
200. *Incontestable Proofs, From Internal Evidence, that S.W. Nicoll, Esquire, is Not the Author of a Vindication of Mr Higgins, From the Charges of Corrector*, York: W. Storrey, c.1816, p. 97; Gray, *A History*, pp. 17–18, 29, 36.
201. *SC on the State of Madhouses*, 1814–15, p. 20.
202. SLH, General Committee, 13 June 1816, 14 January 1819. Her length of service hardly compared, however, with the St Luke's master Thomas Dunston, who served for almost fifty years.
203. General Committee, 14 January, 14 July 1808, 12 January, 13 July 1809, 10 January 1811, 9 July 1812, 12 January, 14 January, 8 July 1813, 12 January, 14 July 1814, 12 January, 13 July 1815, 11 January, 11 July 1816, 10 July 1817, 9 July 1818, 8 July 1819.
204. *Copy of a Letter Pricked with a Pin, by Hugh Williams, Broker, No.19 Cannon-street, Manchester; to the Revd. Dr Bayley; on the 54th Day of his Confinement in Bondage, in the Lunatic Hospital, Manchester*, Manchester: B. Radford, 1801, p. 3, copy in British Library, Thomason Tracts, E.2179 (2).
205. *Report of the Committee of Inquiry*, pp. 35–39; *SC on the State of Madhouses*, 1814–15, evidence of Godfrey Higgins, pp. 2, 4, 8, evidence of Dr Charles Best, pp. 143–34. The role of steward was, on paper, comparable to that of master or governor. See Ch. 7 for events at York.

206. Porter contended that Hanoverian asylums were part of the world of Old Corruption 'where the fabric was honeycombed with venality, peculation, petty oppression, neglect, chicanery, bullying, profiteering, cruelties, nepotism.' — R. Porter, 'In the Eighteenth Century Were English Lunatic Asylums Total Institutions ?', *Ego (Bulletin of the Department of Psychiatry, Guy's Hospital)*, Spring 1983, 12–34; W.D. Rubinstein, 'The End of "Old Corruption" in Britain', *Past and Present* 101, 1983, 55–86.

Chapter 4

1. P. Borsay, *The English Urban Renaissance; Culture and Society in the Provincial Town, 1660–1770*, Oxford: Oxford University Press, 1989, pp. 204–11, 227–28, 317; J. Pickstone, *Medicine and Industrial Society; A History of Hospital Development in Manchester and its Region, 1752–1946*, Manchester: Manchester University Press, 1985, p. 11.
2. I. Loudon, *Medical Care and the General Practitioner, 1750–1850*, Oxford: Clarendon, 1986; I. Waddington, *The Medical Profession in the Industrial Revolution*, Dublin: Gill and Macmillan, 1994, pp. 1–30; J. Lane, *A Social History of Medicine; Health, Healing and Disease in England, 1750–1950*, London: Routledge, 2001, Ch.1; A. Digby, *Making a Medical Living; Doctors and Patients in the English Market for Medicine, 1720–1911*, Cambridge University Press, 1994, pp. 170–72; S. C. Lawrence, *Charitable Knowledge; Hospital Pupils and Practitioners in Eighteenth-Century London*, Cambridge University Press, 1996; R. Porter, 'William Hunter: a Surgeon and a Gentleman', in W.F. Bynum and R. Porter (eds.) *William Hunter and the Eighteenth-Century Medical World*, Cambridge University Press, 1985, pp. 7–34.
3. For the career of one of the most successful physician mad-doctors, see J. Andrews and A. Scull, *Undertaker of the Mind; John Monro and Mad-Doctoring in Eighteenth-Century England*, London: University of California Press, 2001, and its sequel *Customers and Patrons of the Mad-Trade; the Management of Lunacy in Eighteenth-Century London*, London: University of California Press, 2003.
4. For the significance of the Edinburgh Medical School at this period, see C. Lawrence, 'Ornate Physicians and Learned Artisans: Edinburgh Medical Men, 1726–1776', in Bynum and Porter, *William Hunter and the Eighteenth-Century Medical World*, pp. 153–76.
5. The following, other than where otherwise stated, is summarized from two main sources — J. Nichols, *Literary Anecdotes of the Eighteenth Century*, London: Nichols, Son, and Bentley, 1812, Kraus Reprint, New York, 1966, Vol. 4, pp. 599–611; A. Suzuki, 'William Battie', *Oxford Dictionary of National Biography* [ODNB], Oxford University Press, 2004. Online. Available at http://www.oxforddnb.com/view/article/1715. See also the detailed critical appraisal in Andrews and Scull, *Undertaker of the Mind*, pp. 49–53.
6. The exact dates for Battie's commencement of his practices in Uxbridge and London are unclear.
7. There is strong evidence that Battie's river-side house was actually at Marlow in Buckinghamshire — Nichols, *Literary Anecdotes*, Vol. 4, p. 607. It is possible, as Suzuki suggests, that he had two country houses.
8. Nichols, *Literary Anecdotes*, Vol. 4, pp. 606–07, 727.
9. *Journal of the House of Commons*, 22 February 1763, p. 488; *Gentleman's Magazine* 23, 1763, p. 126; Andrews and Scull, *Undertaker of the Mind*, pp. 70, 120–27. To the impressionable young medical student Thomas Arnold

and his contemporaries, though, Battie was 'a haughty, self conceited, over-bearing Person' — Linnaean Society, *Correspondence of Richard Pulteney*, 26 December 1762, Arnold to Pulteney.

10. R. Hunter and I. Macalpine, *Three Hundred Years of Psychiatry, 1535–1860*, London: Oxford University Press, 1963, p. 402.

11. SLH, General Court Book, 31 October 1750.

12. SLH, General Court Book, 12 April 1764.

13. W.S. Lewis, *Horace Walpole's Correspondence*, Oxford University Press, 1965, Vol. 32, pp. 314–15; Andrews and Scull, *Undertaker*, p. 154.

14. Hunter and Macalpine, *Three Hundred Years of Psychiatry*, p. 404.

15. This section is drawn from the following:— Nichols, *Literary Anecdotes*, Vol. 9, Additions to Third Volume, pp. 525–27; 'A Memoir of the Life of Alexander Hunter, M.D.', in A. Hunter, *Silva; or, a Discourse of Forest-Trees, and the Propagation of Timber in His Majesty's Dominions*, York: Wilson and Sons, Fourth Edition, 1812, xi–xii; A. Digby, 'Hunter, Alexander (1729?–1809)', *ODNB*. Online. Available at http://www.oxforddnb.com/view/article/14213.

16. Biographical details are taken from P. Carpenter, 'Thomas Arnold: A Provincial Psychiatrist in Georgian England', *Medical History* 33, 1989, 199–216, and from Carpenter, 'Thomas Arnold (c.1742–1816)', *ODNB*. Available at http://www.oxforddnb.com/view/article/685.

17. It was quite common for the proprietorship of private madhouses to pass down through successive generations of families, and for lay proprietors to ensure medical training and qualification for their sons — see W. L. Parry-Jones, *The Trade in Lunacy; a Study of Private Madhouses in England in the Eighteenth and Nineteenth Centuries*, London: Routldge Kegan Paul, 1972, pp. 74–95.

18. Carpenter, 'Thomas Arnold', pp. 201–10. For the quarrels between Arnold and Vaughan, see below.

19. LCRO, Leicester Infirmary Minutes, 13 D 54/2, 18 June 1795, 23 June 1796, 19 September 1797, 19 June 1800. Dr Thomas Graham Arnold seems to have had a rather erratic tenure at the infirmary — he resigned in June 1796, and was reappointed in September 1797, before his final resignation in June 1800. He then moved to Stamford and practiced there — *Gentleman's Magazine* 86, 1816, p. 378. Dr William Withering Arnold was named after his father's friend William Withering, a leading physician in Birmingham.

20. Carpenter, 'Thomas Arnold', pp. 210–11; Leicester Infirmary Minutes, 13 D 54/3, 22 September, 15, 31 October, 17 November 1815.

21. *Gentleman's Magazine* 86, 1816, p. 378.

22. Biographical details, unless otherwise stated, are taken from — W.W. Currie, *Memoir of the Life, Writings, and Correspondence of James Currie, M.D.,F. R.S., of Liverpool*, London: Longman, Rees, Orme, Brown, and Green, 1831; *Dictionary of National Biography (DNB)*, Vol. 34, pp. 341–43; M. DeLacy, 'Currie, James (1756–1805)', *ODNB*. Online. Available at http://www.oxforddnb.com/view/article/6954.

23. Currie, *Memoir of the Life, Writings, and Correspondence*, pp. 10–27.

24. Ibid., pp. 28–42.

25. Ibid., p. 27.

26. Ibid., pp. 43–51; *DNB*, Vol. 13, p. 341. According to DeLacy, *ODNB*, Currie's M.D. was awarded by Glasgow University.

27. Currie, *Memoir of the Life*, pp. 51–57.

28. Ibid., pp. 61–67.

29. Ibid., pp. 75–83, 137. Dangerous ill health, in the form of consumption, returned soon after his marriage. Currie's description of his illness and its

eventual treatment with gentle rides on horse-back, after the apparent failure of a range of depleting physical treatments, was recounted in Erasmus Darwin's *Zoonomia* — reproduced in Currie, *Memoir of the Life*, pp. 84–92. According to the *DNB*, Vol. 13, p. 341, his illness was pleurisy, 'with blood-spitting', and he had to go away to Bristol for a lengthy recuperation.

30. J. Currie, *Medical Reports on the Effects of Water, Cold and Warm, as a Remedy in Fever and Other Diseases*, Liverpool: J. M'Creery, 1797. Further editions appeared in 1798, 1804, and 1805.

31. Currie's interest may well have been excited by a frightening incident in 1780, shortly after he completed his medical training. Walking among the ruins of an old churchyard in Dumfries-shire, he was startled by a half-naked female with an 'expression of countenance that had in it nothing earthly', who sprang up with a 'hideous laugh' before running off into the adjoining woods. He later discovered that he had encountered a 'poor unhappy maniac known by the name of Susanna', who roamed the surrounding country and lived in the woods — Currie, *Memoir of the Life,* p. 53; National Library of Scotland, Archives, MS 14835, fo.66.

32. Currie, *Memoir Of the* Life, p. 69.

33. *Gore's Liverpool General Advertiser*, 20 August, 15 October, 1789; *Williamson's Liverpool Advertiser*, 24 August, 19 October, 2 November 1789. His influential letters were reproduced in J. Currie, *Medical Reports on the Effects of Water, Cold and Warm, as a Remedy in Fever and Febrile Diseases*, Vol. II, London: Cadell and Davies, 1805, Appendix II, pp. 19–43. They were included in the Appendix to W.W. Currie, *Memoir of the Life*, Vol. I. They have also been cited by various historians of psychiatry, including Hunter and Macalpine, *Three Hundred Years of Psychiatry*, pp. 517–20.

34. LRO, 614 INF 1/2, 28 March 1805.

35. *DNB*, Vol. 13, p. 343.

36. Most of the biographical information on Ferriar, unless otherwise stated, is taken from *DNB*, Vol. 18, pp. 389–90, and K.A. Webb, 'Ferriar, John (1761–1815), *ODNB*. Online. Available at http://www.oxforddnb.com/view/article/9368.

37. J. Ferriar, *Medical Histories and Reflections*, London: Cadell and Davies, 1792–98.

38. Ferriar, *Medical Histories*, 1792, pp. 171–86, Vol. 2, 1795, pp. 33–48, 81–115.

39. Ferriar, *Medical Histories and Reflections*. In the first volume Ferriar is styled 'Physician to the Manchester Infirmary, and Lunatic Hospital'; in the second 'Physician to the Manchester Infirmary, Dispensary, Lunatic Hospital, and Asylum', reflecting the division of the lunatic hospital according to financial and social class considerations.

40. Unless otherwise stated, the information on which this section is based is from: *DNB*, Vol. 52, pp. 259–60; H. Brock, 'Simmons, Samuel Foart (1750–1813)', *ODNB*. Online. Available at http://www.oxforddnb.com/view/article/25565.

41. W. Munk, *The Roll of the Royal College of Physicians of London*, London: The College, 1878, Vol. II, p. 320.

42. R. Kilpatrick, '"Living in the Light"; Dispensaries, Philanthropy and Medical Reform in Late Eighteenth-Century London', in A. Cunningham and R. French (eds.), *The Medical Enlightenment of the Eighteenth Century*, Cambridge University Press, 1990, pp. 254–80. Kilpatrick, pp. 257, 271, argues that Dissenters tended to dominate the running of dispensaries in London.

43. SLH, General Court Book, 19 April 1764, 31 October, 8 November 1781. Brock, in *ODNB* incorrectly states that Foart Simmons was elected physician to Bethlem Hospital.

44. SLH, General Committee Book, 12 September 1805, 14 January 1808, 4 March 1811.
45. General Committee Book, 4, 14 March 1811; *Gentleman's Magazine* 81, 1811, pp. 284, 388.
46. I. Macalpine and R. Hunter, *George III and the Mad Business*, London: Allen Lane / Penguin, 1969, pp. 131–45, 161–65.
47. A. Aspinall (ed.), *The Correspondence of George, Prince of Wales 1770–1812*, London: Cassell, 1968, Vol. 5, p. 89; Aspinall (ed.), *The Later Correspondence of George III*, Cambridge University Press, 1968, p. 185. Cited in Macalpine and Hunter, *George III and the Mad Business*, pp. 134–35.
48. Macalpine and Hunter, pp. 143–45, 161–55; British Library, Additional Manuscripts, 41,735, Willis Papers, ff.1–8, 19–23, 35–36, 43–44, 50–58, 65–66.
49. T. Percival, *Medical Ethics; or a Code of Institutes and Precepts, Adapted to the Professional Conduct of Physicians and Surgeons*, Manchester: S. Russell, 1803, pp. 33-34.
50. Loudon, *Medical Care and the General Practitioner*; Waddington, *The Medical Profession in the Industrial Revolution*.
51. Digby, *Making a Medical Living*, pp. 170–76; Lawrence, *Charitable Knowledge; Hospital Pupils and Practitioners*, pp. 56–70, 301–04.
52. Lawrence, 'Ornate Physicians and Learned Artisans', p. 156; Lane, *A Social History of Medicine*, p. 12; Digby, *Making a Medical Living*, p. 172; Borsay, *The English Urban Renaissance*, pp. 205–07, 225–28, 232–37. For an extensive analysis of provincial physicians and 'medico-gentility', see M. Brown, '"For the Dignity of the Faculty"; Fashioning Medical Identities, York, c.1760–c.1850', University of York, PhD thesis, 2004.
53. Linnaean Society, Pulteney Correspondence, 3 April 1767, Arnold to Pulteney.
54. Pulteney Correspondence, 2 April 1767, Dr John Sutton to Pulteney. Sutton, an established Leicester physician, was not impressed, regarding 'such Appearances' as being 'Farcical'. He had earlier been responsible for offering young Arnold some 'sage Advice' on approaching Dr Vaughan, following his arrival in Leicester — 23 December 1766, Sutton to Pulteney.
55. Digby, *Making a Medical Living*, pp. 125, 171–72; A. Borsay, *Medicine and Charity in Georgian Bath; a Social History of the General Infirmary, c.1739–1830*, Aldershot: Ashgate, 1999, pp. 115–18.
56. Lawrence, 'Ornate Physicians and Learned Artisans', pp. 170–72.
57. Percival, *Medical Ethics; Memoirs of the Life and Writings of Thomas Percival*, Bath: Rochard Cruttwell, 1807, ccix.
58. Percival, *Medical Ethics*, p. 1. The context for Percival's work was the bitter internal struggle within the Manchester Infirmary, in which he and Ferriar had been embroiled — J. V. Pickstone, 'Thomas Percival and the Production of Medical Ethics', in R. Baker, D. Porter and R. Porter, *The Codification of Medical Morality*, Vol. I, *Medical Ethics and Etiquette in the Eighteenth Century*, Dordrecht: Klewer Academic, 1993, pp. 161–78.
59. Percival, *Medical Ethics*, p. 1.
60. Ibid., pp. 10–11.
61. Ibid., p. 26.
62. Ibid., pp. 44–45.
63. *Gore's Liverpool General Advertiser*, 20 August 1789; *Williamson's Liverpool Advertiser*, 24 August 1789.
64. A. Hunter, M.D., *The Buxton Manual: or, a Treatise on the Nature and Virtues of the Waters of Buxton, to Which is Prefixed.an Account of the*

External and Internal Use of Natural and Artificial Warm Waters Among the Antients, York, 1797, Sixth Edition., Preface dated 1765.

65. A. Hunter, *Men and Manners, or, Concentrated Wisdom*, York: T. Wilson and R. Spence, 1808, Third Edition., p. 201, no.1142.

66. Hunter, *Men and Manners*, p. 78, no.414.

67. *Ibid.*, p. 82, no.442.

68. *A Letter From a Subscriber to the York Lunatic Asylum, to the Governors of That Charity*, York: Wilson, Spence and Mawman, 1788, p. 8, Appendix I, p. 25, Appendix II, pp. 28–30; A. Hunter, *The History of the Rise and Progress of the York Lunatic Asylum*, York, 1792, pp. 3, 7.

69. W. Mason, *Animadversions on the Present Government of the York Lunatic Asylum in Which the Case of Parish Paupers is Distinctly Considered in a Series of Propositions*, York: Blanchard, 1788, pp. 33–36; J. Gray, *A History of the York Lunatic Asylum*, York: W. Hargrove and Co., 1815, pp. 14–20; A. Digby, *From York Lunatic Asylum to Bootham Park Hospital*, York: University of York, Borthwick Papers No.69, 1986, pp. 7–13; M.Brown, 'Rethinking Early Nineteenth-Century Asylum Reform', *The Historical Journal* 49, 2006, 425–52.

70. *A Letter From a Subscriber*, pp. 8–10, 23; Hunter, *The History*, pp. 1–5.

71. Hunter, *The History*, pp. 14–15.

72. J. Gregory, *Observations on the Duties and Offices of a Physician; and on the Method of Prosecuting Enquiries in Philosophy*, London: W. Strahan and T. Cadell, 1770, pp. 38–39.

73. Digby, *Making a Medical Living*, p. 176. For later examples, see L. D. Smith, '*Cure, Comfort and Safe Custody'; Public Lunatic Asylums in Early Nineteenth Century England*, London: Leicester University Press, 1999, pp. 66–69, 262–68.

74. Andrews and Scull, *Undertaker of the Mind*, pp. 52–59; R. Hunter and I. Macalpine, 'Introduction' to facsimile edition of W. Battie, *A Treatise on Madness*, and J. Monro, *Remarks on Dr Battie's Treatise on Madness*, London: Dawson, 1962.

75. Andrews and Scull, *Undertaker*, pp. 70–72.

76. See Ch.2 for the early development of the Newcastle Lunatic Hospital.

77. P. M. Horsley, *Eighteenth-Century Newcastle*, Newcastle: Oriel Press, 1971, p. 124. Hall (1733–93) was the son of a barber-surgeon. He was appointed physician to the Newcastle Infirmary in 1771. He became the city's leading physician, and prominent in local cultural life as president of the Literary and Philosophical Society.

78. J. Hall, *A Narrative of the Proceedings Relative to the Establishment &c of St Luke's House*, Newcastle: J. White and T. Saint, 1767, pp. 4–9; *Newcastle Courant*, 17 May 1766.

79. Hall, *A Narrative*, pp. 8–17.

80. *Newcastle Courant*, 17, 24 May, 28 June, 9 August 1766.

81. Horsley, *Eighteenth-Century Newcastle*, pp. 113, 119. Lambert was the most prominent surgeon in Newcastle, with a widespread reputation and extensive private practice. He had been closely involved in the founding of the Newcastle Infirmary in 1751 and was one of its surgeons from the outset.

82. Hall, *A Narrative*, pp. 17–25.

83. *Ibid.*, p. 36; *Newcastle Courant*, 19 September, 3, 10, 17, 24, 31 October, 7, 14, 21, 28 November, 5, 12, 19 December 1767, 30 January, 31 December 1768.

84. Horsley, *Eighteenth-Century Newcastle*, p. 122. Dr Adam Askew (1694–1773) had been appointed senior physician to the Newcastle Infirmary when

it opened in 1751; he was described as having a 'certain brusqueness of manner'; K. Wilson, *The Sense of the People; Politics, Culture and Imperialism in England, 1715–1785*, Cambridge University Press, 1995, pp. 81, 353–34, 358. Dr John Rotheram was a physician to the Newcastle Infirmary. He was a noted radical leader in Newcastle, being chairman of the 'Revolution Society' and later a prominent member of the Newcastle Protestant Association. Henry Gibson, one of the other surgeons involved in the St Luke's House disputes, was also particularly prominent in radical activities in the city.

85. Hall, *A Narrative*, pp. 30–31.
86. Ibid., pp. 32–34.
87. J. Hall, M.D., *An Answer to Dr Rotheram's Letter*, Newcastle Upon Tyne: J. White and T. Saint, 1767; *Newcastle Courant*, 26 September 1767.
88. Hall, *A Narrative*, pp. 4, 8–9, 18, 38.
89. Ibid., pp. 15, 18, 24, 29, 37.
90. Ibid., p. 30.
91. Pulteney Correspondence, 23 December 1766, Dr John Sutton to Pulteney.
92. Pulteney Correspondence, 3 April 1767, Arnold to Pulteney.
93. Carpenter, 'Thomas Arnold', pp. 204–05. It would appear that there had been a serious dispute between Arnold and Vaughan over Infirmary matters as early as 1772 — P. Langford, *Public Life and the Propertied Englishman, 1689–1798*, Oxford: Clarendon, 1991, p. 497.
94. *Leicester and Nottingham Journal*, 19 June 1784.
95. Carpenter, 'Thomas Arnold', pp. 205–6. The quarrels were serious enough to descend into physical violence.
96. J. Throsby, *The History and Antiquities of the Ancient Town of Leicester*, Leicester: J. Brown, 1791, p. 314; LCRO, 13 D 54/1, Infirmary Governors Minutes, 21 June 1781, 20 June 1782, 19 June 1783, 17 June 1784.
97. J. Throsby, *Select Views in Leicestershire*, Leicester, 1789, Vol. II , p. 35; *Leicester and Nottingham Journal*, 7 May, 18 June, 10 September 1785; *Leicester Journal*, 14 March 1794.
98. Carpenter, pp. 209–10.
99. Hunter and Macalpine, *Three Hundred Years of Psychiatry*, p. 672.
100. LCRO, 13 D 54/3, 22 September 1815.
101. Carpenter, pp. 199–203.
102. W. Gardiner, *Music and Friends; or, Pleasant Recollections of a Dilettante*, London: Longman, Orme, Brown, and Longman, 1838, p. 409.
103. Carpenter, p. 202.
104. Pickstone, 'Thomas Percival and the Production of Medical Ethics', pp. 167–72; Pickstone and Butler, 'The Politics of Medicine in Manchester, 1788–92'.
105. SCRO, Q/A1c, Manchester Infirmary Rules, 1791. See Ch.5.
106. MRI, Weekly Board, 7, 28 September 1801, 8 November 1802. See Ch.7.
107. LRO, 614 INF 1 /2, 7 January, 2 April 1810. Brandreth retired from the Infirmary shortly afterwards, to be replaced by his son Dr Joseph Pilkington Brandreth —1, 19 October 1810; 614 INF 6/1, 'Liverpool Royal Infirmary – Rules and Orders', 1813, pp. 25–26.
108. T. Renwick, *A Letter to the Trustees of the Liverpool Infirmary*, Liverpool; T. Kaye, 1826, pp. 4–8. For the problems of 1825–26, see Ch. 7.
109. For the conflicts surrounding the introduction of 'Non-Restraint', see Smith, *'Cure, Comfort and Safe Custody'*, Ch. 8, and also L.D. Smith, 'The "Great Experiment": the Place of Lincoln in the History of Psychiatry', *Lincolnshire History and Archaeology* 30, 1995, 55–62.

110. *Rules for the Lunatic Asylum at Lincoln, November 4th, 1819*, Lincoln: William Brooke, 1819, pp. 11–12; *Rules of the Lincoln Lunatic Asylum*, Lincoln: W. Brooke, 1832, pp. 15–16.
111. Sir F. Hill, *Georgian Lincoln*, Cambridge University Press, 1966, pp. 198–99, 216, 250–53, 260, 277–81. Charlesworth even fought a duel in 1826 with Colonel Charles Sibthorp, who subsequently became the city's MP, apparently over an asylum-related matter. On being offered the option of withdrawing, Charlesworth had responded 'that if my coffin stood on one side of me, and riches, friends and honour on the other, so circumstanced I would turn to my coffin rather than make a concession the breadth of a hair.' — Hill, p. 278.
112. Lincoln Local Studies Library, 'At a General Board of Governors, Lincoln Lunatic Asylum, 13 October, 1828'; Lincs Archives, LAWN 1/1/2, Lincoln Lunatic Asylum, Committee Minutes, 19 May 1823, 27 March, 28 April, 5 October 1827.
113. E. P. Charlesworth, M.D., *Remarks on the Treatment of the Insane and the Management of Lunatic Asylums, Being the Substance of a Return From the Lincoln Lunatic Asylum, to the Circular of His Majesty's Secretary of State: With a Plan*, London: C & J Rivington, 1828.
114. *Lincoln Herald*, 28 November, 5 December 1828, 2, 9, 23 January, 10 April, 14, 21, 28 August, 4, 11, 18 September 1829; *Proceedings of the General Quarterly Board of the Lincoln Lunatic Asylum, Held on October 13, 1830*, Lincoln, 1830, pp. 19–20, 24–25.
115. *Lincoln Herald*, 9, 16, 23, 30 October, 6, 13, 20 November 1829.
116. *Proceedings of the General Quarterly Board of the Lincoln Lunatic Asylum*, pp. 3–7, 10–11, 18 — Fisher had called Charlesworth 'a mean, cowardly, ungentlemanly thing in the shape of a man'.
117. *Proceedings of the General Quarterly Board*, pp. 13, 20.
118. Ibid., pp. 8–9, 12–24, 28–33, 40–48, 51–52.
119. Lincs Archives, LAWN 1/1/3, 13 October 1830.
120. LAWN 1/1/3, 15 November 1830, 15 October 1832; Smith, '*Cure, Comfort and Safe Custody*', pp. 265–67.
121. Gregory, *Observations on the Duties and Offices of a Physician*, p. 175. Gregory was Professor of the Practice of Physic at Edinburgh University, and will have directly influenced several of the people discussed in this chapter.
122. Borsay, *The English Urban Renaissance*, pp. 204–07, 226–29; Brown, 'For The Dignity of the Faculty; Fashioning Medical Identities, York, c.1760-c.1850', Ch. 3; K. Wilson, 'Urban Culture and Political Activism in Hanoverian England: the Example of Voluntary Hospitals', in E. Hellmuth (ed.), *The Transformation of Political Culture; England and Germany in the Late Eighteenth Century*, Oxford: Oxford University Press, 1990, pp. 165–67, 177–82.
123. Suzuki, 'Battie, William', *ODNB*. According to Nichols, *Literary Anecdotes*, Vol. 4, p. 606, it was in 1749 that Battie 'obliged the learned world with a corrected version of his favourite Isocrates'.
124. Hunter and Macalpine, 'William Battie, M.D., F.R.S., Pioneer Psychiatrist'; British Library, Additional Manuscripts, MSS 4300, f.190, letter 29 January 1752.
125. Nichols, *Literary Anecdotes*, Vol. 4, p. 607. According to Nichols' correspondent, building was one of Battie's 'whims'; he had contrived to construct a 'very faulty' riverside house at Marlow without a staircase, and without any means to prevent the regular flooding of the lower parts. He had also wasted £1,500 in an abortive scheme to draw river barges by horse power, which brought him into confrontation with the bargemen.

126. British Library, Add. MSS 35057, f.50, letter dated 3 January 1777.
127. An erstwhile inmate of one of Simmons' private madhouses was particularly disparaging about his attainments, suggesting that: 'A man, under the appellation of a Fellow of the Royal Society, may be as ignorant as a Goth, yet he will be looked upon as a Colossus of learning; he may be as unfeeling as a Vandal, yet he will be counted as humane as an Apostle.' — Richard Brothers, *A Letter From Mr. Brothers to Miss Cott, the Recorded Daughter of David, and Future Queen of the Hebrews, With an Address to the Members of His Britannic Majesty's Council, and Through Them to All Governments and People on Earth*, London: G. Riebau, 1798, p. 23.
128. Simmons was part of a corresponding network of dissenting physicians, which also included William Cullen, Thomas Percival, and James Currie - Kilpatrick, ' "Living in the Light"; Dispensaries, Philanthropy and Medical Reform'; F. M. Lobo, 'John Haygarth, Smallpox, and Religious Dissent in Eighteenth-Century England', in Cunningham and French (eds.), *The Medical Enlightenment of the Eighteenth Century*, pp. 217–53. His connection with Percival was influential in obtaining membership of the Manchester Literary and Philosophical Society, of which Currie and Ferriar were also members.
129. Munk, *The Roll of the Royal College of Physicians of London*, Vol. II, p. 320.
130. Lane, *A Social History of Medicine*, p. 15; S. Lawrence, *Charitable Knowledge*, pp. 255–56; Kilpatrick, ' "Living in the Light" ', p. 279.
131. Lawrence, *Charitable Knowledge*, pp. 259, 274.
132. Kilpatrick, pp. 277–79; Lawrence, p. 269.
133. Brown, ' "For the Dignity of the Faculty',", pp. 90–97, deals in some detail with Hunter's gentlemanly activities and aspirations.
134. Nichols, *Literary Anecdotes*, Vol. 9, p. 526.
135. Brown, ' "For the Dignity of the Faculty',", pp. 95–98. After three successful editions the book was re-titled *The Buxton Manual: Or a Treatise on the Nature and Virtue of the Waters of Buxton, to Which is Prefixed, an Account of the External and Internal Use of Natural and Artificial Warm Waters*, York: G. Peacock, 1797, Sixth Edition. Hunter dedicates this volume to the architect John Carr, who designed many prominent buildings including the York Asylum. In the preface, he assures his readers that his only motive for publication was 'a sincere desire to contribute to the ease and satisfaction of the infirm.'
136. Hunter, *Silva: Or a Discourse of Forest Trees and the Propagation of Timber in His Majesty's Dominions*; Brown, ' "For the Dignity"', pp. 104–07.
137. Brown, pp. 108–09; Nichols, *Literary Anecdotes*, Vol. 9, p. 526.
138. A. Hunter, *Terra: a Philosophical Discourse on the Earth Relating to the Culture and Improvement of it for Vegetation and the Propogation of Plants as it was Presented to the Royal Society by J. Evelyn Esq*, York, A. Ward, 1778; Nichols, *Literary Anecdotes*, p. 526; Digby, 'Hunter, Alexander', *ODNB*.
139. A. Hunter, *Culina Famulatrix Medicinae; Or, Receipts in Modern Cookery*, York: Wilson and Spence, 1804.
140. A. Hunter, *Men and Manners, or, Concentrated Wisdom*, 1808 Edition.
141. Ibid., p. 18, no.41.
142. Ibid., p. 86, no.464.
143. Ibid., p. 108, no.590.
144. Ibid., p. 150, no.847.
145. A. Hunter (ed.), *Georgical Essays*, London, 1770; Brown, ' "For the Dignity',", pp. 101–03; Digby, 'Hunter, Alexander'.

146. Nichols, p. 526.
147. W.W. Currie, *Memoir of the Life, Writings, and Correspondence of James Currie*, Vol. I, pp. 64–65.
148. J. A. Shepherd, *A History of the Liverpool Medical Institution*, Liverpool: Liverpool Medical Institution, 1979, p. 44; British Library, Additional Manuscripts, 35644, f.171.
149. *DNB*, Vol. 13, p. 342; W.W. Currie, *Memoir of the Life*, Vol. I, pp. 67, 71, Vol. II, pp. 47–96.
150. Lobo, 'John Haygarth', pp. 218, 225; Kilpatrick, '"Living in the Light"', p. 257.
151. W.W. Currie, *Memoir of the Life*, Vol. II, p. 87, no.21, 26 December 1792, Currie to Percival.
152. *DNB*, p. 342; DeLacy, 'Currie, James', *Oxford DNB*.
153. DeLacy, 'Currie, James'; J. Currie, *The Works of Robert Burns: With an Account of his Life*, London: Cadell and Davies, 1800.
154. *A Letter, Commercial and Political, Addressed to the Rt. Hon. William Pitt....by Jasper Wilson*, London: G.G.J. and J. Robinsons, 1793. DeLacy, *Oxford DNB*, suggests that William Wilberforce assisted Currie in distributing the pamphlet in London.
155. W.W. Currie, Vol. I, pp. 163, 195–96.
156. *DNB*, p. 342.
157. Currie, *Medical Reports on the Effects of Water, Cold and Warm, as a Remedy in Fever and Other Diseases*.
158. De Lacy, 'Currie, James'.
159. Ibid.
160. W.W. Currie, Vol. I, pp. 109–10.
161. Ibid., pp. 39–40.
162. Ibid., pp. 112–26; J. Pollock, *Wilberforce*, Tring: Lion Publishing, 1977, pp. 104, 123, 131.
163. W.W. Currie, p. 127.
164. W.W. Currie, *Memoir of the Life*, Vol. II, p. 50, no.9, 16 January 1788, Currie to Percival.
165. W.W. Currie, Vol. II, pp. 56–57, no.11, 7 February 1790, Currie to Percival. He made a similar point to Percival in the wake of the Priestley riots in Birmingham, pp. 67–68, no.14 — 'I wish the management of the public mind were better understood by the friends of freedom: if they wish to advance far, they must not advance too fast.'
166. D. Turley, 'British Anti-Slavery Reassessed', in A. Burns, and J. Innes, *Rethinking the Age of Reform; Britain 1780–1850*, Cambridge University Press, 2003, pp. 188–90.
167. *DNB*, Vol. 18, p. 378; Webb, 'Ferriar, John', *ODNB*; E. M. Brockbank, *John Ferriar; William Osler*, London: William Heinemann, 1950, pp. 13–14.
168. John Ferriar, *Illustrations of Sterne, with Other Essays and Verses*, Manchester, 1798; Brockbank, *John Ferriar*, pp. 18–25
169. Webb, 'Ferriar, John'.
170. T. Arnold, *Observations on the Management of the Insane; and Particularly on the Agency and Importance of Humane and Kind Treatment in Effecting Their Cure*, London: Richard Phillips, 1809.
171. Ibid.; *Gentleman's Magazine* 86, 1816, p. 378; Carpenter, 'Thomas Arnold', p. 207.
172. Gardiner, *Music and Friends*, p. 410; A. Temple Patterson, *Radical Leicester*, Leicester: University College, 1954, p. 68; Carpenter, p. 207.

173. Pulteney Correspondence, Arnold to Pulteney, 26 December 1762, 3 April 1763, 3 April 1767, 18 November 1784, 16 May 1785, 25 July 1791, 6 May 1798.
174. Temple Patterson, *Radical Leicester*, p. 68; Carpenter, p. 207.
175. *Gentleman's Magazine* 86, 1816, p. 378.
176. These points are highlighted by Andrews and Scull in their penetrating studies of John Monro — *Undertaker of the Mind*, pp. 8, 19–20; *Customers and Patrons of the Mad-Trade*, p. 42.
177. *An Account of the Rise, and Present Establishment of the Lunatick Hospital in Manchester*, Manchester: J. Harrop, 1771, pp. 5, 7, 9; J. Aikin, *Thoughts on Hospitals*, London: Joseph Johnson, 1771, p. 69.
178. SCRO, QAIc, Box 1, Manchester Lunatic Hospital and Asylum, Rules, pp. 10–11.
179. Dr Thomas Arnold effectively managed the asylum, whilst also being the proprietor of a large madhouse in Leicester which would have catered for all the prospective private patients.
180. G.O. Paul, *Observations on the Subject of Lunatic Asylums, Addressed to a General Meeting of Subscribers to a Fund for Building and Establishing a General Lunatic Asylum, Near Gloucester*, Gloucester: D. Walker, 1812, p. 26.
181. LRO, 614 INF 6/1, Liverpool Infirmary, Rules and Orders (1813), pp. 26–27.
182. DCRO, 3992/F/H14/8, 'Table of Rules for the Admission and Discharge of Patients', 3992/F/H26, 'Statues and Constitution of the Lunatic Asylum... Near Exeter' (1804), p. 20
183. *Statutes and Constitutions of the Lunatic Asylum in the Parish of St Thomas, Near Exeter, with the Rules and Orders for the Government and Conduct of the House*, Exeter: S. Hedgeland, 1824, Fourth Edition, pp. 19–20. The house apothecary was also receiving payments, at half the rate of the physicians.
184. *A Letter From a Subscriber*, p. 12; Hunter, *The History of the Rise and Progress of the York Lunatic Asylum*, pp. 25–26, in which Hunter reproduced the relevant extracts from the Manchester Lunatic Hospital Rules.
185. *A Letter From a Subscriber*, p. 11; *Report of the Committee of Inquiry in to the Rules and Management of the York Lunatic Asylum*, York: Thomas Wilson and Sons, 1814, pp. 29, 33; Gray, *A History of the York Lunatic Asylum*, p. 14.
186. *Report of the Committee of Inquiry*, p. 33; Gray, *A History.*, pp. 15–17.
187. Gray, pp. 17–18; Mason, *Animadversions on the Present Government of the York Lunatic Asylum*, pp. 33–37. See also Chapter 7.
188. *Report of the Committee of Inquiry*, pp. 29, 33.
189. G. Higgins, *A Letter to the Right Honourable Earl Fitzwilliam, Respecting the Investigation Which has Lately Taken Place into the Abuses at the York Lunatic Asylum*, Doncaster: W. Sheardown, 1814, p. 21. Higgins estimated that Hunter had earned more than £30,000 from the asylum.
190. C.N. French, *The Story of St Luke's Hospital*, London: Heinemann, 1951, p. 33.
191. SLH, General Committee Book, 4 March 1811, 11 January 1816.
192. Andrews and Scull, *Undertaker of the Mind*, pp. 120, 123–27, 143–46; Hunter and Macalpine, *Three Hundred Years of Psychiatry*, p. 403; W.S. Lewis, *Horace Walpole's Correspondence*, Oxford University Press, 1965, Vol. 33, pp. 77-78.
193. Andrews and Scull, *Undertaker*, p. 154; Hunter and Macalpine, *Three Hundred Years*, pp. 201, 402; Nichols, *Literary Anecdotes*, Vol. 4, p. 609. According to Nichols, Battie acquired Wood's Close in 1758, but ownership was registered under another name. Hunter and Macalpine suggest that

Islington Road was acquired around 1751 and Wood's Close (an existing madhouse dating back to early in the century) in 1754; however, they do not indicate their sources.

194. R. Porter, *Mind Forg'd Manacles: A History of Madness in England From the Restoration to the Regency*, Cambridge University Press, 1987, p. 131.

195. Lewis, *Horace Walpole's Correspondence*, Vol. 33, p. 315, letter to the Countess of Upper Ossory.

196. J. Barrell, *Imagining the King's Death: Figurative Treason, Fantasies of Regicide 1793–1796*, Oxford University Press, 2000, pp. 504–47. Dr Thomas Monro of Bethlem was also involved in the Brothers case. Brothers was determined by both of them to be insane.

197. *A Letter From a Subscriber to the York Lunatic Asylum* p. 12.

198. *Copy of a Letter From Mr. Brothers, Who will be Revealed to the Hebrews, as Their King and Restorer to Dr Samuel Foart Simmons, M.D.*, London: A. Seale, 1802; Brothers, *A Letter From Mr. Brothers to Miss Cott*, pp. vii, 14, 18–20, 23; Barrell, *Imagining the King's Death*, pp. 534–36. Brothers, believing himself the King of the Hebrews with the destiny of returning them to Jerusalem, felt highly aggrieved with Simmons both for having deemed him a lunatic and for incarcerating him.

199. Brothers, *A Letter From Mr Brothers to Miss Cott*, vii, pp. 14, 18. Brothers described Simmons as 'decrepid in his judgment' and 'weak in his intellect', and his behaviour 'ruffian-like'. Brothers also characterized him as 'a gentleman of his rank in life, set off by the advantage of a carriage, and moving in the genteel sphere of a physician'.

200. BPP 1814-15, Vol. IV, *Report from the Select Committee on Madhouses in England*, p. 137, evidence of Dr Alexander Sutherland. It is not certain, though likely, that Simmons had also owned Blacklands House. Sutherland remained at St Luke's until 1841. He was born in London, the son of a Scottish apothecary. He studied medicine at Edinburgh, graduating in 1805 — Munk, *The Roll of the Royal College of Physicians of London*, Vol. III, pp. 68–69.

201. In addition to the men considered in this chapter, these included John Monro, Nathaniel Cotton, Anthony Addington, Francis Willis, Joseph Mason Cox, Edward Long Fox, and William Perfect – Andrews and Scull, *Undertaker of the Mind*, pp. 179–85; Andrews and Scull, *Customers and Patrons of the Mad-Trade*, pp. 42–44; Parry-Jones, *The Trade in Lunacy*, pp. 75–77, 91–92, 112–15, 172; Hunter and Macalpine, *Three Hundred Years of Psychiatry*, pp. 411, 425–26, 501–02, 510, 514, 594–95; S. Burgoyne Black, *An 18th Century Mad-Doctor: William Perfect of West Malling*, Sevenoaks: Darenth Valley Publications, 1995.

202. Hall, *A Narrative of the Proceedings Relative to the Establishment of St Luke's House*, pp. 8–9; *Newcastle Courant*, 17 May 1766.

203. *Newcastle Courant*, 3, 10, 17, 24, 31 October 1767 — the advert continued for several months; Hall, *A Narrative of the Proceedings*, pp. 25, 36. For the scales of charges in madhouses, see Parry-Jones, *The Trade in Lunacy*, pp. 124–27.

204. *Newcastle Courant*, 29 October – 31 December 1768.

205. *A Letter From a Subscriber to the York Lunatic Asylum, to the Governors of That Charity*, II, 5 January 1788, p. 28.

206. Gray, *A History*, pp. 20–21.

207. *York Courant*, 4 November 1793. Hunter was the co-proprietor along with another York physician, Dr Beckwith.

208. J. Reinarz, *The Birth of a Provincial Hospital: the Early Years of the General Hospital, Birmingham, 1765–1790*, Dugdale Society, Occasional Papers, no. 43, 2003. Arnold later commented of Ash that 'like most unhappy People in

his Situation he had not Resolution to persevere in any Course of Medicine'
— Pulteney Correspondence, 16 May 1785, Arnold to Pulteney. Ash was subsequently under the care of Dr John Monro.

209. Carpenter, 'The Private Lunatic Asylums of Leicestershire', *Transactions of
the Leicestershire Archaeological and Historical Society* 61, 1987, 34–42;
Carpenter, 'Thomas Arnold', pp. 201–13

210. Carpenter, 'Thomas Arnold', pp. 209, 211.

211. See above, Ch.2.

212. This will be further considered in chapter 5.

213. Andrews and Scull, *Undertaker of the Mind*, pp. 48–51, 281–82. Although
Battie was not born into a wealthy family, he had the advantage that his
father was a Church of England vicar.

214. Lawrence, 'Ornate Physicians and Learned Artisans', pp. 153, 169–75.

215. Andrews and Scull, *Customers and Patrons of the Mad-Trade*.

Chapter 5

1. P. Michael, *Care and Treatment of the Mentally Ill in North Wales 1800–
2000*, Cardiff: University of Wales Press, 2003; D. Wright, *Mental Disability in Victorian England: the Earlswood Asylum 1847–1901*, Oxford:
Clarendon, 2001; P. Bartlett, *The Poor Law of Lunacy; the Administration
of Pauper Lunatics in Mid-Nineteenth-Century England*, London: Leicester
University Press, 1999; J. Melling and B. Forsythe, *The Politics of Madness;
the State, Insanity and Society in England, 1845–1914*, Abingdon, Routledge, 2006; F. Crompton, 'Needs and desires in the Care of Pauper Lunatics:
Admissions to Worcester Asylum, 1852–72, in P. Dale and J. Melling, *Mental
Illness and Learning Disablility Since 1850; Finding a Place for Mental Disorder in the United Kingdom*, Abingdon, Routledge, 2006, pp. 46–64.

2. There are extensive records available in relation to admissions and discharges
of patients at St Luke's Hospital. Fairly full records are available for York
Lunatic Asylum (1777–1825). Limited admission records have survived for
the Manchester Lunatic Hospital (years 1773–77) and the Exeter Lunatic
Asylum (1801–05). I have been unable to locate similar records for the other
lunatic hospitals.

3. J. Andrews, 'Bedlam Revisited: A History of Bethlem Hospital c.1634–1770',
University of London, unpublished PhD, 1991, pp. 412–548; J. Andrews, A.
Briggs, R. Porter, P. Tucker, and K. Waddington, *The History of Bethlem*,
London: Routledge, 1997, pp. 315–47.

4. R. Porter, *Mind Forg'd Manacles; A History of Madness in England From the
Restoration to the Regency*, Cambridge, University Press, 1987, pp. 119–20,
161–68; P. Bartlett and D. Wright (eds.), *Outside the Walls of the Asylum:
the History of Care in the Community 1750–2000*, London: Athlone, 1999;
Michael, *Care and Treatment of the Mentally Ill in North Wales*, pp. 8–18;
P. Rushton, 'Lunatics and Idiots: Mental Disability, the Community and the
Poor Law in North-East England, 1600–1800', *Medical History* 32, 1988,
34–50; A. Suzuki, 'Lunacy in Seventeenth- and Eighteenth-Century England:
Analysis of Quarter Sessions Records', Part I, *History of Psychiatry* 2, 1991,
437–56, Part II, *History of Psychiatry* 3, 1992, 29–44.

5. W. Battie, *A Treatise on Madness*, London: J. Whiston and B. White, 1758,
pp. 68–69. For the issue of separation, see below, Ch. 6.

6. W. L. Parry-Jones, *The Trade in Lunacy; a Study of Private Madhouses in
England in the Eighteenth and Nineteenth Centuries*, London: Routledge
Kegan Paul, 1972, pp. 13–14, 29–30, 36–39, 45–46.

7. J. Rule, *Albion's People: English Society 1714–1815*, Harlow: Longman, 1992, pp. 1–6.
8. Porter, *Mind Forg'd Manacles*, pp. 160–68; E. Hare, 'Was Insanity on the Increase?', *British Journal of Psychiatry* 142, 1983, 439–55; A. Scull, 'Was Insanity Increasing ? A Response to Edward Hare', *British Journal of Psychiatry* 144, 1984, 432–36.
9. SLH, General Court Book, 26 June 1751, 17 August 1752, 6 August 1753.
10. SLH, Incurable Patient Book, 28 June 1754 onwards.
11. SLH, General Court Book, 5 February 1756, 9 February 1763, 6 February 1765.
12. General Court Book, 5 February 1772.
13. General Court Book, 2 August 1775, 11 August 1779, 11 February 1784, 7 February 1787.
14. General Court Book, 7 February 1787.
15. General Court Book, 4 February 1789, 2 February 1791.
16. Andrews et al., *A History of Bethlem*, p. 401. Bethlem contained 266 patients in 1800. Its numbers had fallen to 119 in 1814, prior to the hospital's move to Southwark.
17. BPP 1807, Vol. II, *Select Committee on the State of Criminal and Pauper Lunatics*, p. 21; BPP 1814–15, Vol. IV, *Select Committee on the State of Madhouses*, p. 126.
18. General Court Book, 9 February 1815, 8 February 1816, 12 February 1818, 11 February 1819, 10 February 1820; BPP 1816, Vol. VI, *Select Committee on Madhouses*, p. 34 —Thomas Dunston said he had 'never known such a thing for years', and attributed the falling numbers and vacant places to 'the institutions in the country'.
19. L. D. Smith, *'Cure, Comfort and Safe Custody'; Public Lunatic Asylums in Early Nineteenth-Century England*, London: Leicester University Press, 1999, pp. 20–36. Asylums opened in Bedford and Nottingham in 1811, Norfolk in 1814, Lancaster in 1816, Stafford and Wakefield in 1818, Bodmin in 1820, and Gloucester in 1823.
20. General Court Book, 8 February 1821.
21. BPP 1826–27, Vol. VI, *Report from Select Committee of the State of Pauper Lunatics in Middlesex and on Lunatic Asylums*, p. 56.
22. Calculations made from the Curable Patients Books.
23. *SC on Criminal and Pauper Lunatics*, 1807, p. 21.
24. Ibid. The higher incidence of female admissions to St Luke's was to persist, and was remarked upon by Charles Dickens following his visit to the hospital in 1851 — 'A Curious Dance Round a Christmas Tree', 17 January 1852, cited in E. Showalter, *The Female Malady; Women, Madness and English Culture, 1830–1980*, London: Virago, 1987, p. 51.
25. Andrews et al, *The History of Bethlem*, p. 330.
26. Porter, *Mind Forg'd Manacles,* p. 163. Showalter contended that, by the mid-nineteenth century, women constituted the majority of patients in public lunatic asylums — *The Female Malady*, p. 3.
27. *York Courant*, 23 September 1777; York Central Library, Bowen MSS, Burgh to Wilberforce, 10 November 1791.
28. *A Letter From a Subscriber to the York Lunatic Asylum, to the Governors of That Charity*, York: Wilson, Spence and Mawman, 1788, p. 7; Royal Commission on Historical Monuments in England, *An Inventory of the Historical Monuments in the City of York*, Vol. IV, *Outside the City Walls East of the Ouse*, London: HMSO, 1974, pp. 47–48; *A Description of York Containing Some Account of its Antiquities, Public Buildings, &c*, York: J. and G. Todd, 1811, p. 70 — according to this, the new building was opened in 1800.

29. G.O. Paul, *Observations on the Subject of Lunatic Asylums, Addressed to a General Meeting of Subscribers to a Fund for Building and Establishing a General Lunatic Asylum, Near Gloucester*, Gloucester: D. Walker, 1812, pp. 29,34. According to Paul, the overall numbers had increased from seventy-two in 1792 to 174 in 1810. Within those figures, there had been a trebling in the numbers of both private patients (twenty-two to sixty) and paupers (thirty-two to ninety-nine). The numbers of charitable patients had remained static.

30. University of York, Borthwick Institute, BOO 6/2/1/1–3, York Lunatic Asylum admission books. These show that from 1777–1820, 1562 males were admitted and 1290 females.

31. J. Gray, *A History of the York Lunatic Asylum*, York: W. Hargrove and Co., 1815, pp. 38–41, 55.

32. *A Description of York Containing Some Account of its Antiquities Public Buildings &c.*, York: J. and G. Todd, 1821, p. 93; A. Digby, *From York Lunatic Asylum to Bootham Park Hospital*, York: University of York, Borthwick Papers No.69, 1986, pp. 24–25.

33. MRI Archives, Annual Reports, 1765–67.

34. Annual Reports, 1772–89; National Monuments Record Centre, BF102063, Manchester Royal Infirmary, p. 11; J. Pickstone, *Medicine and Industrial Society; A History of Hospital Development in Manchester and its Region, 1752–1946*, Manchester: Manchester University Press, 1985, p. 15.

35. Annual Reports, 1800–14; Warneford Hospital Archives, W. P. 5, xv, letter 7 April 1818 from Mr Taylor; W. Brockbank, *Portrait of a Hospital, 1752–1948; to Commemorate the Bi-centenary of the Royal Infirmary Manchester*, London: Heinemann, 1952, p. 60.

36. MRI Archives, Lunatic Hospital Admissions Register 1773–77. The register shows seventy-five males and seventy-seven females admitted between February 1773 and July 1777.

37. Annual Reports, 1812–13, 1813–14. In 1818, the accommodation provided for sixty males and forty females (see note 35).

38. J. Hall, *A Narrative of the Proceedings Relative to the Establishment &c of St Luke's House*, Newcastle: J. White and T. Saint, 1767, p. 17.

39. Paul, *Observations on the Subject of Lunatic Asylums*, p. 26; Newcastle City Library, 'An Account of Patients Admitted, Discharged, and Remaining at the Lunatic Hospital, Newcastle Upon Tyne, From July 18th, 1764, to July 18th, 1817'.

40. W. Parson and W. White, *History, Directory and Gazetteer of the Counties of Durham and Northumberland*, Leeds, 1827, Vol. 1, lxxxii-iii.

41. LRO, 614 INF 5/2, Liverpool Infirmary, Annual Report, 1789–90; James Currie, *Medical Reports on the Effects of Water, Cold and Warm, as a Remedy in Fever and Febrile Diseases*, Vol. II, London: Cadell and Davies, 1805, p. 43. According to Currie, there was accommodation for sixty-four patients.

42. Annual Reports, 1793–1815.

43. Annual Reports, 1818–27. It would appear that the Liverpool Asylum was acting as an admission facility where people were assessed before transfer to the county pauper asylum.

44. Annual Report, 1831.

45. LCRO, Leicester Infirmary, Annual Reports, 1794–95.

46. Leicester Infirmary, Annual Reports, 1796–1814.

47. Leicester Infirmary, Annual Reports, 1815–30.

48. Herefordshire CRO, 560/25, Hereford Infirmary, Governors Meetings, 11 April 1793.
49. SCRO, Q/AIc, Box 1—letter 10 March 1812, from Rev. James Manning; 'General Meeting of Governors of Exeter Lunatic Asylum, Held at Exeter Castle 11 April 1804'; DCRO, 3992 F/H13, Sixth Annual Report (1807).
50. *Statutes and Constitutions of the Lunatic Asylum in the Parish of St Thomas, Near Exeter, with the Rules and Orders for the Government and Conduct of the House*, Exeter: S. Hedgeland, 1824, Fourth Edition, p. 7.
51. Lincoln Local Studies Library, 'The Third Report of the Lincoln Lunatic Asylum'.
52. *State of the Lincoln Lunatic Asylum, 1832*, Lincoln: W. Brooke and Sons, 1832, p. 16; Lincolnshire Archives, Lincoln Lunatic Asylum, Sixteenth Report, 1840, p. 69.
53. *An Account of the Origin, Nature and Objects of the Asylum on Headington Hill, Near Oxford*, Oxford: J. Munday and Son, 1827, p. 20; B. Parry-Jones, *The Warneford Hospital, 1826–1976*, Oxford: Holywell Press, pp. 13, 17; D. Bowes, 'Who Cares for the Insane? A Study of Asylum Care in Nineteenth Century Oxfordshire', unpublished M.A. thesis, Oxford Brookes University, 2000, pp. 11, 19.
54. B. Abel-Smith, *The Hospitals 1800–1948*, London: Heinemann, 1964, p. 1.
55. These figures include the Newcastle Lunatic Hospital.
56. See Ch. 7.
57. The Nottingham Asylum (opened in 1811) contained, in 1826, twenty-nine charity patients and four private patients; by 1836 these numbers had risen respectively to thirty-nine and seven — *Nottingham Journal*, 21 October 1826; Nottingham Reference Library, qL3648, Twenty-sixth Annual Report (1836). The Stafford Asylum (opened in 1818) contained, at the end of 1830, twenty-four charity and twenty-seven private patients — SCRO, D550/63, 8 January 1831. The Cornwall Asylum at Bodmin (opened in 1820) had capacity for ten charity patients and thirty private patients — Cornwall CRO, DDX 97/1, 1 February 1820. The Gloucester Asylum (opened in 1823) contained, at the end of 1830, four charity and twenty-one private patients — Gloucs CRO, HO 22/8/1, Seventh Annual Report (1830), p. 3.
58. 12 Anne, c.23; 17 Geo. II, c.5; K. Jones, *A History of the Mental Health Services*, London: Routledge & Kegan Paul, 1972, pp. 25–28; Parry-Jones, *The Trade in Lunacy*, p. 7; Richard Hunter and Ida Macalpine, *Three Hundred Years of Psychiatry, 1535–1860*, London: Oxford University Press, 1963, pp. 299–301, 615.
59. 14 Geo.III, c.49; Jones, *A History of the Mental Health Services*, pp. 31–33; Parry-Jones, *The Trade in Lunacy*, pp. 9–10; Hunter and Macalpine, *Three Hundred Years of Psychiatry*, pp. 451–56; D. Wright, 'The Certification of Insanity in Nineteenth-Century England and Wales', *History of Psychiatry* 9, 1998, 267–90.
60. 48 Geo.III, c.96; 51 Geo.III, c.79; 55 Geo.III, c.46; 59 Geo.III, c.127; Wright, 'The Certification of Insanity', pp. 272–74.
61. For Bethlem's admission procedures, see Andrews et al, *The History of Bethlem*, pp. 317–32.
62. SLH, 'Instructions to such Persons who apply for the Admission of Patients into St Lukes Hospital for Lunaticks' (c.1751); *Reasons for the Establishing, and Further Encouragement of St Luke's Hospital for Lunaticks. Together With the Rules and Orders for the Government Thereof*, London: J. March and Son, 1790, pp. 41–43.

63. Newcastle City Library, Local Tracts, 111A, 'Rules of the Hospital for Luna-ticks, for the Counties of Northumberland, Newcastle Upon Tyne, and Dur-ham', pp. 2–3; *Newcastle Courant*, 25 June 1763.

64. MRI Archives, 'An Account of the Proceedings of the Trustees of the Pub-lic Infirmary, in Manchester'; Cheadle Royal Hospital, 'Lunatick Hospital, in Manchester, December 10, 1766'; *An Account of the Rise, and Present Establishment of the Lunatick Hospital in Manchester*, Manchester: J. Har-rop, 1771, pp. 8–9, 21.

65. *Rules for the Government of the Lunatic-Hospital & Asylum in Manches-ter* (n.d., c.1816) — copy in Hunter Collection, University of Cambridge Library.

66. SCRO, QAIc, Box 1, Leicester Lunatic Asylum, Rules, p. 7; LRO, 614 INF 5/2, Liverpool Infirmary, Annual Report, December 31, 1796, to Decem-ber 31, 1797; 614 INF 6/1, 'Liverpool Royal Infirmary — Rules and Orders' (1813), p. 25. Similar requirements were also laid down for admission to the Exeter Lunatic Asylum except that the bond had to come from 'two substan-tial House keepers', one of whom resided in Exeter - *Statutes & Constitu-tions of the Lunatic Asylum Near Exeter*, 1824, pp. 15–17.

67. *York Courant*, 30 September 1777.

68. *A Letter From a Subscriber to the York Lunatic Asylum*, p. 23; A. Hunter, *The History of the Rise and Progress of the York Lunatic Asylum*, York, 1792, p. 16.

69. *The Rules and Regulations of the York Lunatic Asylum, With a List of the Governors, &c.&c*, York: Thomas Wilson & Sons, 1820, pp. 31–32.

70. 'Rules of the Hospital for Lunaticks, for the Counties of Northumberland, Newcastle Upon Tyne, and Durham', p. 2.

71. 'Lunatick Hospital, in Manchester, December 10, 1766.'

72. Hunter, *The History of the Rise and Progress*, p. 20; Digby, *From York Lunatic Asylum to Bootham Park Hospital*, pp. 12–13.

73. *Reasons for the Establishing, and Further Encouragement of St Luke's Hos-pital for Lunaticks*, 1790, pp. 42–43.

74. *The Rules and Regulations of the York Lunatic Asylum*, pp. 29–32.

75. Andrews et al, *The History of Bethlem*, p. 317; London Metropoltan Archives, 0/184/1, 'Instructions to such Persons who apply for the Admission of Patients into St Luke's Hospital for Lunaticks'; *Reasons for the Establish-ing, and Further Encouragement of St Luke's Hospital for Lunaticks*, 1790, p. 41.

76. *A Letter From a Subscriber*, p. 22.

77. At Leicester it would appear that private patients were steered toward Arnold's madhouse.

78. London Metropolitan Archives, 0/184/1.

79. SLH, House Committee Minute Books, 1751–58.

80. House Committee Minutes, 9, 30 August, 6, 20 September 1751, 14 Febru-ary, 15 May, 29 September, 20 October, 8 December 1752, etc.

81. House Committee Minutes, 23 August, 8 November 1751, 3, 10 January, 15, 29 May, 17 July, 6 October, 3 November, 15 December 1752, 16 March 1753, 25 January 1754, etc.

82. House Committee Minute Books, 1758–65, 1765–72, 1772–78.

83. *York Courant*, 30 September 1777.

84. Borthwick Institute, L/3/1, 'York Lunatic Asylum', 1 January 1788; Hunter, *The History of the Rise and Progress*, p. 17.

85. *Rules for the Government of the Lunatic Asylum in Hereford*, Hereford, 1799, p. 6.

86. DCRO, 3992 / F / H13, Eleventh Report, 1812.
87. R. Porter, 'Shaping Psychiatric Knowledge: the Role of the Asylum', in Porter (ed.), *Medicine in the Enlightenment*, Amsterdam: Rodopi, 1995, pp. 255–73,
88. Andrews, 'Bedlam Revisited', pp. 453–54; Andrews et al, *A History of Bethlem*, pp. 329–30.
89. SLH, 'Instructions to such Persons who apply for the Admission of Patients into St Lukes Hospital for Lunaticks'; House Committee Minutes, 1751–78.
90. House Committee Minutes, 29 September, 3, 24 November, 1, 8, 29 December 1752, 1 February 1754, 21, 28 November 1755. Numerous similar cases were reported over the following years.
91. House Committee Minutes, 29 September, 27 October 1752, 22, 29 June, 20 July 1753, 18 January, 1 February, 1 March 1754, 18 March, 15 April, 20 May 1757. Other similar cases were reported over the following years.
92. J. Ibbotson D.D., *The Case of Incurable Lunaticks, and the Charity Due to Them, Particularly Recommended*, London: J. Whiston and B. White, 1759; J. Andrews, 'The Lot of the "Incurably" Insane in Enlightenment England', *Eighteenth Century Life* 12, New Series 1, 1988, 1–18.
93. Andrews, 'The Lot of the "Incurably" Insane', p. 7.
94. A. Highmore, *Pietas Londiniensis; the History, Design, and Present State of the Various Public Charities in and Near London*, London: Richard Phillips, 1810, p. 174; SLH, General Court Book, 13 February 1754; Incurable Patient Book, 28 June 1754.
95. General Court Book, 11 February 1755, 5 February 1756, 9 February 1763, 6 February 1765, 7 February 1787.
96. General Court Book, 3 February 1790, 16 June 1794, 7 February 1799, 9 January 1800.
97. SLH, General Committee Book, 9 February 1809, 8 February 1810, 10 January 1811, 11 February 1819, 10 February 1820.
98. Highmore, *Pietas Londiniensis*, p. 175; BPP 1814–15, Vol. IV, *Select Committee on the State of Madhouses*, p. 127.
99. *Newcastle Courant*, 25 June 1763.
100. Newcastle City Library, 'An Account of Patients Admitted, Discharged, and Remaining at the Lunatic Hospital from July 18th, 1764, to July 18th, 1817'.
101. *A Letter From a Subscriber to the York Lunatic Asylum*, p. 22.
102. *Report of the Committee of Inquiry into the Rules and Management of the York Lunatic Asylum*, York: Thomas Wilson and Sons, 1814, Appendix B, p. 30.
103. *Statutes and Constitutions of the Lunatic Asylum Near Exeter*, 1824, p. 4; DCRO, 3992/F/H13, Eleventh Annual Report, 1812.
104. Melling and Forsythe, *The Politics of Madness*, Ch.5.
105. C. Philo, 'Journey to the Asylum: a Medico-Geographical Idea in Historical Context', *Journal of Historical Geography* 21, 1995, 148–68.
106. Ibid., p. 158.
107. Andrews, 'Bedlam Revisited', pp. 429–32; Andrews et al, *History of Bethlem*, pp. 323–26.
108. SLH, 'Instructions to such Persons who apply for the Admission of Patients into St Lukes Hospital for Lunaticks'.
109. 'Lunatick Hospital, in Manchester, December 10, 1766'; *York Courant*, 15 September 1772; *An Earnest Application to the Humane Public, Concerning the Present State of the Asylum Erected Near York for the Reception of Lunatics*, York, 1777, p. 3.

110. SLH, Curable Patients Books, 1751–1820. An alternative analysis has been carried out by Mr Robert Leon, the voluntary archivist of St Luke's, which includes all of modern Greater London within the London figures. Consequently his figures for London are higher and for the home counties are lower. (Private correspondence, 30 November 2001).
111. This was the first time since 1788 that London admissions were below one hundred.
112. The 'home counties' have been deemed here to comprise the non-metropolitan parts of Middlesex, Surrey, and Kent, as well as Essex, Hertfordshire, Berkshire and Buckinghamshire.
113. In the year 1820 the numbers admitted from the home counties (ninety-five) were for the first time virtually the same as those admitted from London, making up almost forty per cent.
114. SLH, Incurable Patients Book.
115. A county asylum was established in Bedfordshire in 1812.
116. There were some admissions from far-flung districts, including Dorset, Herefordshire, Shropshire, Cornwall, the Channel Islands, and various Welsh counties. There was only one recorded from Scotland. The occasional admissions from overseas included Antigua, Norway, and New Providence.
117. *Newcastle Courant*, 25 June 1763.
118. MRI Archives, Lunatic Hospital Admissions Register, 1773–77.
119. Pickstone, *Medicine and Industrial Society*, pp. 11–13.
120. University of York, Borthwick Institute, BOO 6/2/1/1-3, Admissions Books, 1777–1824. There were some admissions where place of origin was not specified, and these have not been included in the figures. Mostly the numbers are small, but between 1781–90 there were forty-two, and between 1791–1800 there were 107. It can reasonably be assumed that the great majority of these came from Yorkshire.
121. *An Earnest Application to the Humane Public*, p. 6; W. Mason, *Animadversions on the Present Government of the York Lunatic Asylum in Which the Case of Parish Paupers is Distinctly Considered in a Series of Propositions*, York: Blanchard, 1788, p. 31; *Observations on the Present State of the York Lunatic Asylum*, York: R & J Richardson, 1809, pp. 3, 9.
122. Borthwick Institute, L/3/1, 'York Lunatic Asylum, January 1, 1788'; Hunter, *The History of the Rise and Progress*, p. 14; Mason, *Animadversions*, p. 31.
123. It is noteworthy that admissions from Lincolnshire ceased in 1821, following the opening of the Lincoln Lunatic Asylum.
124. DCRO, 3992/F/H13, Sixth Report (1807).
125. DCRO, 3992/F/H21.
126. LRO, 614 INF 1/1, Liverpool Infirmary, Board of Governors, 2 March 1795, 7 January 1799, 3 April 1809; 614 INF 2/1, Board of Economy Minute Book, 22 October, 17 December 1812, 1 July 1813.
127. BPP 1807, Vol. II, *Select Committee on the State of Criminal and Pauper Lunatics*, pp. 6-7, 19, 27.
128. Philo, 'Journey to the Asylum', pp. 155–56.
129. Rule, *Albion's People*, pp. 50–84; J.C.D. Clark, *English Society 1688–1832*, Cambridge University Press, 1985, pp. 68–87; H. Perkin, *The Origins of Modern English Society*, London: RKP Ark Edition, 1985, pp. 18–26; E. P. Thompson, 'Eighteenth-century English Society: Class Struggle Without Class?', *Social History* 3, 1978, 133–65; P. Borsay, *The English Urban Renaissance; Culture and Society in the Provincial Town, 1660-1770*, Oxford: Oxford University Press, 1989, pp. 204–05, 222–23, 225–29, 284–46.

130. M. Fissell, *Patients, Power and the Poor in Eighteenth-Century Bristol*, Cambridge: Cambridge University Press, 1991, pp. 112–16; K. Wilson, *The Sense of the People; Politics, Culture and Imperialism in England, 1715–1785*, Cambridge: Cambridge University Press, 1995, pp. 73–80; P. Langford, *Public Life and the Propertied Englishman, 1689–1798*, Oxford: Clarendon, 1991, pp. 494–500; A. Borsay, *Medicine and Charity in Georgian Bath; a Social History of the General Infirmary, c.1739–1830*, Aldershot: Ashgate, 1999, pp. 253–84.

131. L.D. Smith, 'Levelled to the Same Common Standard? Social Class in the Lunatic Asylum, 1780–1860', in O. Ashton, R. Fyson, S. Roberts (eds.), *The Duty of Discontent: Essays for Dorothy Thompson*, London: Mansell, 1995, pp. 142–66.

132. SLH, House Committee Minutes, 30 July, 6 September 1751; W. Harrison, *A New and Universal History, Description and Survey of London and Westminster*, London: 1778, p. 544.

133. SLH, General Committee Book, 11 August 1808, 12 January, 9 February 1809.

134. *SC on the State of Lunatics of Criminal and Pauper Lunatics*, 1807, p. 21.

135. SLH, Curable Patients Books, 1751–75.

136. SLH, General Committee, 14 April, 10 November 1814.

137. *Newcastle Courant*, 25 June 1763; 'An Account of Patients Admitted, Discharged, and Remaining at the Lunatic Hospital, Newcastle upon Tyne, From July 18th, 1764, to July 18th, 1817.'

138. *Gore's Liverpool General Advertiser*, 15 October 1789; T. Renwick, *A Letter to the Trustees of the Liverpool Infirmary*, Liverpool; T. Kaye, 1826, p. 11; Liverpool Archives, 614 INF 1/1, 2 March 1795.

139. Manchester Infirmary, Weekly Board, 30 October 1775.

140. Liverpool Archives, 614 INF 2/1, 22 October, 17 December 1812.

141. SCRO, Q/AIc, Box 1, letter 10 March 1812, Manning to Charles Aylesbury.

142. Warneford Hospital Archives, Oxford, W. P. 5, xvii, letter 20 April 1820.

143. Smith, 'Levelled to the Same Common Standard?', pp. 145–48; *An Account of the Origin, Nature and Objects of the Asylum on Headington Hill*, pp. 4–6.

144. *York Courant*, 15 January 1788.

145. *York Courant*, 15 January 1788; Mason, *Animadversions*; York Central Library, Bowen MSS, letter 10 November 1791, Burgh to Wilberforce; Gray, *A History of the York Lunatic Asylum*, pp. 17–19; *Observations on the Present State of the York Lunatic Asylum*, 1809, pp. 3, 6, 8–9, 15.

146. *Report of the Committee of Inquiry*, p. 48.

147. *An Account of the Rise*, p. 5; *An Earnest Application to the Humane Public*, p. 4.

148. *An Account of the Rise*, pp. 10–11;

149. *Report of the Committee of Inquiry*, pp. 28–29; *A Letter From a Subscriber*, p. 22; Hunter, *The History of the Rise and Progress*, p. 16.

150. Paul, *Observations on the Subject of Lunatic Asylums*, pp. 29–30.

151. *A Letter From a Subscriber*, p. 8; *Sotheran's York Guide, Including a Description of the Public Buildings, Antiquities, &c.&c. in and About that Ancient City*, York: Wilson, Spence, and Mawman, 1796, pp. 59–60.

152. Paul, *Observations on the Subject of Lunatic Asylums*, pp. 29–30.

153. *Report of the Committee of Inquiry*, p. 8.

154. Paul, *Observations*, p. 50.

155. SCRO, Q/AIc, Box 1, letter 11 March 1812, Squires to Aylesbury.

156. DCRO, 3992/F/H 26, 'The Plan of the Intended Lunatic Asylum'; 3992 F/ H13, Annual Reports, 1807, 1820, 1823.
157. *A Letter From a Subscriber*, pp. 8, 12–13, 19–20; *York Courant*, 22 January 1788; Hunter, *The History of the Rise and Progress*, pp. 1–3, 7.
158. *Gore's Liverpool General Advertiser*, 24 August, 2 November 1789.
159. *An Abstract of Proceedings Relative to the Institution of a General Lunatic Asylum in or Near the City of Gloucester*, Gloucester: R. Raikes, 1794, pp. 3, 10–13; G.O. Paul, *A Scheme of an Institution and a Description of a Plan for a General Lunatic Asylum for the Western Counties to be Built in or Near the City of Gloucester*, Gloucester, 1796, pp. 2–4; Paul, *Observations*, pp. 33–34, 47–48; *SC on the State of Criminal and Pauper Lunatics*, 1807, pp. 18–19.
160. Manchester Infirmary, Annual Reports, XXXI, 24 June 1782 to 24 June 1783.
161. Borthwick Institute, L/3/1, 'York Lunatic Asylum', 1 January 1788; Paul, *Observations*, pp. 30–31; *Report of the Committee of Inquiry*, pp. 50–52.
162. *Exeter Flying Post*, 2 April 1795; DCRO, 3992/F/H26, 'The Plan of the Intended Lunatic Asylum'; SCRO, Q/AIc, Box 1, 'General Meeting of Governors of Exeter Lunatic Asylum, held at Exeter Castle 11 April 1804'.
163. *Statutes & Constitutions of the Lunatic Asylum Near Exeter*, 1824, p. 31.
164. SCRO, Q/AIc, Box 1, 'Rules for the Government of the Manchester Lunatic Hospital and Asylum', p. 8; letter, 7 March 1812, Jackson to Aylesbury.
165. LRO, 614 INF 1/1, 2 April 1810; 614 INF 6/1, 'Liverpool Royal Infirmary Rules and Orders, 1813', p. 25.
166. Smith, 'Cure, Comfort and Safe Custody', pp. 40, 74–75, 79, 167–68, 179.
167. *York Courant*, 15 January 1788.
168. Arnold, *Observations on the Management of the Insane*, p. vii.
169. 'Lunatick Hospital, in Manchester, December 10, 1766'.
170. J. Scott, D.D., *A Sermon Preached at York on the 29th of March, 1780, for the Benefit of the Lunatic Asylum*, York: A. Ward, 1780, p. 24.
171. T. Arnold, *Observations on the Management of the Insane*, London: Richard Phillips, 1809, pp. vi, 8.
172. D. H. Tuke, *Chapters in the History of the Insane in the British Isles*, London: Kegan Paul, Trench & Co., 1882, p. 89.
173. J. Ferriar, *Medical Histories and Reflections*, London: Cadell and Davies, 1792, Vol. 1, pp. 175, 179; J. Currie, *Medical Reports on the Effects of Water, Cold and Warm, as a Remedy in Fever and Other Diseases*, Second Edition, London: Cadell and Davies, 1798, pp. 140–46.
174. *SC on the State of Madhouses*, 1814–15, p. 4; *York Herald*, 2 April 1814; G. Higgins, *The Evidence Taken Before a Committee of the House of Commons Respecting the Asylum at York; With Observations and Notes, and a Letter to the Committee &c.&c.&c.*, Doncaster: W. Sheardown, 1816, p. 47.
175. Gray, *A History of the York Lunatic Asylum*, Appendix, pp. 18–20, 42–44.
176. Higgins, *The Evidence Taken Before a Committee of the House of Commons*, Appendix 1, p. 2.
177. *An Appendix to a Book Lately Published, Entitled,"Incontestable Proofs, &c.&c.", (in Which the Publications of Mr Higgins and Others on the York Lunatic Asylum are Not Sparingly Criticised,) Containing Observations on the Reports, Expences, & Incidents, That Have Occurred in That Asylum Within the Last Two Years*, York: W. Storry, 1818, viii.
178. *SC on the State of Madhouses*, 1814–15, p. 132.

179. SLH, General Committee Book, 10 March 1808. The governors granted her the large sum of £20 to enable her to go and recuperate at the sea-side.

180. General Committee Book, 13 October 1814. He had to be granted £10 to go to the country to recover.

181. Manchester Infirmary, Weekly Board, 7 March 1774; *General Evening Post*, 26 February 1774.

182. S. Tuke, *Practical Hints on the Construction and Economy of Pauper Lunatic Asylums*, York: William Alexander, 1815, pp. 15, 26.

183. *SC on Pauper Lunatics in Middlesex and on Lunatic Asylums*, 1826–27, p. 57.

184. *SC on the State of Madhouses*, 1816, p. 34.

185. Paul, *Observations on the Subject of Lunatic Asylums*, p. 27.

186. Lincolnshire Archives, LAWN 1/1/1, 28 January 1822.

187. *SC on the State of Madhouses*, 1814–15, pp. 16–17.

188. Manchester Infirmary, Weekly Board, 7 March 1774.

189. Weekly Board, 17 July 1797.

190. *SC on the State of Madhouses*, 1816, p. 29.

191. *An Appendix to a Book Lately Published, Entitled,"Incontestable Proofs, &c.&c."*, vii.

192. *Copy of a Later Pricked With a Pin, by Hugh Williams, Broker,No.19, Cannon-street, Manchester; to the Rev. Dr Bayley; on the 54th Day of his Confinement in Bondage, in the Lunatic Hospital, Manchester*, Manchester: B. Radford, 1801, pp. 2–3. [Copy in British Library, Thomason Tracts, E.2179(2)].

193. SLH, General Committee Book, 9 February 1804.

194. Scott, *A Sermon Preached at York on the 29th of March, 1780*, p. 24.

195. Ferriar, *Medical Histories and Reflections*, Vol. I, p. 177.

196. Ibid., p. 183.

197. J. Ferriar, *Medical Histories and Reflections*, London: Cadell and Davies, Vol. II, 1795, p. 100.

198. Ibid., pp. 89–91, 95–96, 99–100, 107.

199. *SC on the State of Madhouses*, 1816, p. 30.

200. Warneford Hospital Archives, W. P. 5, xv, letter 7 April 1818 from Mr Taylor, Manchester Infirmary.

201. *SC on the State of Madhouses*, 1814–15, p. 16.

202. Warneford Hospital Archives, W. P. 5, xv, letter 7 April 1818.

203. *SC on the State of Madhouses*, 1816, p. 30.

204. A New Governor, *A Vindication of Mr Higgins From the Charges of Corrector: Including a Sketch of Recent Transactions a the York Lunatic Asylum*, York: Hargrove and Co., 1814, p. 37.

205. *SC on the State of Madhouses*, 1814–15, p. 7; Gray, *A History of the York Lunatic Asylum*, pp. 9–14, 18–19, 23–25, 30, 42; *York Herald*, 2 April 1814; A New Governor, *A Vindication of Mr Higgins*, p. 38.

206. *York Herald*, 26 March 1814; *SC on the State of Madhouses*, 1814–15, pp. 1–2, 9;

207. Newcastle City Library, 'An Account of Patients Admitted, Discharged, and Remaining at the Lunatic Hospital, Newcastle Upon Tyne', 1817; *York Courant*, 15 January 1788; Warneford Hospital Archives, W. P. 5, xv, letter 7 April 1818.

208. *SC on the State of Madhouses*, 1816, p. 32.

209. Tuke, *Practical Hints on the Construction and Economy of Pauper Lunatic Asylums*, pp. 14–15.

210. Ibid., p. 26.
211. *SC on Pauper Lunatics in Middlesex*, 1826–27, p. 145.
212. Higgins, *The Evidence Taken Before a Committee of the House of Commons*, Appendix XI, pp. 17–18; *SC on the State of Madhouses*, 1814–15, p. 3 — Godfrey Higgins suggested that there had also been another case involving a woman 'of superior situation in life'.
213. *SC on the State of Madhouses*, 1814–15, p. 2. Backhouse was reported to be now keeping a private madhouse in York. A critic of Higgins strongly refuted his evidence regarding Backhouse — *Incontestable Proofs, From Internal Evidence, that S.W. Nicoll, Esquire, is Not the Author of a Vindication of Mr Higgins, From the Charges of Corrector, in a Letter Addressed to Earl Fitzwilliam, to Which are Added, Some Observations on Mr Higgins's Evidence, Taken Before a Committee of the House of Commons, Respecting the Asylum at York*, York: W. Storrey, c.1816, pp. 85–97.
214. *SC on the State of Madhouses*, 1816, pp. 28, 32. Dowding was listed on the staff in July 1809, but not in January 1811 — SLH, General Committee Book, 13 July 1809, 10 January 1811.
215. J. Howard, *An Account of the Principal Lazarretos in Europe, and Additional Remarks on the Present State of Those in Great Britain and Ireland*, Warrington: William Ayres, 1789, p. 139.
216. Paul, *Observations on the Subject of Lunatic Asylums*, pp. 31–32.
217. S.H. Spiker, *Travels Through England, Wales and Scotland, in the Year 1816*, London: Lackington, Hughes, Harding, Mavor and Jones, 1820, pp. 108–09.
218. *SC on the State of Madhouses*, 1814–15, p. 16.
219. Warneford Hospital Archives, W. P. 5, xv, letter 7 April 1818.
220. Williams, *Copy of a Letter Pricked With a Pin*, pp. 2–3.
221. Higgins, *The Evidence Taken Before a Committee of the House of Commons*, Appendix XI, p. 18.
222. *Gore's General Advertiser*, 5 January 1826; *Liverpool Mercury*, 6, 13 January 1826; *Morning Herald*, 12 January 1826.
223. Renwick, *A Letter to the Trustees of the Liverpool Infirmary*, pp. 12–13.
224. There are, however, some unanswered questions regarding the evident lack of certification for private patients admitted to the York Asylum.
225. See below, Ch. 6.

Chapter 6

1. R. Porter, *Mind Forg'd Manacles; A History of Madness in England From the Restoration to the Regency*, Cambridge, University Press, 1987, Ch. 4.
2. Porter, *Mind Forg'd Manacles*, pp. 4–5; R. Porter, 'Shaping Psychiatric Knowledge: the Role of the Asylum', in Porter (ed.), *Medicine in the Enlightenment*, Amsterdam: Rodopi, 1995, pp. 255–73.
3. W. Battie, *A Treatise on Madness*, London: J. Whiston and B. White, 1758, p. 68.
4. J. Monro, *Remarks on Dr Battie's Treatise on Madness*, London: John Clarke, 1758, preface.
5. W. F. Bynum, 'Rationales for Therapy in British Psychiatry, 1780–1835', in A. Scull (ed.), *Madhouses, Mad–Doctors and Madmen; the Social History of Psychiatry in the Victorian Era*, Philadelphia: University of Pennsylvania Press, pp. 35–57.
6. G. N. Hill, *An Essay on the Prevention and Cure of Insanity*, London: Longman, Hurst, Rees, Orme & Brown, 1814, p. 17.

7. Porter, *Mind Forg'd Manacles*, p. 183; A. Suzuki, 'Anti-Lockean Enlightenment ?; Mind and Body in Early Eighteenth-Century English Medicine', in Porter (ed.), *Medicine in the Enlightenment*, pp. 336–59.

8. J. Currie, *Medical Reports on the Effects of Water, Cold and Warm, as a Remedy in Fever and Other Diseases*, Liverpool: J. M'Creery, 1797, p. 146.

9. J. M. Cox, *Practical Observations on Insanity*, London: Baldwin and Murray, 1804, p. 46.

10. A. Harper, *A Treatise on the Real Cause and Cure of Insanity*, London, C. Stalker, 1789, cited in R. Hunter and I. Macalpine, *Three Hundred Years of Psychiatry, 1535–1860*, London: Oxford University Press, 1963, p. 52.

11. T. Arnold, *Observations on the Nature, Kinds, Causes, and Prevention of Insanity, Lunacy, or Madness*, Vol. II, Leicester: G. Ireland, 1786, p. 88; Suzuki, 'Anti-Lockean Enlightenment ?', pp. 337–78.

12. *Gore's Liverpool General Advertiser*, 15 October 1789; Hunter and Macalpine, *Three Hundred Years*, pp. 517–20.

13. J. Ferriar, *Medical Histories and Reflections*, London: Cadell and Davies, Vol. II, 1795, pp. 5–48; Hunter and Macalpine, pp. 544–46.

14. Battie, *A Treatise on Madness*, pp. 41–58.

15. Arnold, *Observations on the Nature, Kinds, Causes, and Prevention of Insanity*, Vol. II, p. 67.

16. Ibid., p. 67 et seq.

17. Ibid., pp. 158, 183.

18. Ibid., pp. 159, 174.

19. Ibid., pp. 194–99.

20. Ibid., pp. 238–50.

21. Ibid., pp. 80–81, 291-444.

22. Ferriar, *Medical Histories and Reflections*, Vol. II, pp. 93–94.

23. J. Haslam, *Observations on Insanity*, London: Rivington, 1798, pp. 99–103; Cox, *Practical Observations*, pp. 8–12.

24. Porter, *Mind Forg'd Manacles*, p. 183.

25. Battie, *A Treatise*, pp. 43, 59–60.

26. Ibid., p. 44.

27. Ibid., pp. 61, 69.

28. Ibid., p. 72.

29. Arnold, *Observations on the Nature*, Vol. II, pp. 72–4; Hunter and Macalpine, *Three Hundred Years*, p. 469.

30. T. Arnold, *Observations on the Nature, Kinds, Causes, and Prevention of Insanity, Lunacy, or Madness*, Vol. I, Leicester: G. Ireland, 1782, p. 124.

31. Ibid., pp. 125–248.

32. Hunter and Macalpine, *Three Hundred Years*, p. 469.

33. W. Cullen, *First Lines in the Practice of Physic*, Edinburgh: Elliot, 1784, cited in Hunter and Macalpine, p. 477.

34. J. Hall, *A Narrative of the Proceedings Relative to the Establishment &c of St Luke's House*, Newcastle: J. White and T. Saint, 1767, p. 23.

35. BPP 1814–15, Vol. IV, *Report from the Select Committee on the State of Madhouses in England*, p. 136.

36. Battie, *A Treatise*, pp. 2, 75, 92, 98–99.

37. Monro, *Remarks on Dr Battie's Treatise*, p. 50.

38. Cox, *Practical Observations*, pp. 76–81.

39. *SC on the State of Madhouses*, 1814–15, p. 136.

40. Ferriar, *Medical Histories and Reflections*, Vol. II, pp. 94–95.

41. Ibid., p. 106.

42. J. Ferriar, *Medical Histories and Reflections*, London: Cadell and Davies, Vol. I, 1792, pp. 172-74; Vol. II, p. 102.
43. Ibid., p. 95.
44. Ibid.,pp. 95–96. He did elsewhere express reservations about the efficacy of tartar emetic — Vol. I, pp. 172–73.
45. Ferriar, *Medical Histories*, Vol. II, pp. 96–97.
46. Ibid., p. 99
47. Ibid., pp. 99–102.
48. Ibid., pp. 102–06.
49. Ibid., p. 106.
50. Cox, *Practical Observations*, p. 90.
51. Ferriar, *Medical Histories*, Vol. I, pp. 173, 181.
52. Currie, *Medical Reports on the Effects of Water*, pp. 140–41.
53. Ferriar, *Medical Histories*, Vol. I, p. 177.
54. Cox, *Practical Observations*, p. 89.
55. Battie, *A Treatise*, pp. 76, 94, 99.
56. Ferriar, *Medical Historties*, Vol. II, pp. 105-06.
57. T. Arnold, *Observations on the Management of the Insane; and Particularly on the Agency and Importance of Humane and Kind Treatment in Effecting Their Cure*, London: Richard Phillips, 1809, pp. 49–53.
58. W.W. Currie, *Memoir of the Life, Writings, and Correspondence of James Currie, M.D.,F.R.S., of Liverpool*, London: Longman, Rees, Orme, Brown, and Green, 1831, Vol. II, no.83, letter 17 July 1790 to Mrs R.G., 'On the Symptoms, Causes, and Treatment of Insanity', p. 298.
59. Ferriar, *Medical Histories*, Vol. I, pp. 173, 177.
60. G.O. Paul, *Observations on the Subject of Lunatic Asylums, Addressed to a General Meeting of Subscribers to a Fund for Building and Establishing a General Lunatic Asylum, Near Gloucester*, Gloucester: D. Walker, 1812, p. 28.
61. Arnold, *Observations on the Management of the Insane*, pp. 51–52.
62. *SC on the State of Madhouses*, 1814–15, p. 136.
63. BPP 1816, Vol. VI, *Select Committee on Madhouses*, p. 30.
64. Currie, *Medical Reports on the Effects of Water*, p. 143.
65. Ferriar, *Medical Histories*, Vol. I, p. 177; Vol. II, pp. 100, 106–07.
66. W.W. Currie, *Memoir of the Life*, Vol. II, p. 299.
67. Currie, *Medical Reports*, pp. 141, 144, 147.
68. Ferriar, *Medical Histories*, Vol. I, pp. 175, 177, 181; Vol. II, pp. 100, 102, 107.
69. Battie, *A Treatise*, p. 95.
70. W. Withering, *An Account of the Foxglove, and Some of its Medical Uses*, Birmingham: Robinson, 1785, cited in Hunter and Macalpine, *Three Hundred Years*, pp. 487–88. Withering had trained at Edinburgh with Thomas Arnold and they became close friends. Arnold's second son, William Withering Arnold, was named after him.
71. Ferriar, *Medical Histories*, Vol. I, p. 176.
72. Currie, *Medical Reports*, pp. 142–44, 147.
73. Cox, *Practical Observations*, p. 85.
74. Hunter and Macalpine, *Three Hundred Years*, pp. 405, 407–10.
75. Battie, *A Treatise*, p. 94.
76. J. Andrews, 'Bedlam Revisited: A History of Bethlem Hospital c.1634–1770', University of London, unpublished PhD, 1991, pp. 307–08; J. Andrews, A. Briggs, R. Porter, P. Tucker, and K. Waddington, *The History of Bethlem*, London: Routledge, 1997, p. 428.

77. *SC on the State of Madhouses*, 1814–15, p. 136.
78. Arnold, *Observations on the Nature*, Vol. II, p. 450.
79. Arnold, *Observations on the Management of the Insane*, pp. 49–52.
80. W.W. Currie, *Memoir of the Life*, Vol. II, p. 298.
81. Ferriar, *Medical Histories*, Vol. I, p. 185.
82. Ferriar, Vol. II, pp. 97–98.
83. DCRO, 3992 F/H6/2, e.g. 28 February 1813; LCRO, Leicester Infirmary, Annual Report, year ending June 1821.
84. Ferriar, Vol. I, p. 181. The application of a seton was a counter-irritant treatment, using a thread passed through the skin.
85. Battie, *A Treatise*, pp. 92, 94. This was one point on which he and his critic Monro were in agreement — Monro, *Remarks on Dr Battie's Treatise*, p. 47.
86. Ferriar, Vol. I, pp. 182–83.
87. SLH, House Committee Minutes, 13 August 1773.
88. SLH, General Committee Book, 1 June 1791, 5 June 1793.
89. *SC on the State of Madhouses*, 1814–15, p. 136.
90. DCRO, 3992 F/H6/1, Housekeeping and Expense Book, Inventory 1803.
91. SCRO, Q/AIc, Box 1, 'General Meeting of Governors of Exeter Lunatic Asylum, held at Exeter Castle 11 April 1804'.
92. Currie, *Medical Reports on the Effects of Water, Cold and Warm, as a Remedy in Fever and Other Diseases*.
93. Currie, *Medical Reports*, Vol. I, pp. 140, 146–47.
94. Ibid., pp. 140–46.
95. Ferriar, *Medical Histories*, Vol. I, pp. 179–81.
96. Ferriar, Vol. II, pp. 103, 107.
97. Currie, *Medical Reports*, Appendix 1, pp. 17–18.
98. Cox, *Practical Observations*, op. cit., p. 92.
99. Cox, *Practical Observations on Insanity*, London: Baldwin and Murray, 1806, Second Edition., pp. 137–76; N. J. Wade, U. Norrsell, 'Cox's Chair: "A Moral and a Medical Mean in the Treatment of Maniacs"', *History of Psychiatry* 16, 2005, 73–88.
100. *SC on the State of Madhouses*, 1814–15, p. 21.
101. Porter, *Mind Forg'd Manacles*, pp. 187–228; Porter, 'Shaping Psychiatric Knowledge: the Role of the Asylum', pp. 257–70. It needs to be stressed that the term 'moral' in treatment or management, as it was used in the eighteenth and nineteenth centuries, referred to what might now be called 'psychological' rather than being a judgmental description relating to the value system. A misinterpretation of terminology has probably contributed to the tendency to over-estimate and even romanticize the significance of the York Retreat in relation to other institutions for the insane.
102. Ferriar, *Medical Histories*, Vol. II, p. 111.
103. Battie, *A Treatise*, p. 68.
104. Ferriar, Vol. II, p. 110.
105. Arnold, *Observations on the Management of the Insane*, pp. 45–48.
106. Paul, *Observations on the Subject of Lunatic Asylums*, pp. 27–28.
107. Porter, *Mind Forg'd Manacles*, p. 155.
108. SLH, General Court Book 1750–79, 'Considerations Upon the Usefulness and Necessity of Establishing an Hospital, by Subscription, as a Farther Provision for Poor Lunaticks'.
109. Arnold, *Observations on the Nature*, Vol. I, p. 9.
110. MRI Archives, 'Lunatick Hospital, in Manchester, December 10, 1766'.
111. Battie, *A Treatise*, p. 69.

112. Arnold, *Observations on the Management*, p. 46.
113. Ibid., pp. 15, 48.
114. SCRO, Q/AIc, 'Rules for the Government of the Lunatic Hospital and Asylum in Manchester', 1791, pp. 13–14; Liverpool Archives, 614 INF 6/1, 'Liverpool Royal Infirmary — Rules and Orders' (1813), p. 28.
115. SCRO, Q/AIC, 'Statutes, Laws, or, Rules for the Government of the Leicester Lunatic Asylum', 1794, p. 9.
116. *Rules for the Government of the Lunatic Asylum in Hereford*, Hereford, 1799, p. 8.
117. *SC on the State of Madhouses*, 1814–15, pp. 16, 151.
118. *SC on Madhouses*, 1816, p. 53.
119. BPP 1826–27, Vol. VI, *Report of the Select Committee on the State of Pauper Lunatics in the County of Middlesex, and on Lunatic Asylums*, p. 113.
120. L. D. Smith, *'Cure, Comfort and Custody'; Public Lunatic Asylums in Early Nineteenth-Century England*, London: Leicester University Press, 1999, pp. 192–94.
121. Porter, 'Shaping Psychiatric Knowledge', pp. 257–67.
122. I. Macalpine and R. Hunter, *George III and the Mad Business*, London: Allen Lane, 1969, pp. 277–78.
123. Ferriar, *Medical Histories*, Vol. II, pp. 108–09; Porter, 'Shaping Psychiatric Knowledge', p. 260.
124. Manchester Lunatic Hospital and Asylum, Rules, 1791, p. 13; *Rules for the Government of the Lunatic Asylum in Hereford*, p. 7; *Statutes and Constitutions of the Lunatic Asylum Near Exeter, with Rules and Orders for the Government and Conduct of the House*, Third Edition, Exeter: Trewman and Son, 1804, p. 22; Liverpool Infirmary, Rules, 1813, p. 28.
125. Leicester Asylum, Rules, 1794, p. 11.
126. Paul, *Observations on the Subject of Lunatic Asylums*, pp. 27–28.
127. Arnold, *Observations on the Management of the Insane*, pp. 10–11.
128. Ibid., pp. 11–12.
129. Ibid., p. 24.
130. Battie, *A Treatise*, p. 69.
131. J. Aikin, *Thoughts on Hospitals*, London: Joseph Johnson, 1771, pp. 66–70.
132. Ferriar, *Medical Histories*, Vol. II, pp. 109, 112.
133. Cox, *Practical Observations*, p. 17. Cox claimed that 'madmen are generally cowards'.
134. D. H. Tuke, *Chapters in the History of the Insane in the British Isles*, London: Kegan Paul, Trench & Co., 1882, p. 90.
135. *SC on the State of Criminal and Pauper Lunatics*, 1807, p. 23.
136. *SC on the State of Madhouses*, 1814–15, p. 133.
137. Manchester Lunatic Hospital, Rules, 1791, p. 13; Hereford Lunatic Asylum, Rules, p. 7; Liverpool Infirmary, Rules, 1813, p. 28; *Statutes and Constitutions of the Lunatic Asylum Near Exeter*, 1804, p. 22.
138. *Quarterly Review*, 1809, Vol. II, p. 176; Arnold, *Observations on the Management of the Insane; and Particularly on the Agency of Humane and Kind Treatment in Effecting Their Cure*.
139. Arnold, *Observations on the Management*, p. 11.
140. Ibid., pp. 39–40.
141. Ibid. pp. 11, 37–38.
142. Ibid., pp. 41–42.
143. Ibid., pp. 54–55.

144. Ferriar, *Medical Histories*, Vol. II, pp. 108–09; Hunter and Macalpine, *Three Hundred Years*, pp. 544–45; Porter, 'Shaping Psychiatric Knowledge', p. 260; A. Digby, *Madness, Morality and Medicine: a Study of the York Retreat, 1796–1914*, Cambridge: Cambridge University Press, 1985, pp. 7, 10.

145. Ferriar, *Medical Histories*, Vol. II, pp. 111–12.

146. Digby, *Madness, Morality and Medicine*, pp. 63–64, 85; S. Tuke, *A Description of the Retreat, an Institution Near York, for Insane Persons of the Society of Friends*, York: W. Alexander, 1813, pp. 157–59.

147. Ferriar, *Medical Histories*, Vol. II, p. 110. Andrew Scull has also drawn parallels between Ferriar's approach and that of the Retreat, highlighting Ferriar's idea of the management of 'hope and apprehension' — *The Most Solitary of Afflictions; Madness and Society in Britain, 1700–1900*, London and New Haven: Yale University Press, 1993, p. 97. Michael Fears also showed Ferriar to have been an early exponent of 'moral treatment' — M. Fears, 'The "Moral Treatment" of Insanity: a Study in the Social Construction of Human Nature', Ph.D thesis, University of Edinburgh, 1978, pp. 83–86.

148. Digby, *Madness, Morality and Medicine*, pp. 42, 50–51; Tuke, *A Description of the Retreat*, pp. 152–56.

149. See for example L.D. Smith, 'To Cure Those Afflicted with the Disease of Insanity; Thomas Bakewell and Spring Vale Asylum', *History of Psychiatry* 4, 1993, 107–27.

150. Arnold, *Observations on the Management*, pp. 43–44.

151. MRI Archives, Manchester Infirmary, Annual Report, 1782–83.

152. DCRO, 3992/F/H26, 'Statutes and Constitutions of the Lunatic Asylum' (1801), p. 11; *SC on the State of Madhouses*, 1814–15, p. 20.

153. Paul, *Observations on the Subject of Lunatic Asylums*, p. 27.

154. A New Governor, *A Vindication of Mr Higgins From the Charges of Corrector: Including a Sketch of Recent Transactions a the York Lunatic Asylum*, York: Hargrove and Co., 1814, p. 37.

155. J. Howard, *An Account of the Principal Lazaretos in Europe, and Additional Remarks on the Present State of Those in Great Britain and Ireland*, Warrington: William Ayres, 1789, p. 139; *SC on the State of Madhouses*, 1814–15, p. 16 — convalescent women were reported to be doing knitting, needlework and lace making.

156. SLH, General Committee Book, 13 June 1799, 11 September 1816.

157. *SC on Criminal and Pauper Lunatics*, 1807, p. 21.

158. *SC on the State of Madhouses*, 1816, p. 33. One long-stay male patient had regularly been involved in assisting the apothecary prepare the medicines — p. 29.

159. *SC on the State of Madhouses*, 1814–15, pp. 136–37.

160. Smith, *'Cure, Comfort and Safe Custody'*, pp. 227–33.

161. Smith, *'Cure, Comfort and Safe Custody'*, Ch. 8.

162. J. Haslam, *Observations on the Moral Management of Insane Persons*, London: H. Hunter, 1817, p. 30.

163. Tuke, *Description of the Retreat*, pp. 97, 142, 163–73. He had little doubt that coercion had its place — 'We cannot, however, anticipate that the most enlightened and ingenious humanity, will ever be able entirely to supersede the necessity of personal restraint.', p. 163.

164. Arnold, *Observations on the Management*, p. 8.

165. Currie, *Medical Reports*, p. 141.

166. Ferriar, *Medical* Histories, Vol. II, p. 109.

167. *Liverpool Mercury*, 20 January 1826, letter from John Davis, former Governor of Liverpool Lunatic Asylum.
168. Manchester Infirmary, Weekly Board, 20 December 1773.
169. *SC on the State of Madhouses*, 1814–15, p. 131.
170. Manchester Lunatic Hospital and Asylum, Rules, 1791, p. 13; Hereford Lunatic Asylum, Rules, p. 8; Liverpool Infirmary Rules, 1813, p. 28.
171. DCRO, 3992/F/H26, 'Statutes and Constitution of the Lunatic Asylum in the Parish of St Thomas Near Exeter', 1801, p. 11.
172. Exeter Lunatic Asylum, Statutes and Constitution, 1801, p. 11; Manchester Lunatic Hospital and Asylum, Rules, 1791, p. 13; Leicester Lunatic Asylum, Rules, 1794, p. 10 — hands as well as feet were to be examined daily; Hereford Lunatic Asylum, Rules, p. 8; Liverpool Infirmary, Rules, 1813, p. 28; *Rules for the Lunatic Asylum at Lincoln*, Lincoln: William Brooke, 1819, p. 10.
173. Andrews, 'Bedlam Revisited', pp. 205–19; M. Winston, ' The Bethel at Norwich: an Eighteenth Century Hospital for Lunatics', *Medical History* 38, 1994, p. 43.
174. C.N. French, *The Story of St Luke's Hospital*, London: Heinemann, 1951, p. 18.
175. Herefordshire CRO, Pateshall MSS, A95/V/Ju/24.
176. DCRO, 3992/F/H6/1, Housekeeping and Expense Book, 1801–06.
177. LCRO, 13 D 54/2, 28 September 1792; E.R. Frizelle, *The Life and Times of the Royal Infirmary at Leicester*, Leicester: Leicester Medical Society, 1988, p. 66.
178. S. Tuke, *Practical Hints on the Construction and Economy of Pauper Lunatic Asylums*, York: William Alexander, 1815, pp. 10, 35, 38–39.
179. *SC on the State of Madhouses*, 1814–15, pp. 13–13
180. Ibid., pp. 136–37. Sutherland also acknowledged the connection between the extent to which 'confinement' was required and the levels of staffing. His views on the selective use of chains according to social class considerations were in close accord with those of Thomas Arnold — see below.
181. Ibid., pp. 16–17.
182. *SC on Criminal and Pauper Lunatics*, 1807, p. 23.
183. *SC on Madhouses*, 1816, p. 32.
184. *SC on Pauper Lunatics in Middlesex*, 1827, p. 57. According to another witness, so-called 'crib patients' were confined in bed constantly from Friday to Monday — p. 90.
185. E. Mackenzie, *A Descriptive and Historical Account of the Town and County of Newcastle Upon Tyne*, Newcastle: Mackenzie and Dent, 1827, Vol. I, pp. 525–26.
186. *SC on the State of Madhouses*, 1814–15, p. 20.
187. Scull, *The Most Solitary of Afflictions*, p. 67.
188. *SC on the State of Madhouses*, 1814–15, pp. 131–33, 136.
189. Arnold, *Observations on the Management*, p. 14.
190. Ibid., pp. 16–17, 54. The inevitable conclusion was that the criteria applied in the Leicester Asylum were different to those in Arnold's madhouse, even though he claimed that the two places were operated on a similar system.
191. *SC on the State of Madhouses*, 1814–15, p. 140; G. Higgins, *The Evidence Taken Before a Committee of the House of Commons Respecting the Asylum at York; With Observations and Notes, and a Letter to the Committee &c.&c.&c.*, Doncaster: W. Sheardown, 1816, p. 47.
192. *Liverpool Mercury*, 13 January 1826.
193. Lincolnshire Archives, LAWN 1/2/1, Lincoln Lunatic Asylum, Director's Journal, 1824–28; R. G. Hill, *Total Abolition of Personal Restraint in the*

Treatment of the Insane. A Lecture on the Management of Lunatic Asylums, and the Treatment of the Insane; Delivered at the Mechanics' Institute, Lincoln, on the 21st of June, 1838, London: Simpkin, Marshall and Co., 1839, Appendix A, pp. 60–63; L.D. Smith, 'The "Great Experiment": the Place of Lincoln in the History of Psychiatry', *Lincolnshire History and Archaeology* 30, 1995, 55–62.

194. Hill, *Total Abolition of Personal Restraint*, pp. 66–73; Lincoln Local Studies Library, 'State of the Lincoln Lunatic Asylum', 1829, pp. 5–6.

195. Hill, op. cit., pp. 70–71; Lincolnshire Archives, LAWN 1/1/2, 9, 16 February, 6 April, 4 May 1829; Smith, 'The "Great Experiment"', p. 57.

196. Smith, 'The "Great Experiment"', p. 57.

197. Hill, *Total Abolition of Personal Restraint*; Lincoln Local Studies Library, 'State of the Lincoln Lunatic Asylum',1831, p. 2, 1832, p. 5; Smith, *'Cure, Comfort and Safe Custody'*, pp. 261–64.

198. Scull, *The Most Solitary of Afflictions*, pp. 87, 92.

199. Digby, *Madness, Morality and Medicine*, pp. 4–18.

Chapter 7

1. See Ch. 2.

2. For the significance of mercantilist ideas in the development of the voluntary hospital movement, see A. Borsay, *Medicine and Charity in Georgian Bath; a Social History of the General Infirmary, c.1739–1830*, Aldershot: Ashgate, 1999, pp. 211–18.

3. Rev. R.B. Dealtry, *A Sermon Preached at York on Wednesday the 10th of April, 1782, for the Benefit of the Lunatic Asylum*, York: A. Ward, 1782, p. 17.

4. University of York, Borthwick Institute, RET 8/1/1/1/3, York Lunatic Asylum, Annual Report, 1813.

5. R. Porter, 'In the Eighteenth Century Were English Lunatic Asylums Total Institutions?', *Ego; Bulletin of the Department of Psychiatry, Guy's Hospital*, Spring 1983, p. 33. The derogatory term 'Old Corruption' has more usually been employed in relation to the wider political system in the eighteenth and early nineteenth centuries — W.D. Rubinstein, 'The End of "Old Corruption" in Britain', *Past and Present* 101, 1983, 55–86; p. Harling, *The Waning of 'Old Corruption'; the Politics of Economical Reform in Britain, 1779–1846*, Oxford: Clarendon Press, 1996.

6. See Ch. 2.

7. K. Jones, *Lunacy, Law and Conscience, 1744–1845. The Social History of the Care of the Insane*, London: Routledge and Kegan Paul, 1955. See also K. Jones, *A History of the Mental Health Services*, London: Routledge and Kegan Paul, 1972, Chs. 4–6.

8. A. Scull, *Museums of Madness; the Social Organization of Insanity in Nineteenth-Century England*, London: Allen Lane, 1979; Scull, *The Most Solitary of Afflictions; Madness and Society in Britain, 1700–1900*, London and New Haven: Yale University Press, 1993; Scull, 'Psychiatry and Social Control in the Nineteenth and Twentieth Centuries', *History of Psychiatry* 2, 1991, 149–69.

9. A. Suzuki, *Madness at Home: the Psychiatrist, the Patient, and the Family in England, 1820–1860*, London and Berkeley: University of California Press, 2006, pp. 14–16, 177–78.

10. M. Brown, 'Rethinking Early Nineteenth-Century Asylum Reform', *The Historical Journal* 49, 2006, 425–52.

11. P. McCandless, 'Insanity and Society: a Study of the English Lunacy Reform Movement, 1815–1870', Ph.D thesis, University of Wisconsin, 1974, pp. 1–90; M. Donnelly, *Managing the Mind: a Study of Medical Psychology in Early Nineteenth Century Britain*, London: Tavistock, 1983.

12. See Ch.5.

13. *The Daily Universal Register*, 2, 3 October 1786; D. H. Tuke, *Chapters in the History of the Insane in the British Isles*, London: Kegan Paul, Trench & Co., 1882, p. 89; L. Smith, 'The Architecture of Confinement: Public Asylum Buildings in England, 1750–1820', in J. Moran and L. Topp (eds.), *Madness, Architecture and the Built Environment*, London: Routledge, 2006, forthcoming.

14. *The Picture of London for 1818*, London: Longman, 1818, p. 202.

15. MRI Archives, Manchester Infirmary, Annual Reports, 1771–72, 1772–73, 1780–81, 1786–87, 1788–89; Royal Commission on the Historical Monuments of England, NBR No: 102063, Manchester, NGR: SJ 843 982, Manchester Royal Infirmary, p. 11, and attached ground plan.

16. MRI Archives, Annual Report, 1782–83.

17. Manchester Infirmary, Weekly Board, 7, 28 September 1801, 8 November 1802; N. Roberts, *Cheadle Royal Hospital: A Bicentenary History*, Altrincham: John Sherratt and Son, 1967, p. 30.

18. Roberts, *Cheadle Royal Hospital*, pp. 43–53.

19. The original building still survives and the availability of unused land close by continues to be evident.

20. W. Mason, *Animadversions on the Present Government of the York Lunatic Asylum in Which the Case of Parish Paupers is Distinctly Considered in a Series of Propositions*, York: Blanchard, 1788, p. 22; York Central Library, Bowen MSS, Burgh to Wilberforce, 10 November 1791.

21. *A Letter From a Subscriber to the York Lunatic Asylum, to the Governors of That Charity*, York: Wilson, Spence and Mawman, 1788, p. 7; *Sotheran's York Guide, Including a Description of the Public Buildings, Antiquities, &c. &c. in and About that Ancient City*, York: Wilson and Spence, 1796, p. 58.

22. *A Description of York Containing Some account of its Antiquities, Public Buildings, &c*, York: J. and G. Todd, 1811, p. 70.

23. Royal Commission on Historical Monuments, NBR No: 60268, York, NGR: SE 610 520; *A Description of York Containing Some Account of its Antiquities Public Buildings &c.*, York: John and George Todd, 1821, p. 93; J. Lane, *A Social History of Medicine; Health, Healing and Disease in England, 1750–1950*, London: Routledge, 2001, p. 104; A. Digby, *From York Lunatic Asylum to Bootham Park Hospital*, York: University of York, Borthwick Papers No.69, 1986, pp. 25–26.

24. J. Hall, *A Narrative of the Proceedings Relative to the Establishment &c of St Luke's House*, Newcastle: J. White and T. Saint, 1767, p. 17; G.O. Paul, *Observations on the Subject of Lunatic Asylums, Addressed to a General Meeting of Subscribers to a Fund for Building and Establishing a General Lunatic Asylum, Near Gloucester*, Gloucester: D. Walker, 1812, p. 26.

25. DCRO, 3992 F/H13, Exeter Lunatic Asylum, Sixth Report, 1807; BPP 1814–15, Vol. IV, *Report from the Select Committee on Madhouses in England*, p. 20.

26. SCRO, Q/A1c, Box 1, letter 10 March 1812 from Rev. James Manning; *Ninth Report of the Commissioners in Lunacy to the Lord Chancellor*, 1855, Appendix (B), 'Hospitals, Their Origins, History and Constitution', p. 49.

27. LCRO, Leicester Infirmary, Annual Reports, 1795–1830.

28. LRO, Liverpool Infirmary, Annual Reports, 1794–1808.

29. *Ninth Report of Commissioners in Lunacy*, Appendix (B), p. 52.
30. Lincolnshire Archives, LAWN 1/1/1, 24 March 1817, 18 February 1820.
31. LAWN 1/1/2, 5 October 1827 (this gives the proposed capacity as 78), 13 October 1828.
32. B. Parry-Jones, *The Warneford Hospital, 1826–1976*, Oxford: Holywell Press, 1976, pp. 8, 13; D. Bowes, 'Who Cares for the Insane? A Study of Asylum Care in Nineteenth Century Oxfordshire', Oxford Brookes University, M.A., 2000, pp. 11–12.
33. *SC on the State of Madhouses*, 1814–15, p. 177.
34. Gloucs CRO, HO22/1/1, 30 October 1823, 19 October 1830.
35. *Staffordshire Advertiser*, 26 September 1818; SCRO, D550/62, Stafford General Lunatic Asylum, Weekly Return Book; Cornwall CRO, DDX 97/1, 1 February 1820 — of the 112 places provided, ten were for subscription patients and thirty for private patients.
36. A. Halliday, *A General View of the Present State of Lunatics and Lunatic Asylums in Great Britain and Ireland*, London: Thomas & George Underwood, 1828, p. 18.
37. C. Stevenson, *Medicine and Magnificence; British Hospital and Asylum Architecture, 1660–1815*, New Haven and London: Yale University Press, 2000, pp. 97, 103; L. D. Smith, *'Cure, Comfort and Safe Custody'; Public Lunatic Asylums in Early Nineteenth Century England*, London: Leicester University Press, 1999, pp. 14, 33
38. SLH, House Committee Minutes, 12 November 1773.
39. W. Harrison, *A New and Universal History, Description and Survey of London and Westminster*, London: 1778, p. 544.
40. SLH, General Committee, 17 December 1813.
41. *SC on the State of Madhouses*, 1814–15, p. 16.
42. Ibid., p. 32.
43. Herefordshire CRO, 560/26, Hereford Infirmary, Governors Minutes, 30 October 1823.
44. LCRO, Leicester Infirmary, Governors Minutes, 13 D 54/3, 22 September, 15, 31 October, 17 November 1815.
45. MRI Archives, Manchester Infirmary, Weekly Board, 7 September 1801.
46. G.O. Paul, *Observations on the Subject of Lunatic Asylums, Addressed to a General Meeting of Subscribers to a Fund for Building and Establishing a General Lunatic Asylum, Near Gloucester*, Gloucester: D. Walker, 1812, pp. 25–27.
47. Tyne and Wear RO, Newcastle Common Council, 1817–24, fos.450–55, 24 June 1824.
48. Newcastle Common Council, 1824–35, p. 119, 27 December 1825.
49. E. Mackenzie, *A Descriptive and Historical Account of the Town and County of Newcastle Upon Tyne*, Newcastle: Mackenzie and Dent, 1827, Vol. I, p. 525.
50. K. Jones, *A History of the Mental Health Services*, London: Routledge & Kegan Paul, 1972, pp. 65–78; R. Hunter and I. Macalpine, *Three Hundred Years of Psychiatry, 1535–1860*, London: Oxford University Press, 1963, pp. 696–704; A. Scull, *Museums of Madness; the Social Organization of Insanity in Nineteenth-Century England*, London: Allen Lane, 1979, pp. 76–82. A recent fundamental re-examination of the York Asylum scandal is to be found in M. Brown, 'Rethinking Early Nineteenth-Century Asylum Reform'. He clearly places the evolution and exposures of the asylum's difficulties, and their subsequent redress, in the context of wider socio-political and ideological struggles in the city and county of York.
51. *SC on the State of Madhouses*, 1814–15, p. 32.

52. Paul, *Observations on the Subject of Lunatic Asylums*, p. 32.
53. S. Tuke, *Practical Hints on the Construction and Economy of Pauper Lunatic Asylums*, York: William Alexander, 1815, pp. 13–14, 35–39.
54. A New Governor, *A Vindication of Mr Higgins From the Charges of Corrector: Including a Sketch of Recent Transactions a the York Lunatic Asylum*, York: Hargrove and Co., 1814, pp. 38–39
55. Ibid., p. 35; *York Herald*, 26 March 1814; *SC on the State of Madhouses*, 1814–15, pp. 1–2, 9–10; G. Higgins, *The Evidence Taken Before a Committee of the House of Commons Respecting the Asylum at York; With Observations and Notes, and a Letter to the Committee &c.&c.&c.*, Doncaster: W. Sheardown, 1816, Appendix 1, Letter from S.W. Nicoll, pp. 1-2; Digby, *From York Lunatic Asylum to Bootham Park Hospital*, pp. 18–19.
56. *York Herald*, 2 April 1814; *SC on the State of Madhouses*, 1814–15, pp. 137, 139, 143.
57. *York Herald*, 1 October 1814; *York Courant*, 3 October 1814; *Report of the Committee of Inquiry in to the Rules and Management of the York Lunatic Asylum*, York: Thomas Wilson and Sons, 1814, pp. 8–9, 49; G. Higgins, *A Letter to the Right Honourable Earl Fitzwilliam, Respecting the Investigation Which Has lately Taken Place into the Abuses at the York Lunatic Asylum*, Doncaster: W. Sheardown, 1814, p. 21 — Higgins claimed that Hunter had earned over £30,000 from the asylum, and that Best had earned £7000 within a few years; Higgins, *The Evidence Taken Before a Committee of the House of Commons*, pp. 49–54, Appendix 1, pp. 3–5.
58. Mason, *Animadversions*, pp. 33–37; J. Gray, *A History of the York Lunatic Asylum*, York: Hargrove and Co., p. 18
59. *Report of the Committee of Inquiry*, pp. 9–11.
60. A New Governor, *A Vindication of Mr Higgins*, p. 8.
61. Ibid., pp. 7, 9.
62. Tyne and Wear RO, Newcastle Common Council, 1810–17, Fo.494, 2 October 1817, 1817–24, fo.306, 26 June 1822, fo.443, 26 April, 24 June 1824.
63. BPP 1816, Vol. VI, *Select Committee on Madhouses*, pp. 29–31; *The Picture of London*, 1818, p. 203; Tuke, *Chapters in the History*, p. 89-91; BPP 1826–27, Vol. VI, *Report of the Select Committee on the State of Pauper Lunatics in the County of Middlesex, and on Lunatic Asylums*, pp. 56–58, 70-73, 90, 103-05, 111–13, 145–46, 167–68, 172–73; W. L. Parry-Jones, *The Trade in Lunacy; a Study of Private Madhouses in England in the Eighteenth and Nineteenth Centuries*, London: Routldge Kegan Paul, 1972, pp. 240–41; J.W. Rogers, *A Statement of the Cruelties, and Frauds Which are Practised in Madhouses*, London: E. Justins, for the Author, 1816, pp. 16–17 — Rogers must have been referring to Dunston when he claimed that 'masters' of public asylums often received a 'douceur' of £500 a year for transferring patients to certain private madhouses. Dunston's son John, who was married to Warburton's daughter, was surgeon both to St Luke's and the Bethnal Green houses, which contained 800 patients in 1827.
64. LCRO, 13 D 54/2/2, 1 February, 17 March 1814.
65. 13 D 54/3, 22 September, 17 November 1815.
66. *Liverpool Mercury*, 6, 13, 20 January 1826; *Morning Herald*, 12 January 1826; T. Renwick, *A Letter to the Trustees of the Liverpool Lunatic Asylum*, Liverpool: T. Kaye, 1826, pp. 3–20.
67. S.W. Nicoll, *An Enquiry into the Present State of Visitation, in Asylums for the Reception of the Insane*, London: Harvey and Darton, 1828, p. 3.
68. L.D. Smith, 'Behind Closed Doors: Lunatic Asylum Keepers, 1800–60', *Social History of Medicine* 1, 1988, pp. 306–07.

69. J. Andrews, 'Bedlam Revisited: A History of Bethlem Hospital c1634–1770', University of London, unpublished PhD, 1991, pp. 299–303.

70. Medicus, *A Short Letter to a Noble Lord, on the Present State of Lunatic Asylums in Great Britain*, Edinburgh, A. Neill, 1806, p. 8.

71. Ibid., pp. 8–9.

72. Tuke, *Practical Hints*, p. 15.

73. Ibid., pp. 26–27.

74. Manchester Infirmary, Weekly Board, 5 April, 25 October, 20 December 1773.

75. *General Evening Post*, 26 February 1774; Manchester Infirmary, Weekly Board, 7 March 1774; W. Brockbank, *Portrait of a Hospital, 1752–1948; to Commemorate the Bi-centenary of the Royal Infirmary Manchester*, London: Heinemann, 1952, pp. 22–23.

76. Weekly Board, 10 April, 4 September 1809; *The Pilot*, 29 August 1809. Browne had been removed from the hospital by his family several days before his death. It was his brother who reported his allegations against Bell. Dr Winstanley said that he had noticed no injuries before Browne left the hospital, inferring that they had taken place subsequently.

77. SLH, House Committee Minutes, 12 June 1761, 24 June 1762.

78. *SC on Madhouses*, 1816, p. 32. The patient became pregnant. The approximate date of the incident can be ascertained from staffing records — SLH, General Committee Book, 13 July 1809, 10 January 1811.

79. SLH, General Committee Book, 6, 13 February, 13 March 1817; C.N. French, *The Story of St. Luke's Hospital*, London: Heinemann, 1951, pp. 45–46.

80. SLH, General Committee Book, 30 January, 12 February 1818.

81. *SC on the State of Madhouses*, 1814–15, p. 2. Godfrey Higgins had suggested that the governors may not have been aware of the circumstances, but that Dr Hunter was aware.

82. *SC on the State of Madhouses*, 1814–15, pp. 3, 7, 139, 144; Gray, *A History of the York Lunatic Asylum*, Appendix, pp. 6–41; *Report of the Committee of Inquiry*, pp. 50–51; Higgins, *The Evidence Taken Before a Committee of the House of Commons*, pp. 42–47, Appendix, pp. 1, 16–18.

83. Gray, *A History*, Appendix, pp. 22–41. Mrs Schorey reported other similar instances, including one where Batty kicked him down the stairs

84. *SC on the State of Madhouses*, 1814–15, p. 138.

85. *Report of the Committee of Inquiry*, pp. 10–11, 46–47.

86. Ibid., pp. 12, 50–51.

87. Ibid., pp. 12–13, 48–49.

88. LCRO, 13 D 54/2, 28 September 1792.

89. 13 D 54/3, 31 October 1815.

90. 13 D 54/3, 15 March, 27 August 1816.

91. 13 D 54/3, 3 June 1817.

92. 13 D 54/3, 5 August, 11 November 1817.

93. 13 D 54/4, 31 December 1822.

94. *Liverpool Mercury*, 6, 13, 20 January 1826; *Gore's General Advertiser*, 5 January 1826; *Morning Herald*, 12 January 1826.

95. Lincs Archives, LAWN 1/1/1, 11 September, 11 December 1820.

96. LAWN 1/1/1, 3 September 1821.

97. LAWN 1/1/1, 27 August 1821, 7 October 1822; LAWN 1/1/2, 14, 21 April, 5, 12 May, 1 October 1823.

98. LAWN 1/1/2, 13 November 1826

99. LAWN 1/1/2, 14 May 1827.

100. LAWN 1/1/2, 17 March 1828.

101. Smith, *Cure, Comfort and Safe Custody*, pp. 150–52.
102. Gray, *A History of the York Lunatic Asylum*, pp. 40–41.
103. SLH, General Committee Book, 9 February 1804. Hughes received a substantial reward of five guineas.
104. *Copy of a Letter Pricked With a Pin, by Hugh Williams, Broker, No.19, Cannon-street, Manchester; to the Revd. Dr Bayley; On the 54th Day of his Confinement, in Bondage, in the Lunatic Hospital, Manchester*, Manchester: B. Radford, 1801, pp. 2–3.
105. Jones, *A History of the Mental Health Services*, pp. 64–100.
106. A. Burns and J. Innes, *Rethinking the Age of Reform; Britain 1780–1850*, Cambridge University Press, 2003. They refer to the evangelical-radical alliances that were interested in 'ending corruption and slavery, promoting education, and improving conditions in prisons and lunatic asylums' — pp. 24–25, also p. 91. For the lunacy reformers see Scull, *The Most Solitary of Afflictions*, pp. 83–87.
107. BPP 1807, Vol. II, *SC on the State of Criminal and Pauper Lunatics*, pp. 6, 19, 21–24.
108. 48 Geo. III, Ca p. 96, *An Act for the Better Care and Maintenance of Lunatics, Being Paupers or Criminals in England*.
109. Smith, '*Cure Comfort and Safe Custody*', pp. 25–26.
110. S. Tuke, *A Description of the Retreat, an Institution Near York, for Insane Persons of the Society of Friends*, York: W. Alexander, 1813.
111. *York Chronicle*, 23, 30 September, 7, 21 October, 11 November 1813; *York Courant*, 11, 18 October 1813; *York Herald*, 16, 23, 30 October 1813.
112. *SC on the State of* Madhouses, 1814–15; *SC on Madhouses*, 1816.
113. Higgins, *The Evidence Taken Before a Committee of the House of Commons*, pp. 44, 58. For a detailed account of the reformers' attack on the asylum, and particularly of Godfrey Higgins' role, see M. Brown, '"For the Dignity of the Faculty"; Fashioning Medical Identities, York, c.1760–c.1850', University of York, PhD thesis, 2004, pp. 139–154, and also Brown, 'Rethinking Early Nineteenth-Century Asylum Reform'.
114. *York Herald*, 2 April 1814; Digby, *From York Lunatic Asylum to Bootham Park Hospital*, p. 16.
115. *Report of the Committee of Inquiry into the Rules and Management of the York Lunatic Asylum*.
116. Gray, *A History of the York Lunatic Asylum*.
117. *A Complete Collection of the Papers Respecting the York Lunatic Asylum, Published Originally in the York Newspapers*, pp. 62–63.
118. *York Courant*, 29 August 1814; Gray, *A History*, pp. 83, 88; C. Atkinson, *Retaliation; or Hints to Some of the Governors of the York Lunatic Asylum*, York: MW. Carrall, 1814, pp. 3–13 — Atkinson felt he had been unjustly treated and blamed for things over which he had no control, having been the victim of 'party spirit' and insult — 'they have actually deprived me, and my wife, and my children of bread. They have branded my name with an indelible mark! They have chastised my finite frailties, with an infinity of punishment.' (p. 13); Digby, *From York Lunatic Asylum*, pp. 20–24. Best's reputation had been further shattered by his inept performance in front of the select committee. He died in the south of France in 1817; Brown, '"For the Dignity of the Faculty"', pp. 152–53.
119. Higgins, *A Letter to the Right Honourable Earl Fitzwilliam*, p. 27.
120. *York Courant*, 29 August 1814; *The Rules and Regulations of the York Lunatic Asylum, With a List of the Governors, &c.&c.*, York: Thomas Wilson and Sons, 1820; Digby, *From York Lunatic Asylum*, pp. 24–25.

121. Digby, *From York Lunatic Asylum*, pp. 24–27; Smith, '*Cure, Comfort and Safe Custody*', pp. 28–29 — both Samuel Tuke and Godfrey Higgins were closely involved with the establishment of the West Riding County Asylum, making use of the York exposures to mobilize support.
122. LCRO, 13 D 54/3, 17 November 1815. The prestige of the committee had been greatly enhanced by the assistance of the eminent physician Sir Henry Halford in its work.
123. Ibid.
124. LCRO, Leicester Infirmary, Annual Reports, 1818–38; E.R. Frizelle, *The Life and Times of the Royal Infirmary at Leicester*, Leicester: Leicester Medical Society, 1988, pp. 70–71; P. Bartlett, *The Poor Law of Lunacy; the Administration of Pauper Lunatics in Mid-Nineteenth Century England*, London: Leicester University Press, 1999, p. 114. A new joint asylum eventually opened in 1837.
125. Tyne and Wear RO, Newcastle Common Council, 1810–17, Fo.494, 2 October 1817.
126. Newcastle Common Council, 1817–24, Fo.443, 26 April 1824, Fos.450–55, 24 June 1824, 1824–35, p. 119, 27 December 1825.
127. Mackenzie, *A Descriptive and Historical Account of the Town and County of Newcastle Upon Tyne*, Vol. II, pp. 525–26.
128. Newcastle Common Council, 1817–24, fos.450–53.
129. Halliday, *A General View of the Present State of Lunatics and Lunatic Asylums*, p. 18;
130. *Rules for the Government of the Lunatic Hospital and Asylum in Manchester*, c.1816 (copy in Hunter Collection, University of Cambridge).
131. *Ninth Report of the Commissioners in Lunacy to the Lord Chancellor*, 1855, Appendix (B), pp. 52–53.
132. Smith, '*Cure, Comfort and Safe Custody*', pp. 31, 75, 261–64.
133. Lane, *A Social History of Medicine*, p. 85; M. Fissell, *Patients, Power and the Poor in Eighteenth-Century Bristol*, Cambridge: Cambridge University Press, 1991, p. 78; K. Wilson, 'Urban Culture and Political Activism in Hanoverian England: the Example of Voluntary Hospitals', in Eckart Hellmuth (ed.), *The Transformation of Political Culture; England and Germany in the Late Eighteenth Century*, Oxford: Oxford University Press, 1990, pp. 165–70; Borsay, *Medicine and Charity in Georgian Bath*, pp. 211–18.
134. E. Raffald, *The Manchester Directory for the Year 1773*, Manchester: Raffald, 1773, p. 77.
135. SLH, General Court Book, 10 February 1762.
136. General Court Book, 5 February 1772.
137. *SC on the State of Criminal and Pauper Lunatics*, 1807, p. 21.
138. *SC on the State of Madhouses*, 1814–15, p. 131.
139. Raffald, *The Manchester Directory for the Year 1773*, p. 77.
140. Raffald, *The Manchester Directory for the Year 1781*, Manchester: Raffald, 1781, p. 103.
141. MRI Archives, 'A Report of the State of the Infirmary, Dispensary, Lunatic Hospital, and Asylum, in Manchester', 25 June 1800 to 24 June 1801.
142. Univ. of York, Borthwick Institute, RET 8/1/1/1/1, report 'York Lunatic Asylum', 1 January 1788.
143. *York Courant*, 1 July 1793.
144. LRO, 614 INF 5/2, Liverpool Infirmary, Annual Report, 3 March 1794–2 March 1795.
145. LRO, 614 INF 5/2, Annual Report, 6 March 1795–15, March 1796.
146. Annual Reports, 1797, 1798, 1799.

147. Annual Reports, 1801, 1802, 1808.
148. Annual Report, 1813.
149. Annual Reports, 1815, 1820, 1821, 1827. In 1820, for example, ninety-nine patients were admitted, thirty-eight were discharged cured, and thirty were sent to the county asylum. This would seem to suggest that the Liverpool Asylum was acting as a temporary holding centre for pauper patients before they were transferred to Lancaster.
150. Newcastle City Library, 'An Account of Patients Admitted, Discharged, and Remaining at the Lunatic Hospital, Newcastle Upon Tyne, From July 18th, 1764, to July 18th, 1817'.
151. *Newcastle Courant*, 25 June 1763.
152. 'An Account of Patients Admitted, Discharged, and Remaining', 1817.
153. DCRO, 3992 F/H13, Exeter Lunatic Asylum, Sixth Report (1807).
154. T. Arnold, *Observations on the Management of the Insane; and Particularly on the Agency and Importance of Humane and Kind Treatment in Effecting Their Cure*, London: Richard Phillips, 1809, pp. 54–55; *Quarterly Review*, Vol. II, 1809, pp. 171–72.
155. LCRO, Leicester Infirmary, Annual Reports, June 1795–1814.
156. Porter, *Mind Forg'd Manacles*, pp. 185–87.
157. Langford, *Public Life and the Propertied Englishman, 1689–1798*, Oxford: Clarendon, 1991, pp. 490–9; Borsay, *Medicine and Charity in Georgian Bath*, pp. 21–49, 253–95; D.T. Andrew, *Philanthropy and Police; London Charity in the Eighteenth Century*, Princeton and Oxford: Princeton University Press, 1989, pp. 47–54.
158. Halliday, *A General View of the Present State of Lunatics and Lunatic Asylums*, p. 18.
159. A New Governor, *A Vindication of Mr Higgins*, pp. 7–9; Nicoll, *An Enquiry into the Present System of Visitation*, pp. 7–13, 60–61.
160. A New Governor, *A Vindication of Mr Higgins*, p. 8.
161. The contrasting perspectives are most clearly represented in Jones, *Lunacy, Law and Conscience*, and Scull, *Museums of Madness*.
162. Brown, 'Rethinking Early Nineteenth-Century Asylum Reform'.
163. See Ch. 4; Leics CRO, 13D54/3, 29 August, 22 September 1815; p. Carpenter, 'Thomas Arnold: A Provincial Psychiatrist in Georgian England', *Medical History* 33, 1989, pp. 209–10.

Conclusion

1. *Gore's Liverpool General Advertiser*, 15 October 1789.
2. P. Langford, *A Polite and Commercial People: England 1727–1783*, Oxford: Clarendon, 1998, pp. 134–41; K. Wilson, *The Sense of the People; Politics, Culture and Imperialism in England, 1715–1785*, Cambridge University Press, 1995, pp. 73–82; J. Woodward, *To Do the Sick No Harm; A Study of the Voluntary Hospital System to 1875*, London: Routledge Kegan Paul, 1974.
3. A. Wilson, 'The Birmingham General Hospital and its Public, 1765–79', in S. Sturdy (ed.), *Medicine, Health and the Public Sphere in Britain, 1600–2000*, London: Routledge, 2002, pp. 85–106.
4. A. Hunter, *The History of the Rise and Progress of the York Lunatic Asylum*, York, 1792, pp. 1–3.
5. MRI Archives, 'An Account of the Proceedings of the Trustees of the Public Infirmary, in Manchester, in Regard to the Admission of Lunaticks into that Hospital', c.1763.

6. L.D. Smith, 'The County Asylum in the Mixed Economy of Care, 1808–1845', in Joseph Melling and Bill Forsythe, *Insanity, Institutions and Society: a Social History of Madness in Comparative Perspective*, London: Routledge, 1999, pp. 33–47.

7. Roy Porter argued that the development of asylums in the private and voluntary sectors had been too piecemeal to constitute a 'system' — *Mind Forg'd Manacles; A History of Madness in England From the Restoration to the Regency*, Cambridge: Cambridge University Press, 1987, p. 156.

8. M. Fissell, *Patients, Power and the Poor in Eighteenth–Century Bristol*, Cambridge: Cambridge University Press, 1991, pp. 110–39; A. Borsay, *Medicine and Charity in Georgian Bath; a Social History of the General Infirmary, c.1739–1830*, Aldershot: Ashgate, 1999, pp. 25–30, 105–117, 253–76.

9. Porter, *Mind Forg'd Manacles*, Chs. 2, 3; A. Scull, *The Most Solitary of Afflictions; Madness and Society in Britain, 1700–1900*, London and New Haven: Yale University Press, 1993, pp. 47–110; W. F. Bynum, 'Rationales for Therapy in British Psychiatry, 1780–1835', *Medical History* 18, 1974, 317–34.

10. This dilemma has continued and recurred in various guises to the present day, and a 'swing of the pendulum' has been apparent in public policy toward people with mental health problems. Its latest manifestation is in the debates and struggles surrounding the introduction of new legislation to replace the 1983 Mental Health Act.

11. Fissell argues that surgeons at the Bristol Infirmary came to take on a role at least equal to that of physicians, but this was never the case in lunatic hospitals — *Patients, Power and the Poor*, pp. 126–39.

12. Hunter, *The History of the Rise and Progress of the York Lunatic Asylum*, pp. 1–2.

13. A. Scull, *Museums of Madness; the Social Organization of Insanity in Nineteenth-Century England*, London: Allen Lane, 1979, pp. 192–98.

14. BPP 1807, Vol. II, *SC on the State of Criminal and Pauper Lunatics*, pp. 14–21; M. Ignatieff, *A Just Measure of Pain: the Penitentiary in the Industrial Revolution 1750–1850*, London: Penguin, 1978, pp. 98–102.

15. A. Burns and J. Innes (eds.), *Rethinking the Age of Reform; Britain 1780–1850*, Cambridge University Press, 2003, p. 13.

16. A. Scull, C. Mackenzie, N. Hervey, *Masters of Bedlam; the Transformation of the Mad-Doctoring Trade*, Princeton: Princeton University Press, 1996, pp. 31–35, 106; Scull, *The Most Solitary of Afflictions*, pp. 115–32.

17. BPP 1814–15, Vol. IV, *SC on the State of Madhouses*, pp. 20–21.

18. Ibid., pp. 178–79.

19. 'The County Asylum in the Mixed Economy of Care, 1808–1845'.

20. SLH, General Committee, 12 May 1814, 24 May, 8 July 1819; Lincolnshire Archives, LAWN 1/1/2, 14 April 1828; *Journal of the House of Lords*, XLIX, 1814, pp. 1089, 1132 (York); LII, 1819, p. 681 (St Luke's); LX, 1828, pp. 182 (Oxford), 208 (Exeter), 242 (Manchester), 293 (St Luke's), 308 (Lincoln).

21. Sir A. Halliday, *A General View of the State of Lunatics and Lunatic Asylums in Great Britain and Ireland*, London: Thomas & George Underwood, 1828, p. 18.

22. It is noteworthy that the Commissioners in Lunacy, established by the legislation of 1845, reintroduced the terminology of 'lunatic hospitals' to categorize the voluntary institutions and to distinguish them from the growing number of county lunatic asylums. Important new voluntary institutions subsequently opened at Stafford, Nottingham and Gloucester in the 1850s, as their joint asylums split into their constituent parts, with the pauper patients remaining

in the older building whilst the charitable and private patients were moved to the new facilities — Leonard D. Smith, *'Cure, Comfort and Safe Custody'; Public Lunatic Asylums in Early Nineteenth-Century England*, London: Leicester University Press, 1999, p. 79.

23. The former asylums at York, Exeter and Lincoln also continued to operate well into the post-war period.

24. C. Philo, *A Geographical History of Institutional Provision for the Insane From Medieval Times to the 1860s in England and Wales; the Space Reserved for Insanity*, Lampeter: Edwin Mellen Press, 2004, Ch.6.

Bibliography

PRIMARY SOURCES

Archives

British Library, Additional Manuscripts
Cheadle Royal Hospital Archives.
Devon County Record Office: records of Exeter Lunatic Asylum.
Herefordshire County Record Office: records of Hereford Infirmary and Lunatic
    Asylum.
Leicestershire and Rutland Archives: records of Leicester Infirmary and Lunatic
    Asylum.
Lincolnshire Archives: records of Lincoln Lunatic Asylum.
Linnaean Society: correspondence of Richard Pulteney.
Liverpool Record Office: records of Liverpool Infirmary and Lunatic Asylum.
London Metropolitan Archives: records of St Luke's Hospital.
Manchester Royal Infirmary Archives.
Nottinghamshire Archives: records of Nottingham General Lunatic Asylum.
Staffordshire County Record Office: records of Staffordshire General Lunatic
    Asylum.
Tyne and Wear Archives: minutes of Newcastle Common Council.
University of York, Borthwick Institute: records of York Lunatic Asylum.
Warneford Hospital (Oxford) Archives.

Government publications

48 Geo. III, Cap. XCVI, *An Act for the Better Care and Maintenance of Lunatics,
    being Paupers or Criminals in England.*
BPP 1807, Vol. II, *Report of the Select Committee into the State of Madhouses.*
BPP 1814–15, Vol. IV, *Report of the Select Committee on the State of
    Madhouses.*
BPP 1816, Vol. VI, *Third Report of the Select Committee on Madhouses.*
BPP 1826–7, Vol. VI, *Report of the Select Committee on the State of Pauper Luna-
    tics in the County of Middlesex, and on Lunatic Asylums.*
Ninth Report of the Commissioners in Lunacy to the Lord Chancellor, 1855.
Journal of the House of Lords, 1814, 1918, 1928.

Newspapers and journals

Exeter Flying Post
Gentleman's Magazine
Gloucester Journal
Gore's Liverpool General Advertiser
Leicester Journal
Lincoln Herald
Manchester Mercury
Newcastle Courant
Nottingham Journal
The Times
York Courant
York Herald

Contemporary books and pamphlets

A Complete Collection of the Papers Respecting the York Lunatic Asylum, Published Originally in the York Newspapers, During the Years 1813, 1814, and 1815, York: York Herald, 1816.

A Description of York Containing Some Account of its Antiquities, Public Buildings, &c, York: J. and G. Todd, 1811.

A Description of York Containing Some Account of its Antiquities Public Buildings &c., York: John and George Todd, 1821.

A Letter From a Subscriber to the York Lunatic Asylum, to the Governors of That Charity, York: Wilson, Spence and Mawman, 1788.

A New Governor, A Vindication of Mr Higgins from the Charges of Corrector: Including a Sketch of the Recent Transactions at the York Lunatic Asylum, York: Hargrove and Co., 1814.

A Picture of London for 1818, London: Longman, 1818.

Aikin, John, *Thoughts on Hospitals*, London: Joseph Johnson, 1771.

An Abstract of Proceedings Relative to the Institution of a General Lunatic Asylum in or Near the City of Gloucester, Gloucester: R. Raikes, 1794.

An Account of the Origin, Nature and Objects of the Asylum on Headington Hill, Near Oxford, Oxford: J. Munday and Son, 1827.

An Account of the Rise, and Present Establishment of the Lunatick Hospital in Manchester, Manchester: J. Harrop, 1771.

An Appendix to a Book Lately Published, Entitled,"Incontestable Proofs, &c.&c.", (in Which the Publications of Mr Higgins and Others on the York Lunatic Asylum are Not Sparingly Criticised,) Containing Observations on the Reports, Expences, & Incidents, That Have Occurred in That Asylum Within the Last Two Years, York: W. Storry, 1818.

An Earnest Application to the Humane Public, Concerning the Present State of the Asylum Erected Near York for the Reception of Lunatics, York: 1777.

Arnold, Thomas, *Observations on the Nature, Kinds, Causes, and Prevention of Insanity, Lunacy, or Madness*, Leicester: G. Ireland, 1782–6.

Arnold, Thomas, *Observations on the Management of the Insane; and Particularly on the Agency and Importance of Humane and Kind Treatment in Effecting Their Cure*, London: Richard Phillips, 1809.

Atkinson, Charles, *Retaliation; or Hints to Some of the Governors of the York Lunatic Asylum*, York: M.W. Carrall, 1814.

Battie, William, *A Treatise on Madness*, London: J. Whiston and B. White, 1758.

Becher, J.T., *Resolutions Concerning the Intended General Lunatic Asylum Near Nottingham*, Newark: S. and J. Ridge, 1810.

Brand, J., *History of Newcastle Upon Tyne*, London: B. White and Son, 1789.

Brothers, Richard, *A Letter From Mr. Brothers to Miss Cott, the Recorded Daughter of David, and Future Queen of the Hebrews, With an Address to the Members of His Britannic Majesty's Council, and Through Them to All Governments and People on Earth*, London: G. Riebau, 1798.

Brothers, Richard, *Copy of a Letter From Mr. Brothers, Who will be Revealed to the Hebrews, as Their King and Restorer to Dr Samuel Foart Simmons, M.D.*, London: A. Seale, 1802.

Charlesworth, E.P., *Remarks on the Treatment of the Insane and the Management of Lunatic Asylums. Being the Substance of a Return from the Lincoln Lunatic Asylum to the Circular of His Majesty's Secretary of State: With a Plan*, London: C. & J. Rivington, 1828.

Copy of a Letter Pricked with a Pin, by Hugh Williams, Broker, No.19 Cannon-street, Manchester; to the Revd. Dr Bayley; on the 54th Day of his Confinement in Bondage, in the Lunatic Hospital, Manchester, Manchester: B. Radford, 1801.

Cox, Joseph Mason, *Practical Observations on Insanity*, London: Baldwin and Murray, 1804.

James Currie, *Medical Reports on the Effects of Water, Cold and Warm, as a Remedy in Fever and Febrile Diseases*, Liverpool: J. M'Creery, 1797; Vol.II, London: Cadell and Davies, 1805.

Currie, W.W., *Memoir of the Life, Writings, and Correspondence of James Currie, M.D., F.R.S., of Liverpool*, London: Longman, Rees, Orme, Brown, and Green, 1831.

Dealtry, Rev. R.B., *A Sermon Preached at York on Wednesday the 10th of April, 1782, for the Benefit of the Lunatic Asylum*, York: A. Ward, 1782.

Duke of Buckingham and Chandos (ed.), *Memoirs of the Courts and Cabinets of George III*, London: Hurst and Blackett, 1855.

Duke of Buckingham and Chandos (ed.), *Memoirs of the Court of England During the Regency*, London: Hurst and Blackett, 1856.

Ferriar, John, *Medical Histories and Reflections*, London: Cadell and Davies, 1792–8.

Ferriar, John, *An Essay Towards a Theory of Apparitions*, London: Cadell and Davies, Warrington: J and J Haddock, 1815.

Gardiner, William, *Music and Friends; or, Pleasant Recollections of a Dilettante*, London: Longman, Orme, Brown, and Longman, 1838.

Gray, Jonathan, *A History of the York Lunatic Asylum*, York: Hargrove and Co., 1815.

Gregory, John, *Observations on the Duties and Offices of a Physician; and on the Method of Prosecuting Enquiries in Philosophy*, London: W. Strahan and T. Cadell, 1770.

Hall, John, *A Narrative of the Proceedings Relative to the Establishment &c of St Luke's House*, Newcastle: J. White and T. Saint, 1767.

Hall, John, *An Answer to Dr Rotheram's Letter*, Newcastle Upon Tyne: J. White and T. Saint, 1767.

Halliday, Sir Andrew, *A General View of the Present State of Lunatics and Lunatic Asylums in Great Britain and Ireland*, London: Thomas & George Underwood, 1828.

Harrison, Walter, *A New and Universal History, Description and Survey of London and Westminster*, London: 1778.

Harvey, Jane, *A Sentimental Tour Through Newcastle; By a Young Lady*, Newcastle: D. Akenhead, 1794.

Haslam, John, *Observations on Insanity*, London: Rivington, 1798.

Haslam, John, *Observations on the Moral Management of Insane Persons*, London: H. Hunter, 1817.

Higgins, Godfrey, *A Letter to the Right Honourable Earl Fitzwilliam, Respecting the Investigation Which Has lately Taken Place into the Abuses at the York Lunatic Asylum*, Doncaster: W. Sheardown, 1814.

Higgins, Godfrey, *The Evidence Taken Before a Committee of the House of Commons Respecting the Asylum at York; With Observations and Notes, and a Letter to the Committee &c.&c.&c.*, Doncaster: W. Sheardown, 1816.

Highmore, Anthony, *Pietas Londinensis: the History, Design and Present State of the Various Public Charities in and Near London*, London: Richard Phillips, 1810.

Hill, George Nesse, *An Essay on the Prevention and Cure of Insanity*, London: Longman, Hurst, Rees, Orme & Brown, 1814.

Hill, Robert Gardiner, *Total Abolition of Personal Restraint in the Treatment of the Insane. A Lecture on the Management of Lunatic Asylums, and the Treatment of the Insane; Delivered at the Mechanics' Institute, Lincoln, on the 21ˢᵗ of June, 1838*, London: Simpkin, Marshall and Co., 1839.

Holme, Edward, *A Directory of the Towns of Manchester and Salford for the Year 1788*, Manchester: J. Radford, 1788.

Howard, John, *An Account of the Principal Lazarretos in Europe, and Additional Remarks on the Present State of Those in Great Britain and Ireland*, Warrington: William Ayres, 1789.

Hunter, Alexander, *The History of the Rise and Progress of the York Lunatic Asylum*, York, 1792.

Hunter, Alexander, *Men and Manners, or, Concentrated Wisdom*, York: T. Wilson and R. Spence, 1808, Third Edition.

Hunter, Alexander, *Silva; or, a Discourse of Forest-Trees, and the Propogation of Timber in His Majesty's Dominions*, York: Wilson and Sons, Fourth Edition, 1812.

Ibbotson, James, D.D., *The Case of Incurable Lunaticks, and the Charity Due to Them, Particularly Recommended*, London: J. Whiston and B. White, 1759.

Incontestable Proofs, From Internal Evidence, that S.W. Nicoll, Esquire, is Not the Author of a Vindication of Mr Higgins, From the Charges of Corrector, York: W. Storrey, c.1816.

Mackenzie, E., *A Descriptive and Historical Account of the Town and County of Newcastle Upon Tyne*, Newcastle: Mackenzie and Dent, 1827

Marsden, John, DD, *A Sermon Preached at York, on Thursday the 27th of March 1783, for the Benefit of the Lunatic Asylum*, York: A. Ward, 1783.

Mason, W., *Animadversions on the Present Government of the York Lunatic Asylum in Which the Case of Parish Paupers is Distinctly Considered in a Series of Propositions*, York: Blanchard, 1788.

Medicus, *A Short Letter to a Noble Lord, on the Present State of Lunatic Asylums in Great Britain*, Edinburgh: A. Neill, 1806.

Memoirs of the Life and Writings of Thomas Percival, M.D, Bath: Richard Cruttwell, 1807.

Monro, John, Remarks on Dr Battie's Treatise on Madness, London: John Clarke, 1758.

Munk, William, *The Roll of the Royal College of Physicians of London*, London: The College, 1878

Nichols, John, *Literary Anecdotes of the Eighteenth Century*, London: Nichols, Son, and Bentley, 1812, Kraus Reprint, New York, 1966.

Nicholl, Samuel W., *An Enquiry into the Present State of Visitation, in Asylums for the Reception of the Insane*, London: Harvey and Darton, 1828.

Noorthouck, John, *A New History of London, Including Westminster and Southwark, to Which is Added, A General Survey of the Whole; Describing the Public Buildings, Late Improvements, &c*, London: R. Baldwin, 1773.

Observations on the Present State of the York Lunatic Asylum, York: R & J Richardson, 1809.

Pargeter, William, *Observations on Maniacal Disorders*, Reading: for the Author, 1792.

Parson, W. and White, W., *History, Directory and Gazetteer of the Counties of Durham and Northumberland*, Leeds, 1827.

Paul, G.O., *A Scheme of an Institution and a Description of a Plan for a General Lunatic Asylum for the Western Counties to be Built in or Near the City of Gloucester*, Gloucester, 1796.

Paul, G.O., *Observations on the Subject of Lunatic Asylums, Addressed to a General Meeting of Subscribers to a Fund for Building and Establishing a General Lunatic Asylum, Near Gloucester*, Gloucester: D. Walker, 1812.

Paul, G.O., *Doubts Concerning the Expediency and Propriety of Immediately Proceeding to Provide a Lunatic Asylum at Gloucester*, Gloucester: D. Walker, 1813.

Percival, Thomas, *Medical Ethics; or a Code of Institutes and Precepts, Adapted to the Professional Conduct of Physicians and Surgeons*, Manchester: S. Russell, 1803.

Proceedings of the General Quarterly Board of the Lincoln Lunatic Asylum, Held on October 13, 1830, Lincoln, 1830.

Raffald, Eliz., *The Manchester Directory, for the Year 1772, Containing an Alphabetical List of the Merchants, Tradesmen, and Principal Inhabitants in the Town of Manchester*, London, Manchester, 1772.

Raffald, E., *The Manchester Directory, for the Year 1781*, Manchester: Raffald, 1781.

Reasons for the Establishment and Further Encouragement of St Lukes Hospital for Lunatics Together with the Rules and Orders for the Government Thereof, London: J. March and Son, 1790.

Remarks on an Appendix to Incontestable Proofs &c.&c., Which Appendix Contains Various Charges Against the Management of the York Asylum, York: R. and J. Richardson, 1818.

Renwick, Thomas, *A Letter to the Trustees of the Liverpool Infirmary*, Liverpool; T. Kaye, 1826.

Report of the Committee of Inquiry in to the Rules and Management of the York Lunatic Asylum, York: Thomas Wilson and Sons, 1814.

Rules of the Lincoln Lunatic Asylum, Lincoln: W. Brooke, 1832.

Rules for the Government of the Lunatic Asylum in Hereford, Hereford, 1799.

Rules for the Lunatic Asylum at Lincoln, November 4th, 1819, Lincoln: William Brooke, 1819.

Scholes's Manchester and Salford Directory, 1794, Manchester: Sowler and Russell, 1794.

Scott, James, D.D., *A Sermon Preached at York on the 29th of March, 1780, for the Benefit of the Lunatic Asylum*, York: A. Ward, 1780.

Sotheran's York Guide, Including a Description of the Public Buildings, Antiquities, &c.&c. in and About that Ancient City, York: Wilson, Spence, and Mawman, 1796.

Spiker, Samuel H., *Travels Through England, Wales and Scotland, in the Year 1816*, London: Lackinton, Hughes, Harding, Mavor and Jones, 1820.

State of the Lincoln Lunatic Asylum, 1832, Lincoln: W. Brooke and Sons, 1832.

Statutes and Constitutions of the Lunatic Asylum Near Exeter, with Rules and Orders for the Government and Conduct of the House, Third Edition, Exeter: Trewman and Son, 1804.

Statutes and Constitutions of the Lunatic Asylum in the Parish of St Thomas, Near Exeter, with the Rules and Orders for the Government and Conduct of the House, Exeter: S. Hedgeland, 1824.

The Rules and Regulations of the York Lunatic Asylum, with a List of Governors, &c.&c., York: Thomas Wilson and Sons, 1820.

Throsby, John, *Select Views in Leicestershire*, Leicester, 1789.

Throsby, John, *The History and Antiquities of the Ancient Town of Leicester*, Leicester: J. Brown, 1791.

Tuke, Daniel Hack, *Chapters in the History of the Insane in the British Isles*, London: Kegan Paul, Trench & Co., 1882.

Tuke, Samuel, *A Description of the Retreat, an Institution Near York, for Insane Persons of the Society of Friends*, York: W. Alexander, 1813.

Tuke, Samuel, *Practical Hints on the Construction and Economy of Pauper Lunatic Asylums*, York: William Alexander, 1815.

Useful Information Concerning the Origin, Nature, and Purpose of the Radcliffe Lunatic Asylum, Oxford: W. Baxter, 1840.

SECONDARY SOURCES

Books

Abel-Smith, Brian, *The Hospitals 1800–1948*, London: Heinemann, 1964.

Andrew, Donna T., *Philanthropy and Police; London Charity in the Eighteenth Century*, Princeton, NJ and Oxford: Princeton University Press, 1989.

Andrews, Jonathan, Briggs, Asa et al., *The History of Bethlem*, London: Routledge, 1997.

Andrews, Jonathan and Scull, Andrew, *Undertaker of the Mind; John Monro and Mad-Doctoring in Eighteenth-Century England*, London: University of California Press, 2001.

Andrews, Jonathan and Scull, Andrew, *Customers and Patrons of the Mad-Trade; the Management of Lunacy in Eighteenth-Century London*, London: University of California Press, 2003.

Baker, Robert, Porter, Dorothy and Porter, Roy, *The Codification of Medical Morality*, Vol.I, *Medical Ethics and Etiquette in the Eighteenth Century*, Dordrecht: Klewer Academic, 1993.

Barrell, John, *Imagining the King's Death; Figurative Treason, Fantasies of Regicide 1793–1796*, Oxford: Oxford University Press, 2000.

Bartlett, Peter, *The Poor Law of Lunacy; the Administration of Pauper Lunatics in Mid-Nineteenth-Century England*, London: Leicester University Press, 1999.

Bartlett, Peter and Wright, David (eds.), *Outside the Walls of the Asylum: the History of Care in the Community 1750–2000*, London: Athlone, 1999.

Black, Shirley Burgoyne, *An 18th Century Mad-Doctor: William Perfect of West Malling*, Sevenoaks: Darenth Valley Publications, 1995.

Borsay, Anne, *Medicine and Charity in Georgian Bath; a Social History of the General Infirmary, c.1739–1830*, Aldershot: Ashgate, 1999.

Borsay, Peter, *The English Urban Renaissance; Culture and Society in the Provincial Town, 1660–1770*, Oxford: Oxford University Press, 1989.

Brockbank, Edward M., *John Ferriar; William Osler*, London: William Heinemann, 1950.

Brockbank, William, *Portrait of a Hospital, 1752–1948; to Commemorate the Bicentenary of the Royal Manchester Infirmary*, London: Heinemann, 1952.

Burns, Arthur and Innes, Joanna (eds.), *Rethinking the Age of Reform; Britain 1780–1850*, Cambridge: Cambridge University Press, 2003.

Bynum, W.F. and Porter, Roy (eds.), *William Hunter and the Eighteenth-Century Medical World*, Cambridge: Cambridge University Press, 1985.

Clark, J.C.D., *English Society 1688–1832*, Cambridge University Press, 1985.

Cunningham, Andrew and French, Roger (eds.), *The Medical Enlightenment of the Eighteenth Century*, Cambridge: Cambridge University Press, 1990.

Digby, Anne, *Madness, Morality and Medicine: a Study of the York Retreat, 1796–1914*, Cambridge: Cambridge University Press, 1985.

Digby, Anne, *From York Lunatic Asylum to Bootham Park Hospital*, York: University of York, Borthwick Papers No.69, 1986.

Digby, Anne, *Making a Medical Living; Doctors and Patients in the English Market for Medicine, 1720–1911*, Cambridge: Cambridge University Press, 1994.

Donnelly, Michael, *Managing the Mind: a Study of Medical Psychology in Early Nineteenth Century Britain*, London: Tavistock, 1983.

Fissell, Mary, *Patients, Power and the Poor in Eighteenth-Century Bristol*, Cambridge: Cambridge University Press, 1991.

Foss, Arthur and Trick, Kerith, *St Andrew's Hospital, Northampton; the First One Hundred and Fifty Years (1838–1988)*, Cambridge: Granta, 1989.

French, C.N., *The Story of St Luke's Hospital*, London: Heinemann, 1951.

Frizelle, E.R., *The Life and Times of the Royal Infirmary at Leicester*, Leicester: Leicester Medical Society, 1988.

Granshaw, Lyndsey and Porter, Roy (eds.), *The Hospital in History*, London: Routledge, 1989.

Hellmuth, Eckart (ed.), *The Transformation of Political Culture; England and Germany in the Late Eighteenth Century*, Oxford: Oxford University Press, 1990.

Hervey, Nicholas, *Bowhill House; St Thomas's Hospital for Lunatics, Asylum for the Four Western Counties, 1800–69*, Exeter: University of Exeter, 1980.

Hill, Sir Francis, *Georgian Lincoln*, Cambridge: Cambridge University Press, 1966.

Horden, Peregrine and Smith, Richard (eds.), *The Locus of Care; Families, Communities, Institutions and the Provision of Welfare Since Antiquity*, London: Routledge, 1998.

Horsley, P.M., *Eighteenth Century Newcastle*, Newcastle: Oriel Press, 1971.

Hunter, Richard and Macalpine, Ida, *Three Hundred Years of Psychiatry, 1535–1860*, London: Oxford University Press, 1963.

Ignatieff, Michael, *A Just Measure of Pain; the Penitentiary in the Industrial Revolution 1750–1850*, London: Penguin, 1978.

Ingram, Allan, *The Madhouse of Language: Writing and Reading Madness in the Eighteenth Century*, London: Routledge, 1991.

Ingram, Allan (ed.), *Patterns of Madness in the Eighteenth Century, A Reader*, Liverpool: Liverpool University Press, 1998.

Jones, Kathleen, *Lunacy, Law and Conscience, 1744–1845, The Social History of the Care of the Insane*, London: Routledge and Kegan Paul, 1955.

Jones, Kathleen, *A History of the Mental Health Services*, London: Routledge & Kegan Paul, 1972.

Lane, Joan, *A Social History of Medicine; Health, Healing and Disease in England, 1750–1950*, London: Routledge, 2001.

Langford, Paul, *A Polite and Commercial People: England 1727–1783*, Oxford: Clarendon, 1989.

Langford, Paul, *Public Life and the Propertied Englishman, 1689–1798*, Oxford: Clarendon, 1991.

Lawrence, Susan C., *Charitable Knowledge; Hospital Pupils and Practitioners in Eighteenth-Century London*, Cambridge: Cambridge University Press, 1996.

Lewis, W.S., *Horace Walpole's Correspondence*, Oxford University Press, 1965.

Loudon, Irvine, *Medical Care and the General Practitioner, 1750–1850*, Oxford: Clarendon, 1986.

McKendrick, Neil, Brewer, John, and Plumb, J.H., *The Birth of a Consumer Society: the Commercialization of Eighteenth-Century England*, London: Europa, 1982.

McLoughlin, George, *A Short History of the First Liverpool Infirmary*, London: Phillimore, 1978.

Macalpine, Ida and Hunter, Richard, *George III and the Mad Business*, London: Allen Lane / Penguin, 1969.

Malcolm, Elizabeth, *Swift's Hospital: a History of St Patrick's Hospital, Dublin, 1746–1989*, Dublin: Gill and Macmillan, 1989.

Markus, Thomas, *Buildings and Power; Freedom and Control in the Origin of the Modern Building Types*, London: Routledge, 1993.

Melling, Joseph and Forsythe, Bill (eds.), *Insanity, Institutions and Society, 1800–1914; a Social History of Madness in Comparative Perspective*, London: Routledge, 1999.

Melling, Joseph and Forsythe, Bill, *The Politics of Madness; the State, Insanity and Society in England, 1845–1914*, London: Routledge, 2006.

Michael, Pamela, *Care and Treatment of the Mentally Ill in North Wales 1800–2000*, Cardiff: University of Wales Press, 2003.

Moran, James and Topp, Leslie (eds.), *Madness, Architecture and the Built Environment*, London: Routledge, 2007, forthcoming.

Oxford Dictionary of National Biography, Oxford: Oxford University Press, 2004.

Owen, David, *English Philanthropy 1660–1960*, London: Oxford University Press, 1965.

Parry-Jones, Brenda, *The Warneford Hospital, 1826–1976*, Oxford: Holywell Press, 1976.

Parry-Jones, William Llewellyn, *The Trade in Lunacy; a Study of Private Madhouses in England in the Eighteenth and Nineteenth Centuries*, London: Routledge Kegan Paul, 1972.

Philo, Chris, *A Geographical History of Institutional Provision for the Insane from Medieval Times to the 1860s in England and Wales: the Space Reserved for Insanity*, Lampeter: Edwin Mellen, 2004.

Pickstone, John, *Medicine and Industrial Society; A History of Hospital Development in Manchester and its Region, 1752–1946*, Manchester: Manchester University Press, 1985.

Pollock, John, *Wilberforce*, Tring: Lion Publishing, 1977.

Porter, Roy, *Mind Forg'd Manacles; A History of Madness in England From the Restoration to the Regency*, Cambridge: Cambridge University Press, 1987.

Porter, Roy (ed.), *Medicine in the Enlightenment*, Amsterdam: Rodopi, 1995.

Reinarz, Jonathan, *The Birth of a Provincial Hospital: the Early Years of the General Hospital, Birmingham, 1765–1790*, Dugdale Society, Occasional Papers, no. 43, 2003.

Richardson, Harriet, (ed.), *English Hospitals 1660–1948*, Swindon: Royal Commission on Historical Monuments in England, 1998.

Roberts, Nesta, *Cheadle Royal Hospital: A Bicentenary History*, Altrincham: John Sherratt and Son, 1967.
Rule, John, *Albion's People: English Society 1714–1815*, Harlow: Longman, 1992.
Scull, Andrew, *Museums of Madness; the Social Organization of Insanity in Nineteenth-Century England*, London: Allen Lane, 1979.
Scull, Andrew, *The Most Solitary of Afflictions; Madness and Society in Britain, 1700–1900*, London and New Haven: Yale University Press, 1993.
Scull, Andrew (ed.), *Madhouses, Mad-Doctors and Madmen; the Social History of Psychiatry in the Victorian Era*, Philadelphia: University of Pennsylvania Press, 1981.
Scull, Andrew, Mackenzie, Charlotte, and Hervey, Nicholas, *Masters of Bedlam; the Transformation of the Mad-Doctoring Trade*, Princeton, NJ: Princeton University Press, 1996.
Shepherd, John A., *A History of the Liverpool Medical Institution*, Liverpool: Liverpool Medical Institution, 1979.
Showalter, Elaine, *The Female Malady; Women, Madness and English Culture, 1830–1980*, London: Virago, 1987.
Smith, Leonard D., *'Cure, Comfort and Safe Custody'; Public Lunatic Asylums in Early Nineteenth Century England*, London: Leicester University Press, 1999.
Stevenson, Christine, *Medicine and Magnificence; British Hospital and Asylum Architecture, 1660–1815*, New Haven and London: Yale University Press, 2000.
Stroud, Dorothy, *George Dance, Architect 1741–1825*, London: Faber and Faber, 1971.
Suzuki, Akihito, *Madness at Home: the Psychiatrist, the Patient, and the Family, 1820–1860*, Berkeley and London: University of California Press, 2006.
Temple Patterson, A., *Radical Leicester*, Leicester: University College, 1954.
Waddington, Ivan, *The Medical Profession in the Industrial Revolution*, Dublin: Gill and Macmillan, 1994.
Wilson, Charles, *England's Apprenticeship*, London: Longman, 1965.
Wilson, Kathleen, *The Sense of the People; Politics, Culture and Imperialism in England, 1715–1785*, Cambridge: Cambridge University Press, 1995.
Woodward, John, *To Do the Sick No Harm; A Study of the Voluntary Hospital System to 1875*, London: Routledge Kegan Paul, 1974.
Wright, David, *Mental Disability in Victorian England: the Earlswood Asylum 1847–1901*, Oxford: Clarendon, 2001.

Articles and chapters in edited volumes

Andrews, Jonathan, 'The Lot of the "Incurably" Insane in Enlightenment England', *Eighteenth Century Life* 12, New Series, 1, 1988, 1–18.
Bailey, Ann, 'The Founding of the Gloucestershire County Asylum, now Horton Road Hospital Gloucester, 1792–1823', *Transactions of the Bristol and Gloucestershire Archaeological Society* 90, 1971, 178–91.
Berry, Amanda, 'Community Sponsorship and the Hospital Patient in Late Eighteenth Century England', in Horden and Smith, *The Locus of Care; Families, Communities, Institutions and the Provision of Welfare Since Antiquity*, 126–50.
Borsay, Anne, 'Cash and Conscience; Financing the General Hospital at Bath c1738–1850', *Social History of Medicine* 4, 1991, 207–29.
Brown, Michael, 'Rethinking Early Nineteenth-Century Asylum Reform', *The Historical Journal* 49, 2006, 425–52.

Bynum, William F., 'Rationales for Therapy in British Psychiatry, 1780–1835', in Scull, *Madhouses, Mad-Doctors and Madmen; the Social History of Psychiatry in the Victorian Era*, 35–57.

Carpenter, Peter, 'The Private Lunatic Asylums of Leicestershire', *Transactions of the Leicestershire Archaeological and Historical Society* 61, 1987, 34–42.

Carpenter, Peter, 'Thomas Arnold: A Provincial Psychiatrist in Georgian England', *Medical History* 33, 1989, 199–216.

Digby, Anne, 'Changes in the Asylum: the Case of York, 1777–1815', *Economic History Review*, Second Series 36, 1983, 218–39.

Fissell, Mary, 'The "Sick and Drooping Poor" in Eighteenth Century Bristol and its Region', *Social History of Medicine* 2, 1989, 35–58.

Hunter, R.A., 'William Battie, M.D., F.R.S., Pioneer Psychiatrist', *The Practitioner* 174, 1955, 208–15.

Kilpatrick, Robert, '"Living in the Light"; Dispensaries, Philanthropy and Medical Reform in Late Eighteenth-Century London', in Cunningham and French, *The Medical Enlightenment of the Eighteenth Century*, 254–80.

Christopher Lawrence, 'Ornate Physicians and Learned Artisans: Edinburgh Medical Men, 1726–1776', in Bynum and Porter, *William Hunter and the Eighteenth-Century Medical World*, 153–76.

Le Gassicke, J., 'History of Psychiatry on Tyneside', in *Medicine in Northumbria; Essays in the History of Medicine in the North East of England*, Newcastle: Pybus Society for the History and Bibliography of Medicine, 1993.

Lobo, Francis M., 'John Haygarth, Smallpox, and Religious Dissent in Eighteenth-Century England', in Cunningham and French, *The Medical Enlightenment of the Eighteenth Century*, 217–53.

Moir, E.A.L., 'Sir George Onisephorus Paul', in H.P.R. Finberg (ed.), *Gloucestershire Studies*, Leicester University Press, 1957, 195–224.

Murphy, Elaine, 'Mad Farming in the Metropolis. Part 1: A Significant Service Industry in East London', *History of Psychiatry* 12, 2001, 245–82.

Philo, Chris, 'Journey to the Asylum: a Medico-Geographical Idea in Historical Context', *Journal of Historical Geography* 21, 1995, 148–68.

Pickstone, John V., 'Thomas Percival and the Production of Medical Ethics', in Baker, Porter and Porter, *The Codification of Medical Morality*, Vol.I, *Medical Ethics and Etiquette in the Eighteenth Century*, 161–78.

Pickstone, J.V., and Butler, S.V., 'The Politics of Medicine in Manchester, 1788–1792: Hospital Reform and Public Health Services in the Early Industrial City', *Medical History* 28, 1994, 227–49.

Porter, Roy, 'Being Mad in Georgian England', *History Today* 31, 1981, 42–8.

Porter, Roy, 'In the Eighteenth Century Were English Lunatic Asylums Total Institutions?', *Ego (Bulletin of the Department of Psychiatry, Guy's Hospital)*, Spring 1983, 12–34.

Porter, Roy, 'William Hunter: a Surgeon and a Gentleman', in Bynum and Porter, *William Hunter and the Eighteenth-Century Medical World*, 7–34.

Porter, Roy, 'The Gift Relation: Philanthropy and Provincial Hospitals in Eighteenth Century England', in Granshaw and Porter, *The Hospital in History*, London: Routledge, 1989, 149–78.

Porter, Roy, 'Shaping Psychiatric Knowledge: the Role of the Asylum', in Porter, *Medicine in the Enlightenment*, 255–73.

Rubinstein, William D., 'The End of "Old Corruption" in Britain', *Past and Present* 101, 1983, 55–86.

Rushton, Peter, 'Lunatics and Idiots: Mental Disability, the Community and the Poor Law in North-East England, 1600–1800', *Medical History* 32, 1988, 34–50.

Smith, L.D., 'Behind Closed Doors: Lunatic Asylum Keepers, 1800–60', *Social History of Medicine* 1, 1988, 301–27.

Smith, L.D., 'The "Great Experiment": the Place of Lincoln in the History of Psychiatry', *Lincolnshire History and Archaeology* 30, 1995, 55–62.

Smith, L.D., 'Levelled to the Same Common Standard? Social Class in the Lunatic Asylum, 1780–1860', in Ashton, Owen, Fyson, Robert and Roberts, Stephen (eds.), *The Duty of Discontent: Essays for Dorothy Thompson*, London: Mansell, 1995, 142–66.

Smith, Leonard, 'The Architecture of Confinement: Public Asylum Buildings in England, 1750 1820', in Moran and Topp, *Madness, Architecture and the Built Environment*, forthcoming.

Stevenson, Christine, 'Carsten Anker Dines With the Younger George Dance, and Visits St Luke's Hospital for the Insane', *Architectural History* 44, 2001, 153–61.

Suzuki, Akihito, 'Lunacy in Seventeenth- and Eighteenth-Century England: Analysis of Quarter Sessions Records', Part I, *History of Psychiatry* 2, 1991, 437–56, Part II, *History of Psychiatry* 3, 1992, 29–44.

Suzuki, Akihito, 'Anti-Lockean Enlightenment?; Mind and Body in Early Eighteenth-Century English Medicine', in Porter, *Medicine in the Enlightenment*, 336–59.

Thompson, E.P, 'Eighteenth-century English Society: Class Struggle Without Class?', *Social History* 3, 1978, 133–65.

Wade, Nicholas and Norrsell, U., 'Cox's Chair: "A Moral and a Medical Mean in the Treatment of Maniacs"', *History of Psychiatry* 16, 2005, 73–88.

Wilson, Adrian, 'The Birmingham General Hospital and its Public, 1765–79', in Strudy, Steve (ed.), *Medicine, Health and the Public Sphere in Britain, 1600–2000*, London: Routledge, 2002, 85–106.

Wilson, Kathleen, 'Urban Culture and Political Activism in Hanoverian England: the Example of Voluntary Hospitals', in Hellmuth, Eckart (ed.), *The Transformation of Political Culture; England and Germany in the Late Eighteenth Century*, Oxford: Oxford University Press, 1990.

Winston, Mark, 'The Bethel at Norwich: an Eighteenth Century Hospital for Lunatics', *Medical History* 38, 1994, 27–51.

Wright, David, 'The Certification of Insanity in Nineteenth-Century England and Wales', *History of Psychiatry* 9, 1998, 267–90.

Unpublished theses

Adams, Jane, 'The Mixed Economy for Medical Services in Herefordshire c.1770–c.1850', University of Warwick, PhD, 2004.

Andrews, Jonathan, 'Bedlam Revisited: A History of Bethlem Hospital c.1634–1770', University of London, PhD, 1991.

Bowes, David, 'Who Cares for the Insane? A Study of Asylum Care in Nineteenth Century Oxfordshire', Oxford Brookes University, M.A., 2000.

Brown, Michael, '"For the Dignity of the Faculty"; Fashioning Medical Identities, York, c.1760–c.1850', University of York, PhD, 2004.

Fears, Michael, 'The "Moral Treatment" of Insanity: a Study in the Social Construction of Human Nature', University of Edinburgh, PhD, 1978.

McCandless, Peter, 'Insanity and Society: a Study of the English Lunacy Reform Movement, 1815–1870', University of Wisconsin, PhD, 1974.

Index